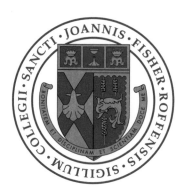

Vascular Surgery

MOSBY'S PERIOPERATIVE NURSING SERIES

Vascular Surgery

Beth Ann MacVittie, RN, MS, CNOR

Primary Service Nurse for Peripheral Vascular Operating Room
University of Rochester Medical Center
Rochester, New York

with 401 illustrations

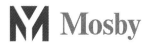 Mosby

St. Louis Baltimore Boston Carlsbad Chicago Naples New York Philadelphia Portland
London Madrid Mexico City Singapore Sydney Tokyo Toronto Wiesbaden

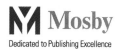
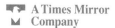

A Times Mirror
Company

Publisher: Nancy L. Coon
Editor: Michael S. Ledbetter
Developmental Editor: Nancy L. O'Brien
Project Manager: Dana Peick
Production Editor: Stavra Demetrulias
Composition Specialist: Wendy Bellm
Designer: Amy Buxton
Manufacturing Manager: Betty Mueller
Cover Photo: Jim Smithers, RN

A NOTE TO THE READER:
The author and publisher have made every attempt to check dosages and nursing content for accuracy. Because the science of pharmacology is continually advancing, our knowledge base continues to expand. Therefore we recommend that the reader always check product information for changes in dosage or administration before administering any medication. This is particularly important with new or rarely used drugs.

Printed in the United States of America
Composition by Mosby Electronic Production
Lithography and Color Film
by Accu-Color, Inc.
Printing/binding by Von Hoffmann

Mosby–Year Book, Inc.
11830 Westline Industrial Drive
St. Louis, Missouri 63146

International Standard Book Number **0-8151-7031-9**

Contributor

Merry Anne Pierson, RN, MSN, CNOR
Staff Nurse General-Vascular Service
St. Thomas Hospital
Nashville, Tennessee

Chapter 1 History and Future of Vascular Surgery

Consultants

Susan Chlebowski, MD
Assistant Professor of Anesthesiology
Chief, Vascular Anesthesia
University of Rochester
Strong Memorial Hospital
Rochester, New York

James A. DeWeese, MD
Chair Emeritus, Division of Cardiothoracic and
    Vascular Surgery
University of Rochester
Strong Memorial Hospital
Rochester, New York

Denise M. Fitzgerald, MS, RN, NP, RVT, CVN
Vascular Nurse Practitioner
University of Rochester
Strong Memorial Hospital
Rochester, New York

Richard M. Green, MD
Chief, Section of Vascular Surgery
University of Rochester Medical Center
Strong Memorial Hospital
Rochester, New York

Karl A. Illig, MD
Assistant Professor of Surgery
University of Rochester Medical Center
Strong Memorial Hospital
Rochester, New York

JoAnne M. McNamara, RN-C, MSN, RVT
Vascular Nurse Practitioner
University of Rochester Medical Center
Strong Memorial Hospital
Rochester, New York

Kenneth Ouriel, MD
Associate Professor of Surgery
Section of Vascular Surgery
University of Rochester Medical Center
Strong Memorial Hospital
Rochester, New York

Merry Anne Pierson, RN, MSN, CNOR
Staff Nurse General-Vascular Service
St. Thomas Hospital
Nashville, Tennessee

Patrick Riggs, MD
Associate Professor of Surgery
Section of Vascular Surgery
University of Rochester Medical Center
Strong Memorial Hospital
Rochester, New York

Cynthia K. Shortell, MD, PC
Clinical Assistant Professor of Surgery and Medicine
Vascular Surgeon Affiliated with
    Rochester General Hospital
University of Rochester Medical Center
Strong Memorial Hospital
Rochester, New York

Reviewers

Barbara Herrmann Cichocki, RN, BSN, CNOR
Perioperative Staff Nurse
Overlook Hospital
Summit, New Jersey

Victora A. Fahey, RN, MSN, CVN
Advanced Practitioner, Vascular Surgery
Northwestern Memorial Hospital
Chicago, Illinois

Patricia L. Griffith, RN, CNOR
Southampton Hospital
Southampton, New York

Michael J. Nugent, RNFA, CNOR
Perioperative Staff Nurse
Thomas Jefferson University Hospital
Philadelphia, Pennsylvania

Janice D. Nunnelee, RN, MSN, CS
University of Missouri-St. Louis
West County Family Practice
St. Louis, Missouri

Patricia C. Seifert, RN, MSN, CNOR, CRNFA
Operating Room Coordinator, Cardiac Surgery
Arlington Hospital, Arlington, Virginia
Alexandria Hospital, Alexandria, Virginia

Carol A. Tyler, RN, BS, CNOR
Staff Nurse III, Operating Room
Evanston Hospital
Evanston, Illinois

Laurel A. Wiersema-Bryant, RN, MSN, CS
Clinical Nurse Specialist
Barnes-Jewish Hospital
St. Louis, Missouri

To my parents, for the lifetime of unconditional love
and encouragement and reading.
And for Joey, my partner in life.

Preface

The vascular patient presents with a myriad of specialized and often complex needs. Most are elderly, many are diabetic, some are very frail. When surgery is indicated, a team approach to their care is essential and especially enhanced by perioperative nursing care. The nursing process is the essential basis for critical thinking, creative planning, and compassionate interventions. The perioperative nurse must be capable of rapidly processing and responding to emergencies or changes in the surgical plan and be able to manage the team members as needed.

This book is intended to be a guide for both experienced and inexperienced perioperative nurses in the various practice settings that serve the vascular patient. It may be helpful to introduce both the basics of vascular surgical nursing and the specifics of surgical procedures and the equipment needed to carry out safe interventions. The collection of anatomy illustrations and photographs of surgery are designed to assist the perioperative nurse in all the phases of perioperative care. Those practitioners who do not spend time in the operating room will gain an expanded understanding of the diagnosis, surgery, and patient experience. The boxed information on preoperative teaching, postoperative care and discharge planning should assist the nurse in providing knowledgeable, safe and comforting patient care.

Some of the unique features of this book include:

- placement of current trends of vascular surgery as a specialty in the context of history.
- a review of the anatomy and physiology focusing on the vascular system with a collection of clear, relevant anatomy illustrations for convenient reference.
- the pathophysiology of the vascular surgical patient.
- diagnostic studies, laboratory values and physical assessment specific to the vascular patient.
- an emphasis on the care and needs of the geriatric and the diabetic patient.
- perioperative nursing care for the preoperative, intraoperative and postoperative periods
- photographs and detailed information on the equipment and instrumentation required for safe vascular surgery.
- fundamental techniques of vascular surgery, scrub nurse skills, and RNFA considerations.
- step-by-step descriptions of the procedures with concise information on expected outcomes and potential complications.
- color photographs of surgical interventions to enhance the procedural descriptions.

Part I: Foundations of Vascular Surgical Nursing, begins with the history of vascular surgery (Chapter 1). This background information assists in placing the current events of vascular surgery in perspective and enhances an appreciation for the process of surgical advances. The second chapter describes the roles of the various health care providers who assist the vascular patients (The Vascular Team). Chapter 3 reviews the relevant anatomy and physiology and provides clear anatomy illustrations that are difficult to find in a single text book. Medications and medical management of vascular disease is covered in Chapter 4. The assessment of the vascular patient includes the history and physical examination, diagnostic procedures and laboratory work as well as a sensitive approach to interviewing and teaching. Chapter 5 includes the studies for diagnosis that the patient may encounter. Knowledge of these tests and procedures will assist the nurse in providing information and support to the patient and family. The complexity of patient needs is emphasized throughout the text but introduced and organized in Chapter 6 (Nursing Diagnoses for the Vascular Patient) and Chapter 7 (Perioperative Nursing Care). There is an emphasis on geriatric patient assessment, interviewing, and laboratory values. Both new and experienced OR personnel will benefit from the photographs and descriptions of the OR environmental considerations, instrumentation, and equipment in Chapter 8. Specific items and methods will vary by region, budget, and surgeon preference, but the intent is that the basics are covered. This may serve as a starting point for teaching or a guide for consideration in expansion of a vascular patient care setting. The foundations half of the text is concluded with a review of vascular prosthetic grafts, their development, care, and handling. This also covers considerations for setting up and planning for the care of a patient with a graft infection.

Part 2: Surgical Interventions covers the most frequently encountered vascular surgical interventions. It begins with Chapter 10, Fundamentals of Vascular Surgery, to provide the reader with an understanding of surgical techniques that may be used in many different procedures and parts of the anatomy. For example, endarterectomy may be the primary procedure as in a carotid endarterectomy. However, an endarterectomy may be performed during the course of an femoral artery reconstructive procedure or on the renal artery during an abdominal aortic resection. These may be unplanned and the intraoperative staff must be prepared to recognize and respond to such procedures by having the necessary equipment and to properly handle pathology specimens. Open procedures (reconstruction, bypasses) versus endovascular or percutaneous techniques (balloon embolectomy, balloon angioplasty) are reviewed. The scrub nurse also needs a repertoire of fundamental techniques and skills in handling vascular grafts, sutures and other specialty supplies. These are discussed and clearly illustrated with color photographs covering the unique skills needed in vascular surgery (e.g., of preparing a suture with pledget material and application of a Rummel tourniquet). There is also a section that describes the fundamental techniques and skills of the RN first assistant (RNFA). This serves as a basis for the RNFA Considerations in the subsequent chapters, which list the specific knowledge and possible duties of an RNFA. The RNFA role is an expanded perioperative practice role that will vary by region, institution, and individual. This text may introduce and help educate others to this important role.

The remaining chapters (11 through 20) are each devoted to a particular surgical intervention that is in the realm of peripheral vascular surgery. The more common procedures are the carotid endarterectomy (Chapter 11), infrainguinal bypass (Chapter 12), aortic aneurysm resection (Chapter 15), arteriovenous fistula creation and revision (Chapter 16), and varicose vein excision (Chapter 19). Again, depending on regional and institutional differences, some of these procedures may be performed by surgeons with other specialty training. Neurosurgeons may perform carotid endarterectomy, general surgeons may perform amputations and varicose vein excision, etc. The intent of this text is to cover a broad and basic range of procedures. Sympathectomies (Chapter 14), first rib resections (Chapter 13) and extraanatomic bypasses (Chapter 17) are not common procedures and are included for reference because they may be infrequently encountered.

The information provided may appear very detailed in some areas. This is to assist those who may need to plan, budget, and set up a vascular OR. There are many ways to achieve the same goal; use this text for reference and as a springboard. Perioperative nurses are a pragmatic and creative lot and no doubt excellent ideas and practices are evolving. Sharing these ideas and learning from our patients and colleagues is professionalism at its best.

Acknowledgements

I never dreamed of writing a book. I often thought I would like to write an article for a nursing journal and someday I will. I can thank Rosemary Roth, friend and mentor of many years, for asking me to help her out by revising a chapter on vascular surgery. That somehow landed me the mixed blessing of this opportunity to write this book (thank you, Michael Ledbetter). The very early support of Jane Rothrock and Trish Siefert gave me courage and very tangible lists of whether and how to begin. The project has taken me so long, that I ask forgiveness if I have left anyone out of my gratitude list.

"My surgeons" (James DeWeese, Richard Green, Ken Ouriel, Patrick Riggs, Cynthia Shortell, and Karl Illig) have taught and tolerated me for years. I am grateful for the many times they patiently assisted the incessant photography by washing and changing gloves, freezing the action for one more shot and placing yet another unrealistic clean towel. Roy, Vic, and Steve did this better than anyone without even being asked! No one helped more than Ken Ouriel with his lightening speed editorial reviews and the loan of the perfect camera for those sudden Kodak moments. Those credited as clinical consultants were much more than manuscript reviewers. Thanks to Sue Chlebowski (my vascular anesthesiologist) for explanations, reams of articles, and passionate care of our patients.

My nursing colleagues and friends have been there for me every step of the way. I cannot thank you enough for changing assignments and shifts to allow me access to the needed photographs. Thanks to Shelley Steinman, Kim O'Connell and Mary Jane Gerstner for reading, ideas, books and articles. Linda Cumbo for being a "hand model" and covering my assignment so I could take those rare pictures. Scott Rosenberg and Chris Martin, the ultimate EEG techs, provided literature, computer assistance and friendship. I am always indebted to my nursing organization, AORN, at both the local and national levels. I credit my involvement with my local chapter for my professional and personal growth and development, enabling me to continue to be a perioperative nurse. Their pride in my progress has been a tangible treasure.

Merry Anne responded to my need when I said "I wish someone would just write this chapter for me," never dreaming it was a possibility (Chapter 1). A true friend! All my friends have lived this book with me despite my terrible neglect of them. Laurie Pask supported with phone calls, sympathy and exercise. The spinners (Meg, Nancy, Joan, Edith, Teddy, Julie and Ann) rode the waves of my successes and failures with me and gave unfailing support and computer HELP!

The photography was a special challenge in coordinating schedule changes, patient permissions and photographers. Royal Chamberlain, Senior Medical Photographer, Strong Memorial Hospital, took the most beautiful procedural photographs. Jim Smithers, photographer and fellow OR nurse, shot the majority of the instrumentation, equipment, and supplies photos. His willingness to work after a long day to move equipment and compose the shots artistically and carefully made all the difference. Dr. Christie Wray generously allowed me to use his camera and film for a series of photographs. Gratia Nagle (fellow author) has been there for me although we have never met. The telephone empathy, advice, and cheerleading of someone who very successfully authored the previous book in this series (Genitourinary Surgery) helped more than I can describe. The additional offer to catch those frustratingly elusive photographs of the AV fistulas has me eternally in your debt. Thank you.

Thanks to Mary Beth Meyers, Ariel Fullington, and Meadox Medicals for an unforgettable tour of the vascular graft production plant. Patty Christian (Meadox Medicals) helped me numerous times with technical information, slides and permissions even when she was extremely busy. Thanks to Laura Fisher of Abbott for financial assistance, providing the opportunity to attend a vascular conference that enhanced my understanding and appreciation of my subject. This allowed me to hear lively panel discussions about the current technologies by vascular surgeons from all regions of the United States.

Company representatives provided me with all kinds of support in the form of literature, phone consultations, brochures and all those beautiful photographs asking only for acknowledgement. Thank you to Bob Bishop (Zimmer), G. Ray Martin (W L Gore), Matt Fahey (Olympus), Shannon Anderson and Mark Anderson (Scanlan International), Sheryl Marrazzo (O R Direct), Chris Clark (Huntleigh Healthcare), Karen Boilsen (Ethicon Endosurgery), Judy E. Lawten (COBE Cardiovascular, Inc.), Sandra Millar (Vascutech), Sheri Timmer (Baxter Cardiovascular), David Blossom (Boston Scientific), and Chris Heiss-Clark (Huntleigh Healthcare).

The support from Mosby was incredible. Thanks to Michael and Teri who got me started. Nancy joined the project at just the right time and deserves a special reward for the unflagging, consistent, and professional support. Her kindness and encouragement during the growing pains of reviews and revisions were above and beyond!

When things seemed the bleakest I had only to think of the generous, enthusiastic outpouring of support and encouragement to realize what an amazing journey this has been. I would not have made it without my partner, Joey, who did all the things that I could not.

Contents

Vascular Surgery

1 History and Future of Vascular Surgery

Merry Anne Pierson

INTRODUCTION

The history of vascular surgery can be traced as far back as 600 to 800 B.C. During this time, an Indian surgeon, Shushruta, not only wrote the first surgical text but was the first to control hemorrhage with hemp fiber ties and to use boiling oil to cauterize bleeding. In the second or third century Antyllus, a Roman surgeon, performed a proximal and distal ligation of an artery to treat an aneurysm by removing its contents (Barker, 1993). Through the years, many attempts were made to repair arteries and veins but these efforts failed because of sepsis and thrombosis.

Vascular surgery, although performed since antiquity, has a very brief history as a self contained and distinct specialty. Most of its development has taken place within the last half of the twentieth century. Early surgeries were of limited scope and usually extremely simple, with disappointing results because only surface lesions could be diagnosed. The historical development of vascular surgery can generally be divided into three distinct sections: (1) arterial, (2) venous, and (3) lymphatic (Szilagyi,1994).

From antiquity through the eighteenth century occasional reports appeared in the medical literature addressing the vascular problems of arterial hemorrhage and, less often, aneurysms. Several methods to control arterial bleeding were attempted over the years, from manual compression to actual ligation of the artery. Ambrose Paré was the first to be credited with the ligation of a vessel as an acceptable mode of treatment. Beginning with the nineteenth century, a progression of successes occurred with the introduction of laboratory techniques for suturing wounds and anastomosing vessels. Improved techniques for suturing arterial wounds using small ivory clamps were first introduced by Gluck in 1882 (Dalton et al, 1993). In 1889 Jassinowsky demonstrated a method for suturing the anastomosis. He avoided penetrating the intima based on the belief that this would cause thrombosis. In 1899 Dorfler demonstrated a technique for suturing that penetrated all the arterial layers using a very fine round needle and extremely fine silk thread (Haimovici, 1984a) .

The most notable contribution in the field of anastomosing and grafting blood vessels was made by Alexis Carrel. In 1902 a brief article described his method of utilizing three stay sutures, a technique now known as *triangulation*. He joined Guthrie in the United States in 1905 and modified his method of anastomosis. Carrel's contributions to the technical aspects of anastomosis can best be summarized as (1) obtaining gentle, temporary hemostasis, (2) careful peeling of the adventitia at the suture site, (3) avoiding tissue dehydration, (4) using three stay sutures (triangulating), (5) using very fine suturing materials, and (6) approximating wide intimal surfaces by everting suture through all layers of the vessel (Haimovici, 1984a).

EARLY SURGICAL CONTRIBUTIONS

Successful management of aneurysms remained an unanswered challenge until the time of Robert Matas (1888-1940). Dr. Matas performed approximately 620 vascular operations. More than 80% of these procedures were arterial ligations with only 15% of these being attempts at some form of vascular restoration. He operated only five times on the diseased abdominal aorta, primarily for aneurysm, with none of the procedures aimed at restoration. Only one patient survived. His major contribution to vascular surgery was the technical development of an effective occlusion of peripheral arterial aneurysms not followed by hemorrhage or recurrence. His technique fell gradually out of use over the next 20 years (Friedman, 1989a).

Autogenous vein use for arterial replacement was attempted by several surgeons. As early as 1906 Goyanes reported the "in situ use" of the popliteal vein to replace a portion of the popliteal artery removed during an aneurysm repair. In 1907 Lexer used a free saphenous vein graft to replace a portion of the axillary artery. In 1947 Cid dos Santos performed the first reconstructive procedure on a human artery by removing the obstructed atherosclerotic segment from a femoral artery (Szilagyi, 1994). The use was quickly extended to the aortoiliac area. Arterial homografts, using the techniques described by Guthrie in the laboratory, quickly followed. Between 1944 and 1949 many successful end-to-end anastomoses were performed to correct thoracic aortic coarctation (Friedman, 1989b).

The first use of a preserved human homograft occurred in 1949, when Gross resected a coarctation of the thoracic aorta and inserted arterial homografts. Other achievements soon followed. In 1951 the first resection and homograft replacement of an abdominal aortic aneurysm (AAA) occurred followed by the first successful resection and replacement of a bifurcated aneurysm in 1952 (Szilagyi, 1994).

The advancement of vascular surgery as a specialty was threatened when postoperative follow-up of arterial homografts proved them to be unstable and unreliable because of degenerative changes. Autologous grafts continue to be used, most notably for peripheral vascular surgeries and coronary artery bypass grafting. Although these early surgeries were successful, the practice of ligating arteries was continued up to the Korean War despite research by DeBakey and Simeone that concluded that suture repair resulted in fewer amputations than ligation (Friedman, 1989c).

During the Korean War the unacceptably high rate of arterial insufficiency following arterial ligation after traumatic injury led to the development of an Army policy known as **Maintenance and/or Restoration** whenever possible (Friedman, 1989c). The use of the now familiar techniques of direct anastomosis, lateral repair, and graft replacement resulted in a 96% success rate. A special team of the **Army Surgical Research Group** was sent to the war zone armed with newly available vascular instruments, antibiotics, blood products, and the military's newest ambulance, the helicopter. **Mobile Army Surgical Hospitals** (MASH units) were then able to repair vascular injuries on site instead of transporting the patient stateside. The first 130 cases performed demonstrated an 89% limb salvage rate, thus leading to a new era in vascular surgery. In 1952, Richard Warren visited Korea and arranged for all MASH hospitals to have the necessary instruments and the surgeons to have the necessary training to perform vascular repair. As a result, out of 304 major vascular repairs during the Korean War, an amputation rate of only 13% was reported versus the 49% amputation rate in World War Two (Friedman, 1989c).

With the outbreak of conflict in Vietnam came the opportunity to advance the lessons learned during the Korean War. The Vietnam Vascular Registry (**Registry of Vascular Injuries**) was formed in 1966 to analyze the treatment of vascular injuries (Friedman, 1989c). Approximately 1000 cases of acute arterial injuries were reviewed. All were managed primarily by vein grafting or end-to-end anastomoses. The limb salvage rate was 87%. The more efficient evacuation of the wounded, the presence of surgeons with the special skills to repair vascular injuries, and increased attempts to repair what historically would have been primary amputations led to the increased success (Friedman, 1989c). Other contributions from the Vietnam Vascular Registry include studies of the complications of vascular repair, specific artery injuries, management of venous injuries, missile emboli, and concomitant fractures with vascular injuries. The knowledge gained from this Registry has greatly influenced the practice of civilian vascular surgery (Friedman, 1989c).

EFFECTS OF PROGRESS IN OTHER FIELDS ON VASCULAR SURGERY

Several factors influenced the slow development of successful results in treating the diseased vascular system. Lack of an effective anticoagulant, limited diagnostic capability, and the lack of a substitute for arterial replacement severely limited progress in this field. Also of major importance were the serious consequences of infection. In addition, the etiology of what is now known as atherosclerosis was completely unknown and often microscopically misinterpreted. The pathology described was derived from inspection of the arteries on autopsy and on amputated limbs. "The essentially segmental nature of the atherosclerotic process did not become obvious until methods were developed to explore the vascular system in its entirety,

first by injection methods in the dissection room and then on living patients via angiography (Szilagyi, 1994, p. 4).

The arrival on the clinical scene of answers to the problems of coagulation, arterial substitution, and the nature of segmental atherosclerosis occurred within a relatively short period of time. Three developments had to occur before vascular surgery could advance. A means to explore the living vascular tree came first.

Arteriography/Angiography

Contrast angiography slowly but successfully became clinically acceptable. The turning point came in 1929 when water soluble organic iodides became available replacing the more hazardous medias used in the past. Three approaches to introducing the contrast media gained general use, direct transcutaneous puncture, i.e., cannulating an artery (1927); translumbar abdominal aortic puncture (1929); and percutaneous arterial catheterization (1953). This last technique, along with the safer radiopaque substances, allowed more precise visualization, especially of the visceral vessels (Szilagyi, 1994).

Anticoagulant Development

Heparin, a safe agent to control blood clotting, was used first in 1937. By 1940 heparin was generally accepted in the treatment of venous thrombosis and was ready to be used as an intervention in the arterial tree. In the same year that heparin began to be used clinically, dicumarol (Coumadin), was also discovered. The use of these anticoagulants in vascular surgery allowed for safer handling of blood vessels by preventing intraoperative and postoperative thrombosis (Szilagyi, 1994). Heparin is widely used intravenously during vascular surgery before temporary occlusion of an artery and as intravascular irrigation during arterial surgery. It is also given subcutaneously before major surgery to prevent venous thrombosis.

Antibiotics

The discovery and development of antibiotics occurred approximately at the same time as the anticoagulants. By controlling infection, a major cause of graft failure, antibiotics had a very beneficial effect on the development of vascular surgery (Szilagyi, 1994).

Other Developments

Blood transfusions and substitutes, coupled with better knowledge of surgery-related metabolic disturbances, greatly influenced the development of vascular surgery. New instrumentation, suture materials, and increasing knowledge of the physiology lead to many advances in techniques and patient monitoring. Without these developments, vascular surgery could not have reached its present state (Haimovici, 1984a).

ARTERIAL SURGERY
Modern Vascular Surgery

The beginnings of the modern era of cardiovascular surgery occurred when Gross successfully ligated a patent ductus arteriosus in 1938, followed in 1944 by Blalock and Taussig reporting the first operation for tetralogy of Fallot by anastomosing the left subclavian to the pulmonary artery by an end-to-side technique. Also in 1944 two physicians in Stockholm succeeded in correcting a coarctation of the aorta. Gross also demonstrated success in correcting coarctation in 1945. Careful laboratory experiments proceeded these important developments (Haimovici, 1984a). These early successes in correcting congenital abnormalities resulted in a great deal of activity throughout the world. An explosion of new methods for investigating and treating cardiac and vascular diseases occurred.

Progress has continued in the diagnostic field, including the advent of "noninvasive" technologies such as ultrasound and ultrasonic duplex scanning. Digital subtraction angiography increased the safety factor of angiography by reducing the concentration of contrast media in vital organs and thus reducing the risk of renal toxicity. Magnetic resonance angiography (MRA), a new technique directly imaging the flow of blood without contrast media, has eliminated the risks associated with contrast media use. MRA is well suited for distal visualization of arteries in severely ischemic limbs. These developments furthered the advances of vascular surgery (Haimovici, 1996a).

Occlusive and Aneurysmal Lesions

Vascular grafting was connected with the early phase of congenital cardiac and vascular surgeries. Indeed, the first arterial transplantation of homografts was accomplished by Gross and his associates in the late 40s, thus beginning the truly modern phase of vascular surgery. In 1951 Dubost and colleagues demonstrated the excisional therapy of treating abdominal aortic aneurysms and replacement with a homograft, beginning the current era of curative aneurysmal surgery. Shortly thereafter, DeBakey and Cooley applied this technique to thoracic aneurysms, leading to its use in all segments of the vascular tree (Haimovici, 1996a; Friedman, 1989d).

The search for an artificial graft material was necessitated by long-term follow-up studies of homograft replacements. The homografts suffered from degenerative changes over time, veins were unsuitable for some arterial replacements, and the supply of homologous tissues grafts was unacceptable. The first successful demonstration of the use of a porous woven conduit of synthetic material, a fabric called Vinyon-N made by Union Carbide for parachutes, occurred in 1949 by Dr. A. Voorhees (Smith, 1993). Other materials had been used historically, including glass, rubber, silicone, and aluminum tubes. Rationale for the use of "plastic tubes" came from Voorhees et al's studies using Vinyon-N and the observation of fibrin plug formation filling the fine mesh holes to clot the graft and allow blood flow. The early problems of this technique included seams created when tailoring the tube in the operating room and cuffing back the tube ends. Edwards and Tapp introduced nylon braided tubes that, when soaked in formic acid could be cut anywhere along their length and easily sutured in place without fraying, solved this problem. Kinking was still the major problem when these grafts were sewn across flexion points in the body. This was soon solved through the crimping process, which allows the graft to flex (Haimovici, 1984a). Intensive investigations began for an "ideal" homograft material. Expanded polytetrafluoroethylene, PTFE, (Gore-Tex or IMPRA), the gluteraldehyde processed umbilical vein homograft (Meadox biograft),velour knit Dacron grafts, and collagen impregnated grafts resulted. The search for the perfect graft material continues (Veith & Haimovici, 1996).

Thromboendarterectomy

Early attempts at removing obstructions in the arterial system by simple thrombectomy were not successful. This technique fell into disuse until J. Cid dos Santos in 1946 attempted thrombectomy with heparin adjunct. In thromboendarterectomy, both the thrombus and the intima and part of the inner media are removed, without the accompanying clotting and reobstruction. This technique remains in use for carotid endarterectomy and some portions of the aortoiliac system and is a valid and useful procedure (Haimovici, 1996b).

The bypass principle

The bypass principle, first advocated in 1931 by Ernst Jeger (Germany) for managing peripheral aneurysms, was not well known (Haimovici, 1996a). Until 1948, the conventional method of excising the lesion and placing a graft was the accepted method for treating these occlusions. J. Kunlin in 1948 reported using this technique in an end-to-side venous graft implantation in a patient with significant fibrotic reaction to a previously grafted site. The rationale of a bypass is based on avoidance of damage to adjacent vessels and nerves and preservation of collateral circulation (Haimovici, 1996a). In the 1950s Robert Linton (Massachusetts General Hospital) further espoused the use of reversed saphenous vein graft as a viable arterial conduit. This resulted in reversed vein grafting as the procedure of choice for reconstructive bypass (Barker, 1993).

Arterial Embolectomy

Arterial embolectomy, one of the earliest known direct arterial procedures, has been performed since 1911. Although refinements in technique and the better use of anticoagulants increased the success rate of this procedure, significant improvement wasn't achieved until 1963 with the introduction of the Fogarty balloon catheter. "This instrument has become an important part of the surgical armamentarium and is used widely in all types of arterial procedures besides embolectomy" (Haimovici, 1996a, p. 4). The invention of the the embolectomy balloon catheter by Dr. Thomas Fogarty is considered a major advancement in technique. The technique has evolved to be used in venous, arterial, and general surgery (Barker, 1993). The name "Fogarty" has become synonymous with balloon embolectomy catheter.

AORTIC ANEURYSM RESECTION AND AORTOILIAC BYPASS

Historically, abdominal aortic aneurysm (AAA) surgery can be traced back to the second century when Antyllus introduced ligation of the aorta above and below the aneurysm and allowed the aorta to granulate closed (Friedman, 1989). Most treatments were palliative and involved some form of ligation of the aorta around the aneurysmal sac. Other methods were tried including Matas' procedure of endoaneurysmorrhaphy in 1888. Of historical interest only, cellophane wrapping of the aneurysm and electrocoagulation were also tried. The modern repair of the aorta is first attributed to René Dubost et al in 1951. With the introduction of fabrics such as Orlon and Teflon in the 1950s the era of prosthetic graft replacement began. In 1957 DeBakey and colleagues introduced knitted Dacron grafts, providing the first effective graft material (Hollier & Wisselink, 1996) (see Chapter 15).

Dissecting Aneurysms

In 1935 Gurin et al first attempted to treat dissecting aneurysms. The second attempt, by Shaw in 1955, emphasized the same technique used by Gurin. In both cases, an opening was made through the intima into the false lumen of the dissecting aneurysm, allowing blood flow to resume to the extremities. This technique came to be known as *fenestration* of the dissected intima. Both patients died within days of surgery because of renal failure (Haimovici,1984a). DeBakey and colleagues performed the first successful dissecting aneurysm repair in 1956. The improvement of medical management of arterial hypertension, the usual cause associated with the condition, has added a nonsurgical solution. Surgery is done when medical intervention fails to control this condition (Haimovici,1996a).

CAROTID ENDARTERECTOMY

Occlusive lesions in the extracranial segments of the internal and external carotid arteries supplying the brain and their impact on blood flow to the brain was described in the early 1800s. In 1914 Hunt again noted the importance of these lesions and their impact on cranial ischemia. However, it wasn't until the development of cerebral angiography, a practical method for diagnosing cerebral arterial disease, that surgical intervention of the carotid artery became a reality (Thompson, 1984). Carrea et al performed the first successful carotid artery reconstruction in Buenos Aries in 1951. The first successful carotid endarterectomy was performed by Michael DeBakey in 1953. The greatest impetus to the development of surgery for carotid occlusive disease was surgery done by Eastcott et al in 1954 (Thompson, 1984). Stroke prevention in symptomatic and asymptomatic patients is the major consideration in diagnosing carotid stenosis. Three separate, randomized, multicenter clinical studies demonstrated that in patients with a 70% to 99% diameter reduction of the internal carotid artery, surgical endarterectomy markedly reduced the follow-up stroke rates (Imparato, 1996) (see Chapter 11).

FEMORAL-POPLITEAL/TIBIAL BYPASS

The year 1947 marked the introduction of thromboendarterectomy by Cid dos Santos. In 1948 Kunlin performed the first bypass graft, thus starting the era of direct revascularization of the lower extremity. Of the two procedures, bypass is the more widely used (Veith & Haimovici, 1996).

Occurrence of occlusive lesions in the femoropopliteal segment affects between 47% and 65.4% of the population over age 60 (Veith & Haimovici, 1996). Longer life spans and better treatment of diseases like diabetes have lead to an older population and an increase in occlusive lesions (see Chapter 12).

EXTRAANATOMIC BYPASSES: FEMOROFEMORAL AND AXILLOFEMORAL BYPASS

In 1952 Freeman and Leeds first described the superficial femoral artery bypass. Blaisdell and Hall in the United States and Louw in South Africa combined Lewis' principle with the idea of a safer, simpler, and quicker procedure to save ischemic limbs in patients too ill to undergo standard aortofemoral procedures. "Almost simultaneously, they performed extracavitary bypasses from the axillary artery to the common femoral artery using synthetic graft material" (Ascer & Veith, 1996, p. 688). McCaughan and Kahn reported two cases of iliac-to-contralateral popliteal crossovers in 1958 (Freidman, 1989e). Popularizing this concept was Vetto, who in 1962 performed subcutaneous crossover femorofemoral grafts in 10 patients with good limb-salvage results (Ascer & Veith, 1996).

Extraanatomic bypasses were also demonstrated to be effective as an alternative to intrathoracic or mediastinal procedures for treating occlusive disease of the arch and its branches. Lyons and Galbraith performed the first extrathoracic bypass in 1956 using a nylon prosthesis to construct a subclavian-carotid bypass. The patient, a 67-year-old man with internal carotid stenosis and transient ischemic attacks, remained asymptomatic 7 months after surgery (Friedman, 1989e). Throughout the 1960s the techniques of extraanatomic bypass were perfected and successes demonstrated in axillofemoral as well as femorofemoral bypass (see Chapter 17).

ARTERIOVENOUS FISTULAE

Guido Guidi (1500-1559), surgeon of Emperor Francis I, is credited with having first described a congenital arteriovenous malformation (Gloviczki & Hollier,1996). Observation of arteriovenous fistulae have been described in the literature since the early 1700s. In a review of the literature through 1914, Callender, a student of Halsted, found approximately 500 arteriovenous fistulae with only 3 being attributed to congenital causes (Gloviczki & Hollier,1996). Experiences with World War Two, the Korean conflict, and Vietnam contributed important information regarding traumatic arteriovenous fistulae. In evaluating data from the Vietnam Vascular Registry, 3.5% of patients had arteriovenous fistulae. An almost equal number had false arterial aneurysms. Studies comparing civilian data with the Registry data demonstrate a similar incidence (Gloviczki & Hollier, 1996).

Vascular Access for Dialysis

The origins of hemodialysis can be traced to the World War Two occupation of the Netherlands by German forces. Dr. Willem Kolff in 1943 developed the first artificial kidney. This original machine was crude and severely limited. The number of treatments done was determined by the number of arterial and venous sites that could be sacrificed for canalization. It was limited solely to acute renal failure where recovery of the kidney was expected (Schanzer and Skladany, 1996). Use of this technique continued to be limited despite the improvements in technology.

The development of an external shunt by Quinton, Scribner, and Dillard in 1960 allowed for repetitive dialysis and opened the field to chronic dialysis treatment. The initial shunts were made of Teflon, a rigid material that limited their performance over time. Silicone replaced Teflon as the tube material, increasing their function. Patency, generally lasting only 3 to 6 months, continued to be a problem. Infection and thrombosis were common, requiring frequent replacement and site change (Schanzer & Skladany, 1996).

Dr. Appel in 1966 first introduced the concept of using a surgically produced arteriovenous fistula. In cooperation with his nephrology colleagues Brescia and Cimino, human trials were begun. They resulted in immediate success, allowing for long-term dialysis with low morbidity. This became the procedure of choice for long term dialysis access (Schanzer & Skladany, 1996).

Both autogenous and homologous materials have been used to create this fistula. One common drawback is the need to let the fistula "mature" before its use. The current approach for temporary dialysis access is to place one of the many intravascular access devices developed for this purpose (Schanzer & Skladany, 1996). Deliberate creation of an arteriovenous fistula for dialysis in end-stage renal failure patients is among the most frequently performed vascular procedures today (see Chapter 16).

VENOUS SURGERY

Venous Interruption

A theory of the pathogenesis of thromboembolism was first presented by Virchow between 1846 and 1856. Spencer, Wells, and Hegan reported the first fatal cases of postoperative pulmonary embolism. The first successful inferior vena caval interruption to prevent embolism was performed by Bottini. In 1906 Trendelenburg ligated the infrarenal vena cava to prevent septic thromboembolism from pelvic and ovarian veins (Greenfield & Proctor, 1996).

In 1934, when autopsy studies associated peripheral vein thrombosis with pulmonary embolism, Homans recommended femoral vein ligation to prevent it. Later, this femoral ligation was associated with failure to prevent pulmonary emboli and development of more emboli. Homans then recommended inferior vena caval (IVC) ligation. Ligation of the IVC, although effective in preventing some pulmonary embolisms, was associated with a 14% mortality rate and a 33% incidence of chronic venous insufficiency (Greenfield & Proctor, 1996).

Plication of the IVC was then trialed to reduce the morbidity associated with ligation. An absorbable suture, first suggested by Dale, was used with the idea that once the risk of embolism had passed the cava would recannulate. A variety of external caval clip devices were tried, with the reduction of long-term mortality, but required general anesthesia in these critically ill patients. During the 1960s intraluminal devices such as the Greenfield filter were introduced. These could be inserted through the femoral or jugular veins under local anesthesia, decreasing the anesthetic risk (Greenfield & Proctor, 1996) (see Chapter 18).

Ligation and Stripping of Varicose Veins

Varicose veins and their treatment have been discussed since antiquity. The first recorded varicose vein treatment is credited to Hippocrates in 370 B.C. The current stab avulsion technique was first used by Galen around 200 A.D. The total removal of the greater saphenous vein by stripping was begun as early as 1844 by Madelung (Germany). Vein ligation and sclerotherapy were advocated in the early 1900s by Tavel. In 1906 Mayo utilized an extraluminal method for vein stripping and in 1906 Babcock (New York) designed the precursor to the current plastic intraluminal vein strippers. Surgical treatment of ligation and stripping has been standard for the last 100 years. Recent studies have questioned this approach (O'Donnell, Jr. & Iafrati, 1996) (see Chapter 19).

THORACIC OUTLET SURGERY

For over 100 years neurovascular compression has been recognized as the cause of a variety of arterial, venous, and neurologic symptoms in the upper extremities. Many treatments and procedures have been attempted based on the location of the compression, which have had varying benefits for the patients. To clearly identify and establish a treatment for these symptoms, this group of compression problems has been named thoracic outlet compression syndrome (TOS). All types of compression in the upper extremities are related to compression of the brachial plexus, the subclavian artery, the subclavian vein, or any combination of the three, between the clavicle and the first rib. Both osseous and soft tissue structures can cause compression of the neurovascular bundles in the shoulder region (Owens, 1984).

As early as the eighteenth century physicians identified a relationship between the cervical ribs and upper extremity neurovascular problems. The first excision of a cervical rib to relieve compression problems occurred in 1861(Owens, 1984). Through the end of the eighteenth century and well into the nineteenth century these compression syndromes were studied. Many reports of relief of symptoms as a result of rib removal, some normal and some abnormal, have been documented. Descent of the clavicle has also been noted to cause the symptoms of compression.

In the discussion of soft tissue structures causing compression, particular mention must be made of the scalenus anticus muscle. From 1905 through the 1930s many reports by Adson and Coffey, Ochsner, DeBakey, and others indicated that symptom relief was obtained when this muscle was divided (Owens, 1984). Development of current theories regarding TOS has followed three arbitrary time periods. The first era known as the cervical rib era, 1740-1920, the second era when other causes were added, 1920-1956, and the third era when TOS became well defined (Sanders & Cooper, 1996) (see Chapter 13).

SYMPATHECTOMY

Sympathectomy has been used in both lower extremity vascular disease and upper extremity disease. Lower extremity sympathectomy, i.e., lumbar sympathectomy, was first performed in 1924 by Julio Diez of Argentina. Two procedures had been tried previously with limited results. In 1899 Jaboulay stripped the arterial adventitia to control leg ulcers. This operation, known as periarterial sympathectomy, was tried again by René Leriche (France). Unfortunately it was based on a misunderstanding of arterial innervation and was not successful. In 1914 Kramer and Todd, followed by many others, correctly described the innervation of the arteries, thus opening the door for effective lumbar sympathectomy (Haimovici, 1996c).

The history of sympathectomy has been tumultuous. When revascularization procedures became widely accepted, the use of sympathectomy declined. But sympathectomy still has indications for use, particularly when peripheral vasospastic disease and extreme occlusive disease are present (Haimovici, 1996c).

Cervical and upper thoracic sympathectomies followed the same historical course of lumbar sympathectomies. Both Jaboulay and Leriche played a part in the early years. The first successful cervical sympathectomy was performed by Kotzareff in 1920. According to Haimovici (1996c), it is well known that cervicothoracic sympathectomy may sometimes fail to offer permanent denervation of the upper extremity. Return of sympathetic activity may be attributed to regeneration of preganglionic fibers and accessory ganglions. Lasting denervation in upper extremities, in some cases, is still difficult to achieve (Haimovici, 1996c) (see Chapter 14).

LAST STAGE RECONSTRUCTION: AMPUTATIONS

Amputation has long been thought of as the last resort. Many types of procedures exist. Syme first performed the procedure that bears his name in 1842 (the Syme amputation removes the foot). Transmetatarsal amputation was first described in 1949. Previously considered to be mutilating and debilitating, amputation, when done as the last stage in the reconstruction of the vascularly impaired limb, creates a new functioning organ of the repaired limb or extremity stump (Haimovici, 1996c). Advances in materials and the understanding of the biomechanics of ambulation have also affected rapid rehabilitation. Detailed criteria for determining the level of amputation have been developed. Cooperation between a diverse group of health care providers is necessary to achieve the best patient results (Haimovici, 1996c) (see Chapter 20).

VASCULAR SURGERY, A SPECIALTY

As progress was made in vascular surgery from 1961 to 1970, it became obvious that special skills and special cognitive and technical preparation were needed in the physician training programs to achieve continued success. These special areas were considered to be the hallmark of a self-contained specialty. By the early 1970s the two vascular societies (the Society for Vascular Surgery and the International Society for Cardiovascular Surgery) recognized that a large portion of surgeons entering the practice of treating vascular disease did not have adequate training in the specialty and were achieving poor patient outcomes (Szilagyi, 1994). The two societies approached the American Board of Surgery with a proposal to develop a specialty for setting standards and supervising the graduate education of vascular residents. The societies felt that this would require lengthening the residency programs by 1 year. This proposal was rejected in 1972. It wasn't until 1982, 10 years later, that the American Board of General Vascular Surgery was established.

Conflict in the specialty areas still existed even as the first examination to establish board certification in Vascular Surgery was being prepared. The American Board of Surgery reasserted in a policy statement that "general surgeons are expected to have detailed knowledge . . . of the preoperative, operative, and postoperative care of patients with diseases of the . . . vascular system" (Szilagyi, 1994).

When the Surgical Residency Review Board performed an inspection of the training programs in 1983 to 1984, only 20 of the inspected programs met the standards for approval as a vascular specialty training program. The reason for so few meeting the criteria was the insufficient vascular experience provided for the general surgery resident. No adequate definition existed for what was "sufficient vascular experience" and the inspecting board refused to define it, although rumors of the minimum requirement being 30 to 40 independent vascular reconstruction operations were frequently heard. No firm guideline had been established as recently as 1994. The problem that has made it difficult for a practicing surgeon to see the logic of the American Board of Surgery's position is a universal agreement of the vascular surgeons that the minimum requirement for gaining competence is a 12-month period, which would mean lengthening the 5-year residency to 6 or severely limiting the residents' exposure to other subdivisions of the general surgery training. In addition, it is felt universally that the minimum requirement for gaining competency in vascular surgery is a range of 80 to 120 independently performed cases. This is not obtainable in the current course of study. The debate continues as the volume of patients requiring vascular intervention grows as a result of the aging of the population (Szilagyi, 1994).

ETHICAL CONSIDERATIONS

With the advent of ever increasing noninvasive diagnostic tools comes the question of which lesions should be treated versus which should not. The underlying philosophy of vascular surgery, to save life and limb by all reasonable means, has a wide range in which it can exert its influence and still remain within the bounds of conventional ethics (Szilagyi, 1994). Tradition has built a list of precepts to guide the vascular surgeon in making decisions regarding how to proceed. The list included the following:

1. An angiogram alone should not be the basis for operating. The starting point of the decision tree should always be the patient's history and a physical examination.
2. Failure to acknowledge the limits of one's abilities is the first step to disaster.
3. Thoughtful consideration must be given to the statistics one believes.
4. Remember that when considering "what price a leg," the price varies depending on the patient's history and previous surgeries.
5. Diagnostic tools do not replace the need for a thorough history and physical examination (Szilagyi, 1994).

Keeping these precepts in mind will assist the surgeon in making decisions of whether to operate or not in an ethical manner.

NEW DEVELOPMENTS FOR THE FUTURE

The continued improvement of noninvasive diagnostic tools, the expansion of less invasive surgery techniques, and continuing research in the vascular field for better arterial substitutes leaves the field of vascular surgery open to many changes in the coming years. In the 1980s and 1990s we have seen such advances as laser technology applied to arterial and venous lesions, special catheters for balloon angioplasty of the vascular tree, and catheters that act like drills for opening lesions. Some of these techniques had lasting effects on the approach to vascular surgery, some did not.

Endovascular grafting of abdominal aortic aneurysms (AAA) is an area under current research. First demonstrated in 1991 by Parodi et al, using stents to secure the transfemorally placed implant, the procedure is gaining recognition as an alternative to traditional aneurysm repair (Edwards et al, 1996). As randomized studies using the graft-placing devices developed by EndoVascular Technologies, Inc., Menlo, Calif., (the only device with FDA approval for clinical trials) continue, the efficacy of transfemoral aortic repair is increasing. Dr. William Edwards, Jr. et al report in their study, published in Annals of Surgery, May, 1996, on the successful use of endovascular grafting in a randomized clinical trial in Nashville, Tenn. Vanderbilt and St. Thomas Hospitals were two of the first 13 clinical sites to participate in a Phase I study of transfemoral placement of endovascular grafts (TPEG) using a tube prosthesis.

The first patient was enrolled in December, 1993, with a total of five patients in the first portion of the study. Four patients had successful procedures. In one patient, they were unable to pass the expandable sheath of the EVT after aggressive dilatation of the iliac artery, requiring open surgery to be performed. Of these four patients, the only female in the study required a femoral/femoral bypass the night of the EVT placement because of ipsilateral iliac artery injury. Another patient developed lymphorrhea, requiring an incision and drainage of the infected lymphocele after 2 months. The four patients were followed for 21.5 months, with no leaks and no enlargement of the aneurysms detected. Standard follow-up includes computed tomography (CT) scan, ultrasound, and abdominal x-ray studies before discharge, at 6 weeks, at 6 months, and annually thereafter (Edwards et al, 1996).

Interventional radiology and specially designed balloon catheters have been used for management of stenotic arterial lesions. Other attempts to find a successful means to recanalize arteries have been made. Papers published in 1964 by Dotter and Judkins and in 1969 by Dotter indicated that new techniques using transluminal approaches were being developed. In 1974 Dotter, Gruntzig, and Hopff introduced a special balloon catheter for dilating occlusive arterial lesions. This was followed by a double balloon catheter developed by Gruntzig (1976) for performing percutaneous transluminal arterioplasty (PTA). Lasers were introduced when early restenosis caused by intimal hyperplasia was encountered. Initially the laser was used to recanalize arterial occlusive segments and as an angioplasty tool. Unfortunately, use of the laser led to a high incidence of arterial wall perforations. Despite adding angioscopy to the protocol for laser use, the perforations continued. Use of the laser proved to be too high risk. Exploration of other technologies for percutaneous revascularization continues (Haimovici, 1996a).

NURSING IMPLICATIONS

The perioperative nurse must have an understanding of vascular disease and its progression to make a comprehensive assessment and develop a plan of care. Considerations should include, but not be limited to, vascular symptoms, medical conditions, nutritional status, use of alcohol and cigarettes, and any existing skin lesions. Identification of peripheral pulses and grading will also assist the nurse with intraoperative tissue perfusion assessment. Verification of the signs and symptoms of peripheral vascular disease, such as muscle and tissue wasting, assist in making decisions for the preoperative, intraoperative, and postoperative plans of care (MacVittie, 1995).

Mental status assessment, emotional state, and level of understanding are all crucial to success. Patients and their caregivers need to be able to identify changes and symptoms that might signify progression of the vascular disease. As vascular surgery has progressed, nursing has played an important role in educating the patient and significant others regarding the symptoms and precautions necessary to ensure success.

Intraoperatively, nursing plays an important role in the outcome of the procedure. Aseptic technique maintenance, tissue perfusion, and skin integrity maintenance, as well as temperature maintenance are all key aspects to ensuring positive outcomes (MacVittie, 1995) (see Chapters 4 to 7).

An interest and desire to participate in a rapidly changing specialty is key to success for the perioperative vascular nurse. As new techniques and procedures for revascularization are developed, the nurse will be challenged to stay abreast of the implications for patients. For instance, the endovascular grafting of AAAs requires two teams of nurses to be available. Whenever this procedure is performed, an operating suite must be prepared to do an emergency open AAA if an adverse situation develops during the endovascular procedure. Constant communication between the team performing the endovascular procedure and the team waiting in the wings in case of emergency is of utmost importance. At any instant the procedure may have to be converted to an open procedure, especially during these early trial periods.

As endoscopic procedures for repairing aneurysms become more common, the perioperative nurse will be faced with another challenge: the need to develop working relationships with radiologists and other specialists. Just as percutaneous transluminal coronary angioplasty became a procedure done in areas outside of the operating room, so may endovascular repair of aneurysms. The perioperative nurse can be of assistance in providing knowledge of aseptic technique, patient advocacy, positioning, and assessment to specialty areas. He or she will also be required to learn about the special skills of other areas.

Endoscopic surgery is gaining increasing popularity with the public. The concept of smaller incisions with the implication of decreased pain, smaller scars, and decreased length of stay is attractive to all involved. Saphenous vein graft harvesting and the creation of arteriovenous fistulas for dialysis are being performed using endoscopic techniques. Industry is working closely with physicians and nurses to develop sophisticated instrumentation such as tunneling light carriers and microclip appliers. Nurses often provide ideas and feedback on the design and handling of new devices.

A thorough knowledge of the impact of new technology on perioperative patient care as well as a commitment to the challenges of a changing environment are essential for the perioperative nurse of tomorrow. Intraoperative duplex scanning is another opportunity for learning new technologies and interacting with other specialties. The ability to adapt current knowledge and skills and apply them in a variety of settings will ensure the role of the perioperative nurse of the future. A specialty nursing organization for vascular nurses, the **Society of Vascular Nursing (SVN)** can best be described by their mission statement. "Founded in 1982, the Society of Vascular Nursing is a not-for-profit international association dedicated to promoting excellence in the compassionate and comprehensive management of persons with vascular disease. Excellence will be attained by providing quality education, fostering clinical expertise and supporting nursing research. The Society will:

- assume a leadership role in defining the vascular component of fundamental nursing education
- establish and implement research-based standards for vascular nursing
- collaborate with other professions to address the unique needs of the vascular patient
- enhance public awareness of vascular disease."

In 1996 the Society of Vascular Nursing established the first examination for national certification in vascular nursing. Those who successfully pass the examination earn the initials CVN after their name.

Box 1-1 History Timeline

200-300	Antyllus ligates an AAA
1759	Hallowell (England) performs first successful arterial surgery for trauma
1877	First vessel anastomosis by Eck, portal vein to IVC in dogs
1888	Matas performs endoaneurysmorrhaphy
1912	Carrel receives Nobel Prize for advances in blood transfusions, vascular suture techniques, and organ transplantation in animals
1916	Heparin isolated; too toxic for clinical use
1924	First lumbar sympathectomy for lower extremity vascular insufficiency by Diez
1931	Jeger advocates arterial bypass principle
1937	Heparin used clinically to control clotting
1947	First meeting of the Society of Vascular Surgery; dos Santos performs successful endarterectomy
1948	Kunlin proposes concept of extraanatomic bypass
1949	First clinical use of streptokinase to dissolve clot in thorax
1950s	Synthetic vascular graft work evolving
	First elective carotid reconstruction by Carrea
	Carotid endarterectomy, separate work by Cooley and DeBakey
	Reversed saphenous vein grafting
1951	Dubost replaces AAA with aortic homograft
1952	Voorhees and Blakemore use synthetic fabric graft on aorta
1955	Intravascular use of streptokinase
1962	Rob (London) performs in situ vein graft with valve disruption for arterial reconstruction
1963	Balloon embolectomy catheter by Thomas Fogarty
1964	First transluminal angioplasty by Dotter
1966	Appel introduces arteriovenous fistulae for hemodialysis
1982	Society of Vascular Nursing founded
1996	National certification examination for vascular nursing established

Modified from Bergan (1991); Barker (1993); Camerota et al (1987); Green & Ouriel (1994); Szilagyi (1994); Schanzer & Skladany (1996).

References

Ascer, E., & Veith, F.J. (1996). Extra-anatomic bypasses. In H. Haimovici (Ed.), *Vascular surgery: Principles and techniques* (pp. 688-699). Cambridge, MA: Blackwell Science.

Barker, W. (1993). A history of vascular surgery. In W.S. Moore (Ed.), *Vascular surgery: A comprehensive review* (pp. 1-15). Philadelphia: W.B. Saunders.

Dalton, M.L., & Connally, S.R. Celiac: The original vascular clamp. *Annals of Vascular Surgery, 391(7):4, 1993.*

Edwards, W. H. Jr., Naslund, T. C., Edwards, W. H. Sr., Jenkins, J. M., & McPherson, K. (1996). Endovascular grafting of abdominal aortic aneurysms: A preliminary study. *Annals of Surgery 223(5):2.*

Friedman, S. G. (1989a). *A history of vascular surgery* (pp. 63-72a). Mount Cask, NY: Futura Publishing.

Friedman, S. G. (1989b). *A history of vascular surgery* (pp. 85-110b). Mount Cask, NY: Futura Publishing.

Friedman, S. G. (1989c). *A history of vascular surgery* (pp. 173-192c). Mount Cask, NY: Futura Publishing.

Friedman, S. G. (1989d). *A history of vascular surgery* (pp. 11-130d). Mount Cask, NY: Futura Publishing.

Friedman, S. G. (1989e). *A history of vascular surgery* (pp. 1-14e). Mount Cask, NY: Futura Publishing.

Friedman, S. G. (1989f). *A history of vascular surgery* (pp. 193-208f). Mount Cask, NY: Futura Publishing.

Gloviczki, P., & Hollier, L. H. (1996). Arteriovenous fistulas. In H. Haimovici (Ed.), *Vascular surgery: Principles and techniques* (pp. 870-892). Cambridge, MA: Blackwell Science.

Greenfield, L. J., & Proctor, M. C. (1996). Venous interruption. In H. Haimovici (Ed.), *Vascular surgery: Principles and techniques* (pp. 1210-1219). Cambridge, MA: Blackwell Science.

Haimovici, H. (1984a). History of vascular surgery. In H. Haimovici (Ed.), *Vascular surgery: Principles and techniques* (p. 3017). Norwalk, CT: Appleton-Century-Crofts.

Haimovici, H. (1996a). An historic overview of vascular surgery: Past record and new trends—a vision for the 1990s. In H. Haimovici (Ed.). *Vascular surgery: Principles and techniques* (pp. 1-10). Cambridge, MA: Blackwell Science.

Haimovici, H. (1996b). Endarterectomy. In H. Haimovici (Ed.). *Vascular surgery: Principles and techniques* (pp. 294-303). Cambridge, MA: Blackwell Science.

Haimovici, H. (1996c). Upper thoracic sympathectomy: Conventional technique. In H. Haimovici (Ed.). *Vascular surgery: Principles and techniques* (pp. 1110-1117). Cambridge, MA: Blackwell Science.

Hollier, L. H., & Wisselink, W. (1996). Abdominal aortic aneurysm. In H. Haimovici (Ed.), *Vascular surgery: Principles and techniques* (pp. 797-827). Cambridge, MA: Blackwell Science.

Imparato, A. M. (1996). Carotid endarterectomy: Indications and techniques for carotid surgery. In H. Haimovici (Ed.), *Vascular surgery: Principles and techniques.* Cambridge, MA: Blackwell Science.

MacVittie, B. A. (1995). Vascular surgery. In Meeker & Rothrock (Ed.), *Alexander's care of the patient in surgery* (pp. 1032-1057). St. Louis: Mosby.

O'Donnell, T. F., & Iafrati, M. D. (1996). Varicose veins. In H. Haimovici (Ed.), *Vascular surgery: Principles and techniques* (pp. 1187-1204). Cambridge, MA: Blackwell Science.

Owens, J. C. D. (1984). Thoracic outlet compression syndrome. In H. Haimovici (Ed.), *Vascular surgery: Principles and techniques* (pp. 877-902). Norwalk, CT: Appleton-Century-Crofts.

Sanders, R. J., & Cooper, M. A. (1996). Venous thoracic outlet syndrome or subclavian vein obstruction. In H. Haimovici (Ed.), *Vascular surgery: Principles and techniques* (pp. 1073-1081). Cambridge, MA: Blackwell Science.

Schanzer, H., & Skladany, M. (1996). Vascular access for dialysis. In H. Haimovici (Ed.), *Vascular surgery: Principles and techniques* (pp. 1028-1041). Cambridge, MA: Blackwell Science.

Smith, R. B. III. (1993). Arthur B. Voorhees, Jr: Pioneer vascular surgeon. *Journal of Vascular Surgery, 18*(3): 343.

Szilagyi, D. E. (1994). Vascular surgery: A propaedeutic of its past, present, and future. In Veith, Hobson, Williams & Wilson (Eds.). *Vascular surgery: Principles and practice* (p. 3). NY: McGraw-Hill.

Thompson, J. E. (1984). Cerebrovascular insufficiency. In H. Haimovici (Ed.). *Vascular surgery: Principles and techniques* (pp. 797-812). Norwalk, CT: Appleton-Century-Crofts.

Veith, F. J., & Haimovici, H. (1996). Femoropopliteal arteriosclerotic occlusive disease. In H. Haimovici (Ed.), *Vascular surgery: Principles and techniques* (pp. 605-631). Cambridge, MA: Blackwell Science.

Bibliography

Dalton, M. L., Canaille, SR, & Sealx, W. C. (1993). The original vascular clamp. *Annals of Vascular Surgery, 7*(4): 391-393.

Dodson, T. F. (1992). Profiles in cardiology: Robert Ritchie Linton. *Clinical Cardiology, 15*(9): 702-704.

Edwards, W. H. Jr., Naslund, T. C., Edwards, W. H. Sr., Jenkins, J. M., & McPherson, K. (1996). Endovascular grafting of abdominal aortic aneurysms: A preliminary study, *Annals of Surgery, 223*(5): 1-5.

Friedmann, P. (1993) Presidential address: Decay and revival of vascular surgery. *Journal of Vascular Surgery, 17*(6): 985-993.

Friedman, S. G., & Friedman, M. S. (1989) Matas, antyllus, and endo-aneurysmorrhaphy. *Surgery, 105*(6): 761-763.

Friedman, S. G. (1989). *A history of vascular surgery.* Mount Cask, NY: Futura Publishing.

Haimovici, H: (1984).*Vascular surgery: Principles and techniques.* Norwalk, CT: Appleton-Century-Crofts.

Haimovici, H. (1996). *Vascular surgery: Principles and practice.* Cambridge, MA: Blackwell Science.

Smith, L. L. (1993). Surgeons and the evolution of vascular surgery. *Archives of Surgery, 128*(9): 957-963.

Smith, R. B. (1993). Arthur B. Voorhees, Jr., pioneer vascular surgeon. *Journal of Vascular Surgery, 18*(3): 341-347.

Wilson, S., Veith, F. J., Hobson, R. W., & Williams, R. A. (1994). *Vascular surgery: Principles and practice.* NY: McGraw-Hill.

2 The Vascular Team

VASCULAR TEAM MEMBERS

Patient

The patient is the most important member of the vascular surgical team. They may choose to be more or less involved, passive or active in their own health care and decision making. The focus of the other team members must remain on the recipient of care. Vascular disease is usually a progressive, multisystem process. Both arterial and venous disorders can be chronic with acute exacerbations. Many patients are smokers and/or diabetics and can be extremely complex patients to care for. The majority of vascular patients are adults and many are elderly with a unique set of needs. Less often, traumatic injuries require venous or arterial repairs. Specific care requirements for the vascular patient are covered in Chapter 7.

Vascular Surgeon

Like many disciplines in the health care professions, vascular surgery is still evolving as a specialty. The American Board of Surgery challenged the idea of vascular surgery being anything other than a part of general surgery. While certification is now granted to recognize the special skills and domain of the specialty, it remains a facet of general surgery. As a result, certified general surgeons may perform vascular surgery (Szilagyi, 1994). As a recognized specialty, vascular surgery has separate board qualifications, approved additional training in fellowships, and an increase in the number of surgeons whose practice is entirely devoted to vascular problems. In many settings, the vascular surgeon may have trained as a cardiovascular surgeon and thus perform cardiac and peripheral vascular procedures.

Anesthesia Providers

Anesthesia allows the surgeon to do surgery in the optimal manner by provision of the most appropriate anesthetic and safe and intensive monitoring as needed. A few of the less invasive procedures, e.g., thrombectomy, percutaneous insertion of a vena cava filter, or revision of an A-V fistula, may require only local anesthesia or monitored anesthesia care. With the use of local anesthesia only or IV conscious sedation, a qualified RN may monitor the patient intraoperatively when she or he does not have the additional duties of performing the circulating role. Most surgical interventions require an anesthesia provider. Their role is to keep the patient comfortable, provide emotional support, monitor the patient throughout the surgery, and ensure safety in the intraoperative and recovery phases.

There are currently three anesthesia care providers: the anesthesiologist, who is an MD with additional residency training in the specialty of anesthesia; a certified registered nurse anesthetist (CRNA); and an anesthesiologist's assistant (AA). The program for anesthesiologists is currently 2 or 3 years long. The CRNA is a registered nurse with a Bachelor of Science degree in nursing or a health-related field, with a minimum of 1 year of critical care experience, and a 2-year nurse anesthesia course of study. Many CRNAs are masters-prepared as well. The AA is usually a physician's assistant (PA) with a pre-med background and 2 years of an anesthesia training program (Hoffer, 1995).

The provision of safe and effective anesthesia is one of the most critical aspects of vascular surgery. Vascular patients usually have cardiac disease and may require extensive screening, preparation, and monitoring. The choice of general or regional anesthesia techniques is largely up to the anesthesia care provider. The patient's life depends on vigilance, expert intervention in case of cardiorespiratory collapse, and appropriate fluid replacement.

Registered Nurse

Because of the diversity of nursing backgrounds, areas of interest and expertise, and the underlying commitment to quality patient care, it is not surprising that the registered professional nurse plays a variety of crucial roles in perioperative care of the vascular patient. Underlying all the phases of perioperative patient care is the provision of psychosocial support, problem solving, and patient education. Perioperative nursing encompasses the preoperative, intraoperative, and postoperative phases of patient care. The RN may be the scrub nurse and in some settings the all-RN staff in the operating room may be cost-effective and flexible for cross-training to other related patient care settings. The Association of Operating Room Nurses (AORN) is one of the largest specialty nursing organizations in the United States. AORN has been the driving force in education, leadership development, and collaboration with government and health care organizations, which has allowed perioperative nursing to develop and achieve excellence in the provision of patient care. Nurses use the six phases of the nursing process of assessment, nursing diagnosis, outcome identification, planning, implementation, and evaluation (Ladden, 1995). The perioperative role can include the skills of the nurse practitioner and clinical nurse specialist, who may perform admission histories and physical examinations, patient education, and discharge planning. A role that is taking on increasing importance is the **case manager**. In the new system of managed care, the case manager directs and supervises the allocation of resources to best meet the needs of the patient in the most cost-effective manner. The skills required for this are not new to nursing, but in the perioperative nurse practitioner and case manager roles they are greatly expanded (Ladden & Keane, 1995).

Chimner and Easterling (1993) describe the implementation of a collaborative care practice model for an inpatient unit utilizing an RN case manager. They successfully used the case manager to coordinate patient needs through educational programs and project teams. They found the collaborative care model resulted in greater patient, nursing, and physician satisfaction. Quality of care improved and patient length of stay decreased.

The AORN Standards and Recommended Practices guide the practice of the circulating nurse in the vascular operating room. The circulating nurse caring for the vascular patient must possess the ability to assess complex patient needs, provide emotional and informational support to both patient and family members, and coordinate the variety of people involved in intraoperative care. It is the registered nurse circulator who is responsible for the smooth coordination of all the personnel who attend the patient in the perioperative setting. She or he is also the key person to communicate and facilitate patient needs and outcome planning. Nursing colleagues in the postoperative care settings who are also practicing perioperative nursing include nurses in the PACU, ICU, ambulatory unit, emergency room, and inpatient units. The OR setting is a unique critical care setting. The patient may be sedated or anesthetized and unaware or unable to recall the events and risks or care rendered. The expert nurse performs nursing functions that may at first seem repetitious and easily learned. However, it is the myriad of abilities, knowledge, and critical thinking skills that are available to be tapped to assist in the unexpected situations, emergencies, and innovations that make the circulating nurse an important patient advocate. The RN acts as a patient advocate by interceding in the physical, spiritual, and ethical decisions that may be made during the perioperative phase. The RN is also called upon to be witness and recorder in the intraoperative setting. Accurate and concise documentation is essential.

Certification in perioperative nursing

Perioperative nurses may choose to become certified to validate and demonstrate their attainment of high professional standards for knowledge and skill. Certification entitles the nurse to use the designation **CNOR** after his or her name. The National Certification Board: Perioperative Nursing (NCB:PNI) is the administrative and policy-setting board for the certification and recertification process.

RN First Assistant (RNFA)

Many institutions are using RN first assistants (RNFA) in surgery. The Association of Operating Room Nurses officially recognized this role in 1983. Currently, many state boards of nursing and credentialing bodies officially recognize the RNFA. The AORN Official Statement on RN first assistants identifies the qualifications for practice (Box 2-1). The RNFA is considered the best qualified nonphysician to serve as a surgical first assistant. The RNFA may be an employee of the institution, a surgeon, or be self-employed. RNFAs are perioperative nurses and as such may function as the circulating or scrub nurse, nurse manager, or nurse educator. They practice interdependently with the surgeon when performing the duties of the RNFA. The RNFA may assist by using the surgical instruments to handle tissue, provide exposure, suture, and provide hemostasis (Rothrock, 1993).

Box 2-1 **Qualifications for the RN First Assistant**

Qualifications for RN first assistants should include, but not be limited to

- certification in perioperative nursing (CNOR)
- documentation of proficiency in perioperative nursing practice as both a scrub and circulating nurse
- ability to apply principles of asepsis and infection control
- knowledge of surgical anatomy, physiology, and operative technique related to the operative prodedures in which the RN assists
- ability to perform cardiopulmonary resuscitation
- ability to perform effectively in stressful and emergency situations
- ability to recognize safety hazards and initiate appropriate preventive and corrective action
- ability to perform effectively and harmoniously as a member of the team
- ability to demonstrate skill in behaviors unique to the RN first assistant (as defined), and
- meet requirements of statutes, regulations, and institutional policies relevant to RN first assistants

From AORN (1997). *AORN Standards, Recommended Practices, and Guidelines* (pp. 23-24). Denver: AORN.

Certification for the RNFA

An RNFA must have already attained the CNOR status in order to take the RNFA certification examination. The National Certification Board: Perioperative Nursing administers and sets policy for this certification as it does for the CNOR process.

Surgical Technologist

Originally a nursing role, the scrub "nurse" role may be delegated to assistive personnel. The scrub nurse or technologist works under the supervision of the RN. The surgical technologist may have a variety of backgrounds and training experiences. Some hospitals provide on-the-job training for the role of the scrub nurse. Other institutions have found it helpful to use licenced practical or vocational nurses in this role. These individuals may have had formal education in basic anatomy and physiology, pathophysiology, pharmacology, and concepts of patient care. Formal training programs for surgical technologists may vary from a number of weeks of training to 1 to 2 years in length and prepare the individual for a variety of tasks in the OR environment. Besides acting as a scrub nurse, surgical technologists may be assigned to ordering and stocking supplies, instrument processing, and other essential tasks. Because of their understanding of the complex instrumentation in today's OR, they excel in caring for and preparing instrument sets for sterilization. They may be assigned to select supplies and instrumentation for case cart systems because of their knowledge and understanding of surgical procedures.

Certification of surgical technologists

Surgical technologists may require certification in many institutions. Current certification processes mandate a formal educational program for eligibility to take the examination. By the year 2000, certification examinations will require an accredited formal training program. As with most certification processes, an individual must be motivated, willing to invest the money and time required for preparation and examination, and attend continuing education classes and seminars to maintain certification. Some employers support certification by reimbursement for the certification process and/or by a wage increase. Certification may be a condition of employment. The Liaison Council on Certification for the Surgical Technologist (LCC-ST) has awarded certification for 20 years (Candidate Information Booklet, 1995).

Vascular Laboratory Technician

There has been an explosion in the noninvasive and invasive techniques and testing procedures for the diagnosis of vascular problems in the past 20 years. Noninvasive vascular laboratories are accepted and used routinely to assess patients preoperatively and postoperatively (Yao, 1994). With the evolution of the laboratory, specially trained personnel are needed. These individuals are registered vascular technologists (RVTs), who may or may not be an RN. Most of the tests are considered subjective and dependent upon the skill of the technician (Blackburn & Peterson-Kennedy, 1994). The RVT is an integral member of the vascular team who provides critical diagnostic and documentation data. They are frequently needed to perform immediate tests in the PACU, ICU, and other critical care areas, the results of which may decide whether a return to the OR is necessary. Duplex ultrasonography with the addition of color imaging to display blood flow shows great promise for immediate evaluation of technical results intraoperatively for the peripheral vascular patient (Bandyk, et al, 1994). Until recently, scanning technology had been limited to cardiac and aortic procedures. Duplex scanning probes that can be used intraoperatively may result in RVTs assisting in the OR on a more frequent and regular basis.

Electroneurodiagnostic Technician and Neurophysiologist

Intraoperative electroencephalography (EEG) is used routinely by some vascular surgeons to monitor patients undergoing carotid endarterectomy. EEG changes occurring when the artery is clamped may determine whether the surgeon uses a shunt. Shunting carries its own set of risks; therefore, an accurate interpretation of the EEG is critical (Nuwer, 1993). This could prevent the patient from having a stroke (see Chapter 11 on carotid endarterectomy). The neurophysiologist is either a physician or a PhD-prepared individual with the ultimate responsibility for EEG interpretation. They are on call to the OR for their presence during carotid clamping.

Technician registration

The techniques used intraoperatively are based on the experiences of EEG monitoring of outpatients (Nuwer, 1993). The EEG technologist has many tasks and responsibilities. The field of EEG has been evolving to encompass a variety of skills and job descriptions. The name *EEG technologist* has changed to *Electroneurodiagnostic technologist.* Standards have been developed by the American Society of Electroneurodiagnostic Technologists (ASET). A technologist becomes registered by successfully passing written and oral examinations after an appropriate training period. The American Board of Registration of Electroencephalographic and Evoked Potential Technologists (ABRET) conducts the examination and awards the R.EEGT and R.EPT credentials. Before 1990 examining and credentialing was by the American Board of Certified and Registered Electroencephalographic Technicians and Technologists (ABCRET) and the successful candidates were designated as CMET, CRET, and CRNT. Educational and job requirements may vary. An entry level technologist must have a high school diploma and preferably college level courses in anatomy and physiology, basic electronics, and medical terminology. Further training in neurodiagnostic studies and procedures performed for critically ill patients or those in settings such as the OR require an individual who can work with minimal supervision and is sensitive in interacting with patients and other health care providers. In setting a patient up for EEG monitoring, the technologist must be technically proficient in applying electrodes according to standards and established guidelines. They need to obtain accurate histories to apply the most appropriate techniques for monitoring. Because it can take 45 minutes to an hour or more to apply the electrodes and perform baseline monitoring, it is important that the individual have the interpersonal skills to explain the procedure to the patient and gain the necessary cooperation to record optimal tracings. It may also be necessary to work with and accommodate the other personnel and activities necessary for preparing the patient for surgery (Carroll, 1994).

The EEG staff must be notified in a timely manner when sending the patient for surgery. The EEG technologist will usually have the patient prepared immediately before surgery, bring the monitoring machine to the holding area, and perform baseline recordings in the holding room. The technologist is responsible for maintaining and transporting the equipment safely. They will also assist in patient transfers so that the electrodes remain intact. A competent EEG technologist has a working knowledge of neuroanatomy, electrical safety, and infection control practices. They must work independently to calibrate and troubleshoot monitoring equipment. They need to recognize EEG patterns and correlate them to changes in medical status. When additional medications are given to the patient during general anesthesia, the technician may be called upon to interpret the resultant brain wave slowing (Carroll, 1994).

Product Representative

The role of the product representative is taking on increasing importance in this time of cost constraints, with the concomitant need to maintain a reduced inventory and remain competitive with the rapid technological advancements. A knowledgeable representative can assist the surgical team in many ways. He or she can provide current product information and alert the team to improvements or problems in a particular item. No one has unlimited resources and product representatives can be helpful when unanticipated usage depletes normal inventory (PAR) levels. They can obtain critical supplies and assist in cost containment by keeping inventory at an acceptable level. Many companies have sophisticated, high quality in-service programs, reference literature, and videos to help the OR staff in the acquisition of knowledge and skills for safe utilization of new equipment and supplies. At times it may be appropriate to permit a product representative into the operating room during surgery when they can help by providing technical information. Policies and procedures must be in place to safeguard the patient's right to privacy. Operating room nurses have had a long, productive working relationship with industry in evaluating the need and appropriateness of OR equipment and supplies. The perioperative nurse is responsible for effective product evaluation for the benefit of the patient and the health care institution. One AORN standard addresses the perioperative nurse's role as a participant in product evaluation. The standard describes the role of the perioperative nurse as one of close, informed involvement. It also recommends that "manufacturers' representatives should provide both clinical and technical data related to new products and medical devices, improvements, packaging, sterilization, and environmental conservation" (Box 2-2). (Recommended Practices for Product Evaluation and Selection for the Perioperative Setting, 1996, p. 239).

Radiology Personnel

The x-ray technician and radiologist are involved in the preoperative phase of surgical patient care by diagnosing vascular disease and assisting in the delineation of its location and severity.

Box 2-2 Influences on Selection of New Technologies

In a thought-provoking editorial, Dr. Gaylord (1991) describes the forces at work that influence the utilization of new technologies or tests. An ideal method for evaluating new methods of patient care is not always left to the health care professionals and regulatory agencies. Government, insurance companies, businesses, the public, and the press all have their own ideas and agendas. High-profile marketing and sensational headlines often have a major influence on how medical decisions are made. Aggressive marketing that attracts major investors may be beneficial for its financial support and may very much determine which technologies are tested widely and first. The consumer plays a much more demanding role in its quest for health care and magazines and newspapers are increasingly influential. Health care providers are increasingly aware that they are at risk of being sued if they do not order a particular diagnostic test or attempt a promising technique. This may not be based on what is the best practice but what is *perceived* as the best practice in a courtroom. Dr. Gaylord describes the physician as having the ultimate responsibility for sound and ethical judgement in selecting new technologies.

Gaylord, G. M. (1991). Vascular interventional radiologists, the development of new technologies, marketing, and the auk. *Radiology, 181*(1): 15-16.

Many vascular problems require angiograms to diagnose arterial lesions. This may require the patient to be hospitalized for a day before surgery. Some arterial lesions may be amenable to radiologic interventions such as balloon angioplasty or the use of urokinase to open an acutely occluded limb. These procedures are appropriately performed in the radiology suite. Interventional radiologists may be needed to perform a retrieval procedure when a complication occurs involving intravascular devices. These include vena cava filters, intravascular stents, or fragments from invasive monitoring equipment. The frequency of these occurrences is increasing (Egglin, et al, 1995). This assistance may protect both the patient and the surgeon or anesthesiologist. X-rays may be needed to assist the surgeon to identify or clarify vessels intraoperatively or to document surgical results for patient follow-up. Endovascular procedures may also be performed in conjunction with a more invasive surgical procedure, requiring that it be scheduled in the OR. Some procedures can be performed in either the operating room or the radiology suite. The increased interest in less invasive procedures and other technologic advances has resulted in a controversy over whether the surgeon or the interventional radiologist is the best person to perform endovascular procedures. The vascular surgeon may be the best judge of patient selection and can convert immediately to an open surgical procedure if necessary. However, the interventional radiologist already has the hand-eye coordination skills needed for placement of endovascular devices using fluoroscopic guidance. Practices vary depending on the setting, local standards, and the individuals involved. Perhaps the best solution is to use the skills of both specialities to provide optimal care. It may be that the surgical environment is the best location for some radiological interventions based on infection control parameters. When radiologists and radiology technicians come to the operating room to assist, it is important that these additional team members adhere to the strict aseptic practices of the OR environment. Monitoring traffic and asepsis is one of the duties of the circulating nurse. Radiology personnel have specialized knowledge of interventional catheters and guidewires and are an excellent resource for both using and purchasing these supplies. Institutions may find it cost-effective to share inventories of some expensive angioplasty balloon catheters and accessories.

Ancillary Personnel

A variety of support staff is required to maintain a safe and efficient surgical environment. Many roles are unique to the institutions and vary according to geographic location and patient population. A large university setting may have additional specially trained individuals for certain tasks, while others must cross-train for skills that are not required on a full-time basis. Some settings may use the services of off-site diagnostic services such as the vascular laboratory. Communities may share the use of diagnostic equipment such as CT or magnetic resonance imaging (MRI) scanners.

In major vascular surgical procedures or procedures that have the potential for large amounts of blood loss, a blood salvage system may be used. There are a variety of products on the market. Some autotransfusion devices require minimal time and in-service training and can be managed by the circulating nurse. Other devices, such as cellsavers, are set up and monitored by either highly skilled cardiopulmonary perfusionists in settings where cardiac surgeries are performed or ancillary staff who are trained to perform this task.

THE TEAM CONCEPT

Description of a Team

A team is comprised of individuals who agree on a common mission, share similar values, and establish mutual goals to achieve their definition of success. The members of a team are willing and able to subordinate personal, individual goals for the common good of the team and its mission. As teams develop, they tend to grow through three stages. Initially, they show traits of dependence and tend to blame others for failures and achievements. Gradually they become independent and characteristically take responsibility for actions and outcomes. The most productive teams reach a state of interdependence in which they work as a unit and work collaboratively with other groups for positive outcomes (Zoglio, 1993). One of the problems encountered in team building is the concept of relinquishing personal goals for the good of the team in a culture that rewards and promotes independence (Elledge & Phillips, 1996). This may be especially difficult in multidisciplinary teams that include physicians who have been socialized into a more authoritarian and hierarchical environment of medicine.

Business has been using the concept of self-directed work teams since the 1950s. This became more widespread and publicized in the late 1980s and 1990s as a result of the pressures generated by a more global economy. Industry was driven to increase worker participation in order to remain competitive. Two of the major influences were the demand for quality and customer service. Successful organizations demonstrated that their viability depended on the commitment and skills of their workforce. People and not machines were responsible for quality. Major companies (Ford Motor Company, General Electric, Xerox) have used work teams with enormous success. Employees exhibited increased pride in their work, increased rewards, took ownership for problem solving, and generally felt empowered (Box 2-3).

Teams change and develop over time as the individuals change and as the needs of the individuals and the team as a whole evolves. A successful team exhibits a number of behaviors that increase effective communication within the team. Successful internal communication may then result in improved communication with those outside their team. Effective communication enhances trust, which facilitates problem solving, constructive feedback, and team functioning (Ryan, 1994). Team meetings to discuss and resolve clinical and role problems can provide a means both to educate and to provide team member support. Team meetings serve to both improve and streamline communication (Chimner & Easterling, 1993). A cohesively functioning team will assist in decreasing stress.

Stressors on the Team

Atkinson and Fortunato (1996) define *stress* as tension that is caused by physical, chemical, or emotional factors. *Eustress* is a positive tension that motivates an individual to productive

> *Box 2-3* **Key Elements of Successful Self-Directed Work Teams**
>
> Goals are understood by all members
> High degree of involvement by all members
> Environment of trust exists
> Communication is open and honest
> Members have a sense of belonging
> Each member is recognized as being unique and valuable
> Creativity and risk taking are encouraged
> Problem solving and analyzing are promoted
> Leadership is participatory

Adapted from Harper, B., & Harper, A. (1992). *Succeeding as a self-directed work team.* NY: MW Corporation.

action. *Distress* is a negative strain that can challenge a person's ability to cope and adapt. Stressors can be divided into intrinsic (internal origin) or extrinsic (external origin). Many stressors account for the strains placed upon a surgical team. Much has been written in the literature about the phenomenon of burnout in the helping professions. There are forces that frustrate, tire, and discourage. The results of unrelieved stress may be seen as decreased productivity, lack of job satisfaction, absenteeism, injury, marital discord, and substance abuse (Wolfgang, 1988). Some factors that contribute to stress are environmental: noise (monitors, suction, telephones, pagers, music, talking [both needed and unnecessary]), temperature, lights, gowns, latex gloves, masks, caps, malfunctioning heat control of room, humidity, surgical procedure (difficult or unexpected findings, blood loss, inadequate anesthesia), equipment (lost, unavailable, broken, inferior, inadequate, late), inadequately trained personnel (nurse, tech, MD, support persons), excessive or inadequate lighting, lack of resources, shared equipment, time constraints (shifts, service allocation of OR time, loss of prime time because of a patient's late arrival at the hospital, difficult preparation, scheduling conflicts, bed shortages, turnover time), and role conflict (money, time off, rewards, goals, ethical and moral issues, blurred vs. shared responsibilities).

Role conflict is a major stressor for nurses. Individuals and groups may have differing expectations of the nurse's role and responsibilities, and these responsibilities may be poorly defined or overlap. Conflicting demands can lead to feelings of stress, guilt, and anxiety. Loyalty to coworkers or an organization may conflict with duty to a patient. This may occur when the organization emphasizes speed and a patient needs extra time. Role conflict and overload may occur when an individual's multiple roles result in time conflicts. This is commonly encountered when demands of home and family compete with professional activities (Gelfant, 1983).

Stress Reduction

Assisting patients in managing health care needs is inherent in the nursing role. Managing stress is an important aspect of providing care. Nurses sometimes need to be reminded by colleagues and managers to utilize caring strategies on themselves to maintain their own health and the ability to continue to provide care to others. Behaviors that can alleviate stress in the OR include maintaining a tasteful sense of humor, practicing respect by saying "please" and "thank you," and providing positive feedback regularly and constructive criticism kindly (Atkinson & Fortunato, 1996).

Nurses can learn to reduce stress by actively seeking out external resources. Many institutions have employee assistance programs to provide support through evaluation and referral for both work and family problems. Professional and adult education programs on stress reduction techniques are increasingly popular and available. Programs on assertiveness training, conflict resolution, or crisis intervention may be helpful. Tap into the skills of other nursing colleagues. Psychiatric consultation liaison nurses (PCLNs) are masters-prepared nurses who specialize in psychiatric and mental health nursing. Their expertise can be used to assist with complex patient problems and staff conflicts (Robinette, 1996).

Striving for balance in one's life will help maintain health by reducing stress. Watch for physical cues that the body sends. Allow time for adequate rest, food, activity, and recreation. Develop relationships and interests that nourish and replenish to counteract stresses and strains. Meditation and mental imagery are tools that can take little time and yet replenish and revitalize (Atkinson & Fortunato, 1996).

Descamps and Thomas (1993) examined the impact of fun on the job on the strain that nurses experience. They focused on the stressors of a heavy workload, inability to adequately provide for patient and family emotional needs, and exposure to death and dying. They found support for their theory that active physical play or "horsing around" significantly lessened the strains of work overload and job dissatisfaction. They recommended that administrators and managers view these behaviors as productive rather than nonproductive.

References

Association of Operating Room Nurses, Inc. (1996). *Standards and recommended practices.* Denver: AORN, Inc.

Atkinson, L. J., & Fortunato N. (1996). *Berry & Kohn's operating room technique* (8th ed.). St. Louis: Mosby.

Bandyk, D. F., Mills, J. L., Gahtan, V., & Esses, G. E. (1994). Intraoperative duplex scanning of arterial reconstructions: Fate of repaired and unrepaired defects. *Journal of Vascular Surgery, 20*(3): 426-423.

Blackburn, D. R., & Peterson-Kennedy, L. (1994). Noninvasive vascular testing. In V. A. Fahey (Ed.), *Vascular nursing* (2nd ed., pp. 73-103). Philadelphia: W. B. Saunders.

Carroll, I. A. (1994). Guideline five: Recommendations for writing job descriptions for technologists and samples. *Journal of Clinical Neurophysiology, 11*(1): 16-27.

Candidate Information Booklet (1995). *National Certification Examination for Surgical Technologists.* The Psychological Corporation. San Antonio: Harcourt Brace.

Chimner, N. E., & Easterling, A. (1993). Collaborative practice through nursing case management. *Rehabilitation Nursing, 18*(4): 226-230.

DesCamp, K. D., & Thomas, C. C. (1993). Buffering nursing stress through play at work. *Western Journal of Nursing Research, 15*(5): 619-627.

Egglin, T.K., Dickey, K. W., Rosenblatt, M., & Pollak, J.S. (1995). Retreival of intravascualar foreign bodies: Experience in 32 cases. *American Journal of Roentgenology, 164*(5): 1259-1264.

Elledge, R. L., & Phillips, S. L. [1996]. *Team building for the future: Beyond the basics.* San Diego: Pfeiffer & Co.

Gaylord, G. M. (1991). Vascular interventional radiologists, the development of new technologies, marketing, and the auk. *Radiology, 181*(1): 15-16.

Gelfant, B. (1983). Nurse role conflict and hospital organizational stress. *Hospital Topics, 61*(1): 22-27.

Harper, B., & Harper, A. (1992). *Succeeding as a self-directed work team.* New York: M W Corporation.

Hoffer, J. L. (1995). Anesthesia. In M. H. Meeker, & J. C. Rothrock (Eds.), *Alexander's care of the patient in surgery* (10th ed., pp.143-181). St. Louis: Mosby.

Ladden, C.S. (1995). Concepts basic to perioperative nursing. In M. H. Meeker, & J. C. Rothrock (Eds.), *Alexander's care of the patient in surgery* (10th ed., pp. 3-18). St. Louis: Mosby.

Ladden, C., & Keane, A. (1995). Perioperative nurse practitioners. *AORN Journal, 61*(6):1067-1071.

Robinette, A. L. (1996). PCLNs: Who are they? How can they help you? *American Journal of Nursing, 96*(7): 48-50.

Rothrock, J. C. (1993). Appendix 1: Definition of RN First Assistant. *The R.N. first assistant: An expanded perioperative nursing role* (2nd ed.). Philadelphia: J. B. Lippincott.

Ryan, T. (1994). All for one and one for all: Team building and nursing. *Journal of Nursing Management, 2*(3):129-134.

Szilagy, D. E. (1994). Vascular surgery: A brief account of its past and present. In F. J Veith, R. W. Hobson, R. A. Williams, & S.E. Wilson (Eds.), *Vascular surgery: Principles and practice* (2nd ed., pp. 3-6). New York: McGraw-Hill.

Wolfgang, A. P. (1988). Job stress in the health professions: A study of physicians, nurses, and pharmacists. *Hospital Topics, 66*(4):24-27.

Yao, J. T. (1994). Noninvasive studies of peripheral vascular disease. In F. J Veith, R.W. Hobson, R. A. Williams, & S.E. Wilson (Eds.), *Vascular surgery: Principles and practice* (2nd ed., pp. 90-97). New York: McGraw-Hill.

Zoglio, S. W. (1993). *Teams at work: 7 keys for success.* Doylestown, PA: Tower Hill Press.

3 Anatomy and Physiology

INTRODUCTION

Basic knowledge of anatomy is essential for all phases of the care of the vascular patient. The circulatory system consists of the arterial, venous, and lymphatic systems. The venous system is the most complex but most attention is directed to the arterial system because it is the basis for most limb-threatening vascular disease and the most amenable to surgical intervention (Figures 3-1 to 3-10). Arteries and veins have three layers:

- tunica intima—innermost
- tunica media—muscular middle
- tunica adventitia—fibrous outer (Figure 3-10)

The **adventitial layer** of a vessel wall consists of collagen and the nutrient vessels (vasa vasorum) (Table 3-1). This layer has three functions: structural, holding the wall to surrounding tissue, and providing the smooth muscle cells with nutrients. The **media** in arteries includes smooth muscle cells with elastic collagen fibers (Callow, 1995). Arteries differ from veins in function and structure. Structurally, arteries have a thicker muscle layer and more elastic fibers and therefore have a thicker wall than veins. The properties of elasticity and distensibility enable the vessels to compensate for changes in blood pressure and volume.

Because of the thicker muscle layer, smaller severed arteries can contract and constrict enough to stop hemorrhage.

Veins are more fragile than arteries and whether traumatic or iatrogenic, venous bleeding can be difficult to control. Veins cannot contract enough to stop hemorrhage. Another difference is the presence of semilunar intimal folds, or **valves**, in veins that prevent back flow. The **tunica intima** or inner layer is a smooth lining layer of endothelial cells. Veins and arteries are nourished by a tiny network of vessels, the vasa vasorum, as well as by the intraluminal blood flow. The vasa vasorum is the collection of arterioles, venules, capillaries, and lymphatics that nourish the adventitia of the vessels. The vasa vasorum is more prevalent in the vein walls than in artery walls but very little else is known about this tiny network (Callow, 1995). Tone in arteries and veins is regulated by the autonomic nervous system with veins having fewer nerve fibers. These nerve fiber endings are found in the adventitial layer (Thibodeau & Patton, 1996). The two systems are connected: arteries (except the pulmonary artery), carrying oxygenated blood, branch into smaller arteries, then arterioles, then capillaries to venules to veins.

Text continued on p. 25

Table 3-1 **Structure of Blood Vessels**

TYPE OF VESSEL	TUNICA INTIMA (ENDOTHELIUM)	TUNICA MEDIA (SMOOTH MUSCLE; ELASTIC CONNECTIVE TISSUE)	TUNICA ADVENTITIA (FIBROUS CONNECTIVE TISSUE)
ARTERIES	Smooth lining	Allows constriction and dilation of vessels; thicker than in veins; muscle innervated by autonomic fibers	Provides flexible support that resists collapse or injury; thicker than in veins; thinner than tunica media
VEINS	Smooth lining with semilunar valves to ensure one-way flow	Allows constriction and dilation of vessels; thinner than in arteries; muscle innervated by autonomic fibers	Provides flexible support that resists collapse or injury; thinner than in arteries; thicker than tunica media
CAPILLARIES	Make up entire wall of capillary; thinness permits ease of transport across vessel wall	(Absent)	(Absent)

From Thibodeau G. A., & Patton K. T. (1996). *Anatomy and physiology* (3rd ed.). St. Louis: Mosby.

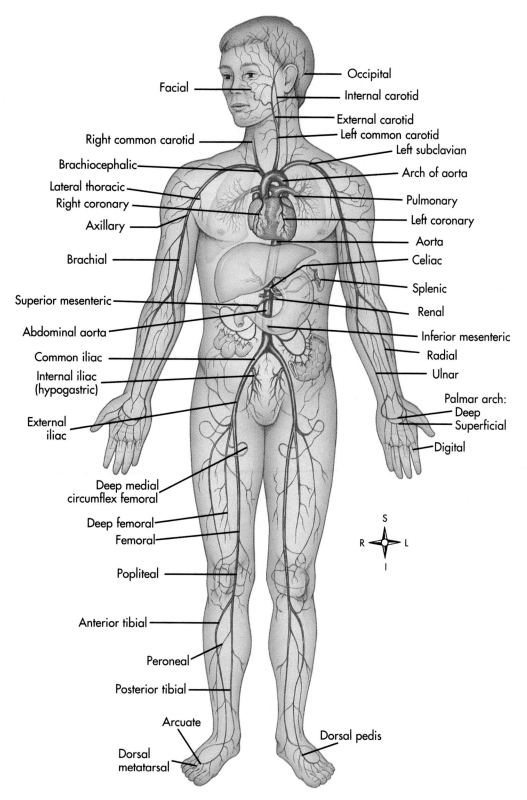

Fig. 3-1 Principal arteries of the body. *(From Thibodeau, G. A., & Patton, K. T. [1996]. Anatomy and physiology [3rd ed.]. St. Louis: Mosby.)*

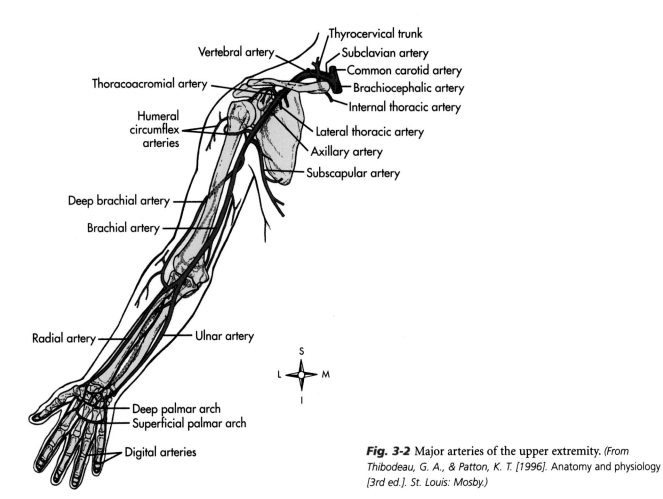

Vertebral artery

Thyrocervical trunk
Subclavian artery
Common carotid artery

Thoracoacromial artery

Brachiocephalic artery
Internal thoracic artery

Humeral circumflex arteries

Lateral thoracic artery
Axillary artery
Subscapular artery

Deep brachial artery

Brachial artery

Radial artery

Ulnar artery

S
L ← → M
I

Deep palmar arch
Superficial palmar arch

Digital arteries

Fig. 3-2 Major arteries of the upper extremity. *(From Thibodeau, G. A., & Patton, K. T. [1996]. Anatomy and physiology [3rd ed.]. St. Louis: Mosby.)*

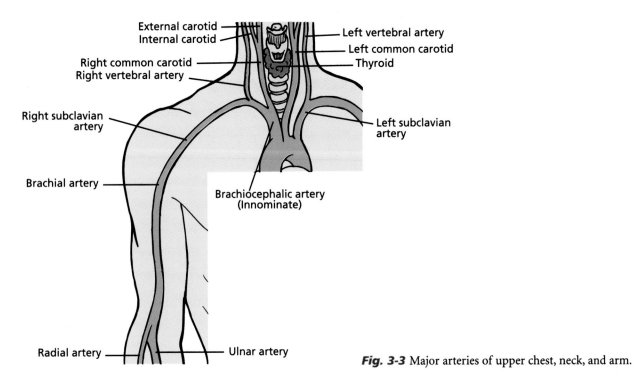

External carotid
Internal carotid

Left vertebral artery
Left common carotid

Right common carotid
Right vertebral artery

Thyroid

Right subclavian artery

Left subclavian artery

Brachial artery

Brachiocephalic artery (Innominate)

Radial artery

Ulnar artery

Fig. 3-3 Major arteries of upper chest, neck, and arm.

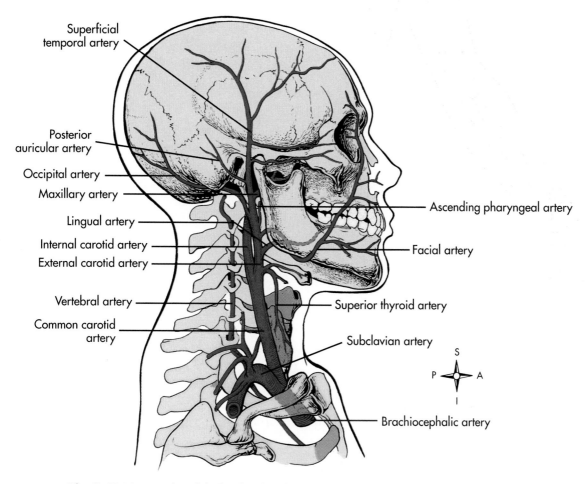

Fig. 3-4 Major arteries of the head and neck. *(From Thibodeau, G. A., & Patton, K. T. [1996]. Anatomy and physiology [3rd ed.]. St. Louis: Mosby.)*

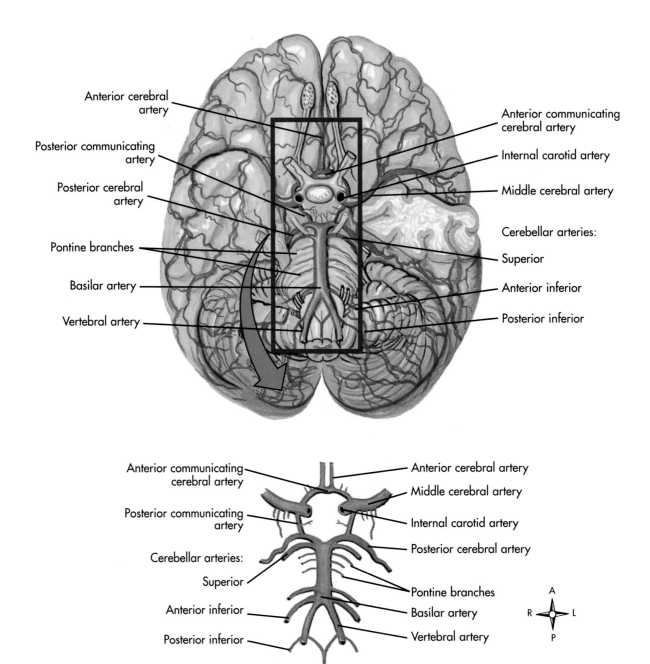

Fig. 3-5 Arteries at the base of the brain. *(From Thibodeau, G. A., & Patton, K. T. [1996]. Anatomy and physiology [3rd ed]. St. Louis: Mosby.)*

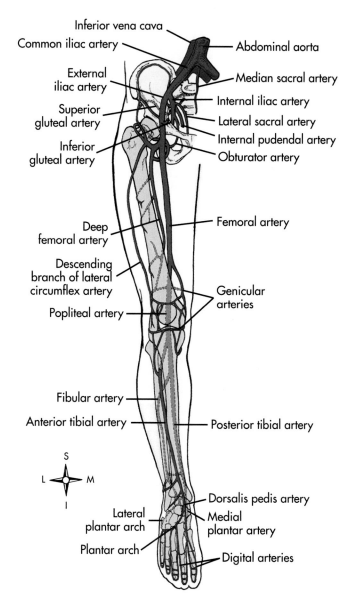

Inferior vena cava

Common iliac artery

External iliac artery

Superior gluteal artery

Inferior gluteal artery

Deep femoral artery

Descending branch of lateral circumflex artery

Popliteal artery

Fibular artery

Anterior tibial artery

Lateral plantar arch

Plantar arch

Abdominal aorta

Median sacral artery

Internal iliac artery

Lateral sacral artery

Internal pudendal artery

Obturator artery

Femoral artery

Genicular arteries

Posterior tibial artery

Dorsalis pedis artery

Medial plantar artery

Digital arteries

S

L — M

I

Fig. 3-6 Major arteries of the lower extremity. *(From Thibodeau, G. A., & Patton, K. T. [1996].* Anatomy and physiology *[3rd ed]. St. Louis: Mosby.)*

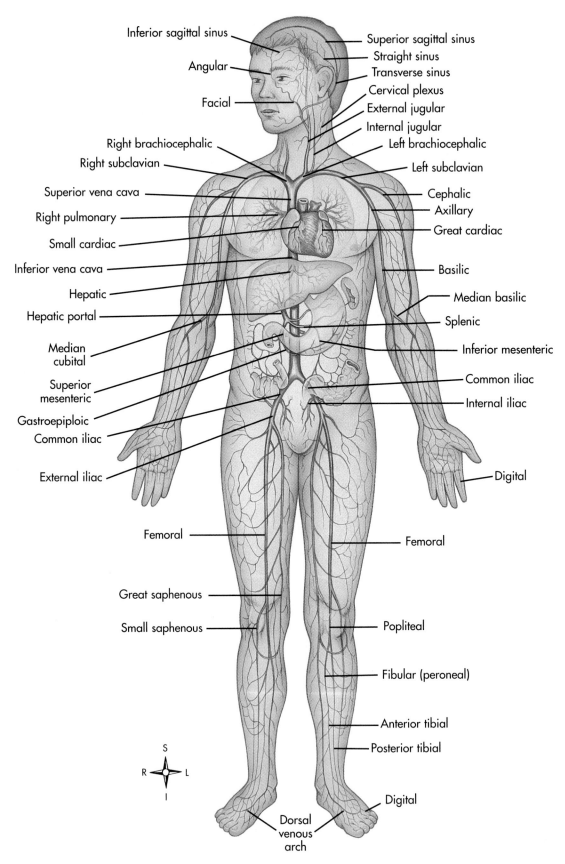

Fig. 3-7 Venous circulation. *(From Cannobio, M. M. [1990]. Cardiovascular disorders. St. Louis: Mosby.)*

Portal vein and tributaries

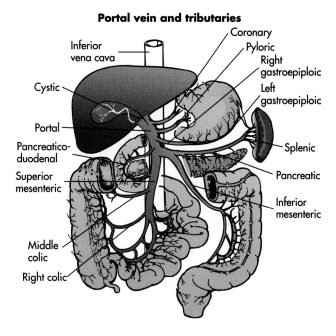

Fig. 3-8 Hepatic portal vein. *(From Beare, P. G., & Myers, J. L. [1998]. Adult health nursing [3rd ed.]. St. Louis: Mosby.)*

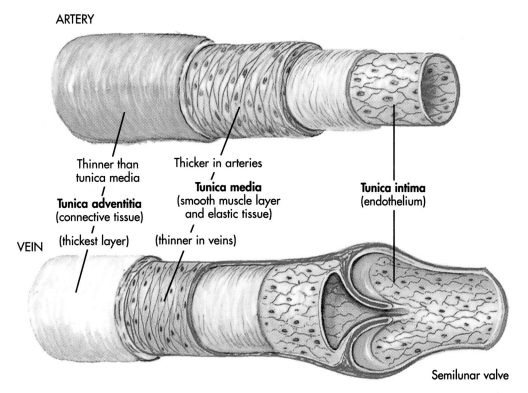

Fig. 3-9 Cross-section of an artery and vein showing the three layers: intima, media, and adventitia. *(From Thibodeau, G. A., & Patton, K. T. [1996]. Anatomy and physiology [3rd ed]. St. Louis: Mosby.)*

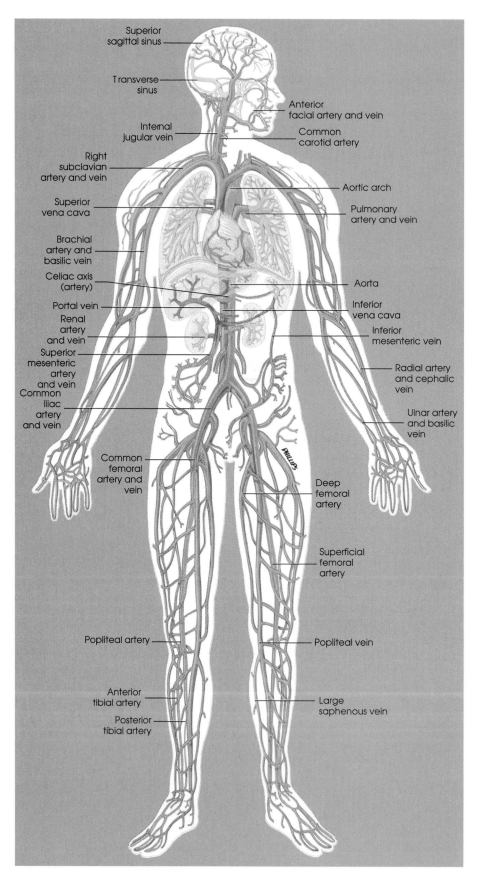

Fig. 3-10 Major arteries and veins. *(From Ballinger, P. W. [1995].* Merrill's atlas of radiographic positions and radiologic procedures *[8th ed.]. St. Louis: Mosby.)*

ARTERIES

During fetal development a number of channels are retained and form main arteries. Peripheral parts persist as capillary channels. Communications between these and nearby capillaries are called **anastomoses**. These also occur between certain large vessels, such as the coronary arteries. In conditions of obstruction to arterial flow, the small vessels and precapillary vessels create collateral circulation. Arteries that supply very mobile structures such as the cheek or tongue and expansible structures, such as the uterus, are very tortuous to permit movement without disruption of the vessel integrity (Basmajian & Slonecker, 1989). **End arteries** are those that do not anastomose with nearby vessels via terminal capillaries. Arteries are classified as elastic or muscular. The large vessels such as the aorta and iliac arteries are elastic. As the arteries decrease in size, the elastic component decreases and the muscle component increases (Callow, 1995).

The smallest vessels of the **arterial** system are the **arterioles**. They are also known as the **resistance arterioles** because their dilation and constriction are responsible for the regulation of flow to the capillaries. They serve to regulate vascular resistance to maintain arterial pressure. Arterioles can do this because their smooth muscle cells, acting as precapillary sphincters, contract and relax at the point just before the origin of the capillary (Figure 3-11, *B* and Table 3-2.)

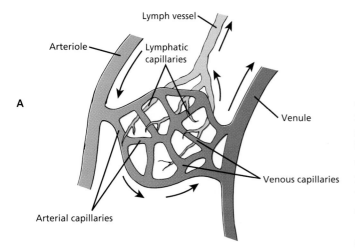

A

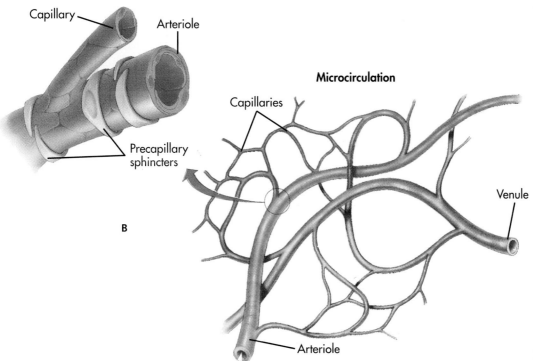

Fig. 3-11 A, Microcirculation involving blood, lymphatic or interstitial fluid, oxygen, and nutrients. **B,** Microcirculation showing pre-capillary sphincters. Hydrostatic pressure falls as blood circulates through the capillary toward the vein. Colloid osmotic pressure from plasma proteins increases and pulls the fluid back into the vessel. The net flow of fluid is outward in the arteriole and inward in the venous side. (**A,** *from Cannobio, M. M. [1990]. Cardiovascular disorders. St. Louis: Mosby.* **B,** *from Thibodeau, G. A., & Patton, K. T. [1996]. Anatomy and physiology [3rd ed.]. St. Louis: Mosby.)*

Table 3-2 **Major Systemic Arteries**

ARTERY*	REGION SUPPLIED	ARTERY*	REGION SUPPLIED
ASCENDING AORTA		**DESCENDING ABDOMINAL AORTA**	
Coronary arteries	Myocardium	Visceral branches	Abdominal viscera
		Celiac artery (trunk)	Abdominal viscera
ARCH OF AORTA		Left gastric	Stomach, esophagus
Brachiocephalic (innominate)	Head and upper extremity	Common hepatic	Liver
Right subclavian	Head, upper extremity	Splenic	Spleen, pancreas, stomach
Right vertebral†	Spinal cord, brain	Superior mesenteric	Pancreas, small intestine, colon
Right axillary (continuation of subclavian)	Shoulder, chest, axillary region	Inferior mesenteric	Descending colon, rectum
Right brachial (continuation of axillary)	Arm and hand	Suprarenal	Adrenal (suprarenal) gland
		Renal	Kidney
Right radial	Lower arm and hand (lateral)	Ovarian	Ovary, uterine tube, ureter
Right ulnar	Lower arm and hand (medial)	Testicular	Testis, ureter
Superficial and deep palmar arches (formed by anastomosis of branches of radial and ulnar)	Hand and fingers	Parietal branches	Walls of abdomen
		Inferior phrenic	Inferior surface of diaphragm, adrenal gland
Digital	Fingers	Lumbar	Lumbar vertebrae and muscles of back
Right common carotid	Head and neck	Median sacral	Lower vertebrae
Right internal carotid†	Brain, eye, forehead, nose	Common iliac (formed by terminal branches of aorta)	Pelvis, lower extremity
Right external carotid†	Thyroid, tongue, tonsils, ear, etc.	External iliac	Thigh, leg, foot
Left subclavian	Shoulder, chest, axillary region	Femoral (continuation of external iliac)	Thigh, leg, foot
Left vertebral†	Spinal cord, brain	Popliteal (continuation of femoral)	Leg, foot
Left axillary (continuation of subclavian)	Shoulder, chest, axillary region	Anterior tibial	Leg, foot
Left brachial (continuation of axillary)	Arm and hand	Posterior tibial	Leg, foot
Left radial	Lower arm and hand (lateral)	Plantar arch (formed by anastamosis of branches of anterior and posterior tibial arteries)	Foot, toes
Left ulnar	Lower arm and hand (medial)		
Superficial and deep palmar arches (formed by anastomosis of branches of radial and ulnar)	Hand and fingers	Digital	Toes
		Internal iliac	Pelvis
		Visceral branches	Pelvic viscera
Digital	Fingers	Middle rectal	Rectum
Left common carotid	Head and neck	Vaginal	Vagina, uterus
Left internal carotid†	Brain, eye, forehead, nose	Uterine	Uterus, vagina, uterine tube, ovary
Left external carotid†	Thyroid, tongue, tonsils, ear, etc.	Parietal branches	Pelvic wall and external regions
		Lateral sacral	Sacrum
DESCENDING THORACIC AORTA		Superior gluteal	Gluteal muscles
Visceral branches	Thoracic viscera	Obturator	Pubic region, hip joint, groin
Bronchial	Lungs, bronchi	Internal pudendal	Rectum, external genitals, floor of pelvis
Esophageal	Esophagus	Inferior gluteal	Lower gluteal region, coccyx, upper thigh
Parietal branches	Thoracic walls (rib cage)		
Intercostal	Lateral thoracic walls (rib cage)		
Superior phrenic	Superior surface of diaphragm		

From Thibodeau G. A., & Patton K. T. (1996). *Anatomy and physiology* (3rd ed.). St Louis: Mosby.
*Branches of each artery are indented below its name.
†See text and/or figures for branches of the artery.

VEINS

Veins vary a great deal in their structure. Age, size, and location affect their structure. The boundaries of the intima, media, and adventitia are not always distinct (Callow, 1995). Veins are more numerous than arteries and their diameters are larger and more variable as they perform at a much lower pressure. Their diameter varies in response to flow demand. Veins are in a partially filled or semicollapsed state most of the time (Figure 3-12). Veins often accompany arteries and their branches. In some areas of the body, such as below the knees and elbows, arteries are followed by paired veins called **venae comitantes**. These are found on either side of the artery and are joined by a network of tiny branches that almost surrounds the artery (Basmajian & Slonecker, 1989). Since the main function of the venous system is to return blood to the heart, competent **valves** are essential (Bishara et al, 1986). These semilunar valves serve to prevent excessive pressure on the vein walls. An imaginary column of blood from the heart to the feet would have tremendous cumulative pressure at the bottom of the column. This pressure is known as **hydrostatic pressure**. The venous valves serve to cut this column into segments and disrupt this cumulative pressure effect (Beare & Myers, 1998). Valves are found in most medium and small veins. Valves are folds of the wall that form paired semilunar pockets or sinuses. The valves closest to the heart are at the terminals of the internal jugular, subclavian, and femoral veins. When the pressure in the thorax increases (abdominal straining or inspiration) the valves prevent the back flow of blood into the limbs, head, and neck. The most numerous valves are found in the limbs because these are the areas subject to the greatest hydrostatic pressure. There are no valves in the portal circulation or in the head. Valves are often located immediately before a branch or tributary of a vessel (Basmajian & Slonecker, 1989).

The location of veins in an individual is more variable than the arteries. For example, the saphenous vein shows a great deal of variation in its branching (Linton, 1938). Veins are often found close to an artery and named similarly (e.g., renal artery and renal vein provide blood flow to and from the kidney). The venous system of the right and left sides of the body are not mirror images of each other. Examples of this can be found by evaluating the inferior and superior vena cavae. They are on the right side of the body; there are no comparable veins on the left side (see Figure 3-7). Another area of interest is the portal circulation. The portal circulation is a part of the venous system (see Figure 3-8). Blood detours from the digestive tract to the liver to be detoxified and processed instead of draining into the main venous system. Blood from the intestine collects in the portal vein and is transported to the liver. This blood continues to collect in veins going to the general circulation to the right atrium. Blood flows from the **celiac artery** to the **hepatic artery** to the liver and from the **gastric arteries** to the stomach. The **superior and inferior mesenteric** arteries supply the large and small intestines. Deoxygenated blood from all these is collected by the **portal vein,** which supplies the liver capillaries with concentrated products of digestion (see Figure 3-9). The portal system delivers higher concentrations of insulin and glucagon to the liver than to the rest of the body (Table 3-3).

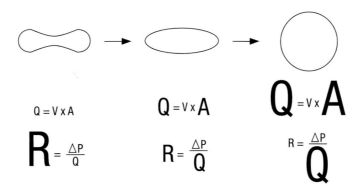

Fig. 3-12 Venous blood flow and physical configuration. When venous flow is low, veins adopt a semicollapsed configuration; in this state, at any given pressure gradient, they offer high resistance. As flow demands increase, a more circular configuration is adopted, thereby decreasing resistance to flow and allowing a higher flow without change in pressure gradient. *Q,* Flow; *A,* cross-sectional area; *R,* resistance; *P,* pressure gradient; *V,* velocity. *(From Criado, E., & Hohnson G. Jr., [1991]). Venous disease.* Current Problems in Surgery, 28(5): 335-400.

Table 3-3 **Major Systemic Veins**

Vein*	Region Drained	Vein*	Region Drained
SUPERIOR VENA CAVA	Head, neck, thorax, upper extremity	**INFERIOR VENA CAVA**	Lower trunk and extremity
		Phrenic	Diaphragm
Brachiocephalic (innominate)	Head, neck, upper extremity	Hepatic portal system	Upper abdominal viscera
Internal jugular (continuation of sigmoid sinus)	Brain	Hepatic veins (continuations of liver venules and sinusoids and, ultimately, the hepatic portal vein)	Liver
Lingual	Tongue, mouth		
Superior thyroid	Thyroid, deep face	Hepatic portal vein	Gastrointestinal organs, pancreas, spleen, gallbladder
Facial	Superficial face		
Sigmoid sinus (continuation of transverse sinus/direct tributary of internal jugular)	Brain, meninges, skull	Cystic	Gallbladder
		Gastric	Stomach
		Splenic	Spleen
Superior and inferior petrosal sinuses	Anterior brain, skull	Inferior mesenteric	Descending colon, rectum
		Pancreatic	Pancreas
Cavernous sinus	Anterior brain, skull	Superior mesenteric	Small intestine, most of colon
Ophthalmic veins	Eye, orbit		
Transverse sinus (direct tributary of sigmoid sinus)	Brain, meninges, skull	Gastroepiploic	Stomach
		Renal	Kidneys
Occipital sinus	Inferior, central region of cranial cavity	Suprarenal	Adrenal (suprarenal) gland
		Left ovarian	Left ovary
Straight sinus	Central region of brain, meninges	Left testicular	Left testis
		Left ascending lumbar (anastomoses with hemiazygos)	Left lumbar region
Inferior sagittal sinus	Central region of brain, meninges		
		Right ovarian	Right ovary
Superior sagittal (longitudinal) sinus	Superior region of cranial cavity	Right testicular	Right testis
		Right ascending lumbar (anastomoses with azygos)	Right lumbar region
External jugular	Superficial, posterior head, neck		
Subclavian (continuation of axillary/direct tributary of brachiocephalic)	Axilla, lower extremity	Common iliac (continuation of external iliac; common iliacs unite to form inferior vena cava)	Lower extremity
Axillary (continuation of basilic/direct tributary of subclavian)	Axilla, lower extremity	External iliac (continuation of femoral/direct tributary of common iliac)	Thigh, leg, foot
Cephalic	Lateral and lower arm, hand	Femoral (continuation of popliteal/direct tributary of external iliac)	Thigh, leg, foot
Brachial	Deep arm		
Radial	Deep lateral forearm		
Ulnar	Deep medial forearm	Popliteal	Leg, foot
Basilic (direct tributary of axillary)	Medial and lower arm, hand	Posterior tibial	Deep posterior leg
Median cubital (basilic) (formed by anastomosis of cephalic and basilic)	Arm, hand	Medial and lateral plantar	Sole of foot
Deep and superficial palmar venous arches (formed by anastomosis of cephalic and basilic)	Hand	Fibular (peroneal) (continuation of anterior tibial)	Lateral and anterior leg, foot
		Anterior tibial	Anterior leg, foot
Digital	Fingers	Dorsal veins of foot	Anterior (dorsal) foot, toes
Azygos (anastomoses with right ascending lumbar)	Right posterior wall of thorax and abdomen, esophagus, bronchi, pericardium, mediastinum	Small (external, short) saphenous	Superficial posterior leg, lateral foot
		Great (internal, long) saphenous	Superficial medial and anterior thigh, leg, foot
		Dorsal veins of foot	Anterior (dorsal) foot, toes
Hemiazygos (anastomoses with left renal)	Left inferior posterior wall of thorax and abdomen, esophagus, mediastinum	Dorsal venous arch	Anterior (dorsal) foot, toes
		Digital	Toes
Accessory hemiazygos	Left superior posterior wall of thorax	Internal iliac	Pelvic region

From Thibodeau G. A., & Patton K. T. (1996). *Anatomy and physiology* (3rd ed.). St Louis: Mosby.

*Tributaries of each vein are indented below its name.

CAPILLARIES

The smallest unit of function in the vascular system is the **capillary.** The work of exchanging nutrients and metabolic wastes is done at this level. This is also known as the **microcirculation** (see Figure 3-11, *A*). Capillaries allow the nutritive substances and oxygen to travel from the blood to the tissue and waste products and carbon dioxide to travel from the tissue to the blood. The cell walls of the capillaries are endothelial and semipermeable. They are permeable to water and crystalloids and impermeable to the proteins of blood plasma and other large molecules (Basmajian & Slonecker, 1989). Capillaries lack media and adventitia. They consist of endothelial cells and a basal lamina. They also have a pericyte cell that is potentially contractile but not considered a muscle cell (Callow, 1995).

ENDOTHELIAL CELLS

Simple squamous epithelial cells, called endothelium in the vascular system, line the capillaries and all vascular structures. **Endothelial cells** are extremely important functionally. They are a physical barrier that keeps the blood within the vessel lumen. Endothelial cells regulate the relaxation and contraction of smooth muscle cells at the local level, secrete substances that resist clotting, and secrete a tissue growth factor (Beare & Myers, 1998). The healthy endothelial lining cells of the blood vessel serve some very complex functions. They remodel the vessel wall when injured, synthesize factors in the coagulation process, and by regulating the vascular tone, they regulate the blood pressure. The endothelial cells are nonthrombogenic; platelets will not adhere to an intact vessel wall. When the endothelial wall is damaged, platelets *do*

adhere. Endothelial cells also secrete components of the fibrinolytic system to maintain homeostasis. Minor injuries heal by the migration of adjacent endothelial cells followed by endothelial cell proliferation. Injuries that penetrate the entire wall cause the migration and growth of smooth muscle cells and adventitial fibroblasts. Both cells synthesize and secrete connective tissue components. Endothelial cells partially induce migration of WBCs to areas of injury (Jaffe, 1992) (Box 3-1).

BLOOD COMPOSITION

The average adult body contains approximately 7 liters of blood that comprises **7% of the total weight** (Basmajian & Slonecker, 1989). Blood **volume** in the body is normally distributed in the following manner: 5% in the capillaries, 7% heart, 9% in the pulmonary vessels, 15% in the arteries, and 64% in the veins (Callow, 1995). The blood consists of plasma and cells (91% water and 9% solids). These solids are proteins, salts, products of digestion, and waste products (oxygen and carbon dioxide), enzymes, and other secretions (Table 3-4). Blood cellular components are red cells (**erythrocytes),** white cells (**leukocytes),** and **platelets** (Figure 3-13 and Table 3-5). Cellular tissues are highly vascular because of the high metabolic demands (muscle, lungs, glands). Fat and bone have a fair vascular supply while connective tissue is only slightly vascular. Structures considered nonvascular include hyaline cartilage, the cornea, and the epidermis. Nervous tissue varies in the amount of blood supplied to it; the gray matter and spinal medulla are cellular and therefore more vascular than white matter and peripheral nerves (Basmajian & Slonecker, 1989).

> *Box 3-1* **Function of Vessel Smooth Muscle Cells**
>
> *Aorta and large arteries:* adjust compliance and peripheral resistance, a factor in cardiac afterload
> *Precapillary level:* changes in vessel diameter regulate blood flow to specific tissues; by changing the total peripheral resistance contributes to regulation of BP
> *Venous wall:* contraction controls the capacity of the cardiovascular system and preload of heart
> *Cutaneous veins:* diameter changes affect the thermoregulation of the skin

From O'Rourke & Vanhoutte, 1992.

Table 3-4 **Composition of Blood Plasma**

COMPONENTS	PERCENTAGE
Water	90%
Solutes	10%
Proteins	6%-8%
Albumin	55% of protein
Globulins	38% of protein
Fibrinogen	7% of protein
Other substances	2%-4%
Organic	
Cholesterol	
Glucose	
Amino acids	
Triglycerides	
Urea, uric acid	
Lactic acid	
Hormones	
Enzymes	
Inorganic ions	
Sodium, chloride, bicarbonate, potassium, calcium, etc.	

From Beare P. G., & Myers J. L. (1998). *Adult health nursing* (3rd ed.). St Louis: Mosby.

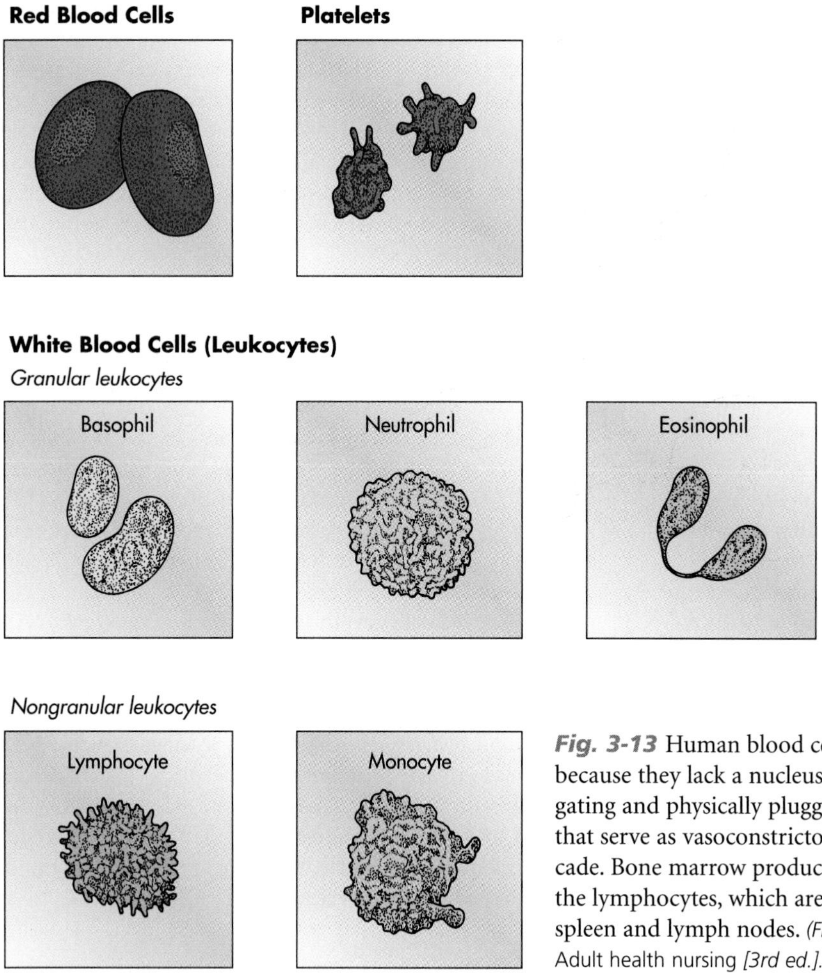

Red Blood Cells

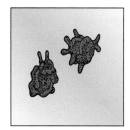

Platelets

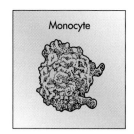

White Blood Cells (Leukocytes)

Granular leukocytes

Basophil	Neutrophil	Eosinophil

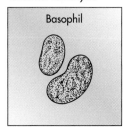
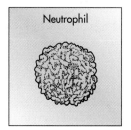
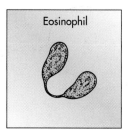

Nongranular leukocytes

Lymphocyte

Monocyte

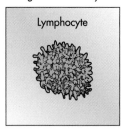
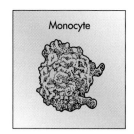

Fig. 3-13 Human blood cells. Platelets are not true cells because they lack a nucleus. They prevent blood loss by aggregating and physically plugging holes, secreting prostaglandins that serve as vasoconstrictors, and initiating the coagulation cascade. Bone marrow produces the majority of the WBCs except the lymphocytes, which are produced in greater quantity by the spleen and lymph nodes. *(From Beare, P. G., & Myers, J. L. [1998]. Adult health nursing [3rd ed.]. St. Louis: Mosby.)*

Table 3-5 **Proportions of Cells in the Blood**

CELLS	PROPORTION
Erythrocytes (red blood cells)	
Hematocrit	42%-45% of blood volume
Count	4.5-5.5 million/mm³
Platelets	
Count	150,000-350,000/mm³
Leukocytes (white blood cells)	
Total count	5000-9000/mm³
Granulocytes	
Neutrophils	65%-75% of all leukocytes
Eosinophils	2%-5% of all leukocytes
Basophils	0.5%-1% of all leukocytes
Agranulocytes	
Lymphocytes	20%-25% of all leukocytes
Monocytes	3%-8% of all leukocytes

From Beare P. G., & Myers J. L. (1998). *Adult health nursing* (3rd ed.). St Louis: Mosby.

HEMOSTASIS

Having an understanding of the clotting mechanism of blood is vital. The blood maintains homeostasis or balance between clot formation and lysis. Injury to a blood vessel surface or to tissue will trigger platelet aggregation (Figure 3-14). This activates either the **intrinsic or extrinsic pathway,** followed by a **common pathway** of hemostasis that results in the formation of fibrin (Figure 3-15 and Table 3-6). A blood vessel responds to injury (trauma or surgery) by constricting and by the formation of a platelet plug. This is the **intrinsic pathway.** The **extrinsic pathway** is activated when the blood plasma (tissue factor, a lipoprotein) reacts with connective tissue cells. Thromboplastin is released when tissue is injured. It reacts with prothrombin in the blood and the process continues down the common pathway to form a fibrin plug. This whole process does not continue indefinitely but is balanced by **fibrinolysis;** this is a hematologic process analogous to clotting and activated by many related factors (Figure 3-16). The fibrin degradation products and antithrombin are anticoagulants (Atkinson & Fortunato, 1996). Many laboratory blood tests are available for the assessment of

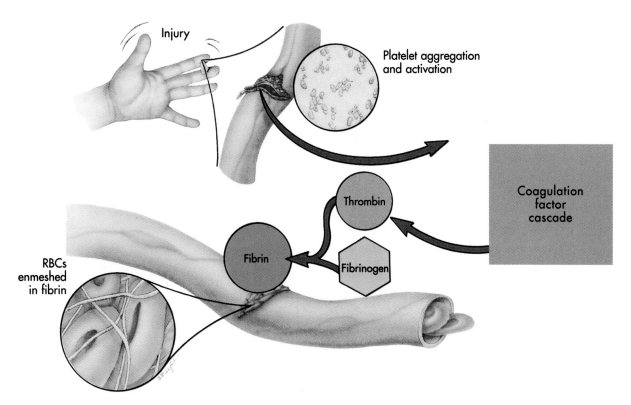

Fig. 3-14 Blood clotting mechanism. *(From Thibodeau, G. A., & Patton, K. T. [1996]. Anatomy and physiology [3rd ed.]. St. Louis: Mosby.)*

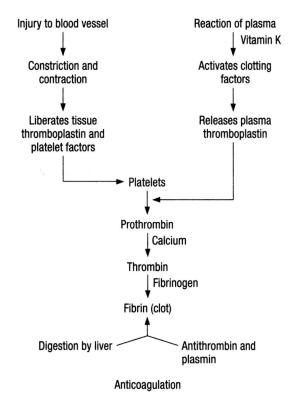

Fig. 3-15 Mechanism of hemostasis. *(From Atkinson, L. J., & Fortunato, N. M. [1996]. Berry & Kohn's operating room technique [8th ed.]. St. Louis: Mosby.)*

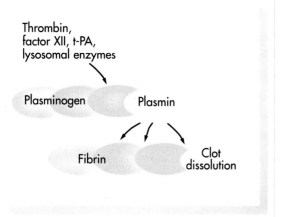

Fig. 3-16 Fibrinolysis. *(From Thibodeau, G. A., & Patton, K. T. [1996]. Anatomy and physiology [3rd ed.]. St. Louis: Mosby.)*

Table 3-6 **Coagulation Factors—Nomenclature and Synonyms**

FACTOR	COMMON SYNONYMS(S)
Factor I	Fibrinogen
Factor II	Prothrombin
Factor III	Thromboplastin
	Thrombokinase
Factor IV	Calcium
Factor V	Proaccelerin
	Labile factor
Factor VI (now obsolete)	None in use
Factor VII	Serum prothrombin conversion accelerator (SPCA)
Factor VIII	Antihemophilic globulin (AHG)
	Antihemophilic factor (AHF)
Factor IX	Plasma thromboplastin component (PTC), Christmas factor
Factor X	Stuart factor
Factor XI	Plasma thromboplastin antecedent (PTA)
Factor XII	Hageman factor
Factor XIII	Fibrin-stabilizing factor

From Thibodeau G. A., & Patton K. T. (1996). *Anatomy and physiology* (3rd ed.). St Louis: Mosby.

Box 3-2 **Tests for Coagulation Abnormalities**

PREOPERATIVE SCREENING
Platelet count (Thrombocyte count)
Detects thrombocytopenia due to drugs, liver disease, or disseminating intravascular coagulopathy (DIC)
Prothrombin time (Protime or PT, International normalized ratio [INR])
11 to 12.5 seconds; 85% to 100%
Anticoagulation 1.5 to 2.5 times control; 20% to 30%
Assesses factors that depend on vitamin K
Assesses extrinsic pathway of coagulation (factors II, VIII, IX, X; produced in the liver)
Partial thromboplastin time (PTT, or activated partial thromboplastin time, aPTT)
Normal PTT is 60 to 70 seconds
aPTT is 30 to 40 seconds
Anticoagulation achieved at 1.5 to 2.5 times the control
Congenital hemostatic defects or effects of heparin

PLATELET FUNCTION
Platelet count
Normal is >150,000 to 400,000/mm^3
Bleeding time
Normal is 1 to 9 minutes
Average time it takes for two forearm scratches to stop bleeding
Anticoagulants increase bleeding time
Platelet aggregation
Normal value dependent on agonist used
Detects specific platelet abnormalities

OTHER TESTS OF PLASMA COAGULATION
Activated clotting time (ACT)
Normal baseline 105 to 167 seconds (may vary with type of activator used)
Bedside assessment of overall blood clotting and heparin anticoagulation
Thrombin Time (TT)
Normal is control +/- 5 seconds
Measures time for plasma to clot after addition of thrombin
Assesses effects of heparin and other thrombin inhibitors and adequacy of fibrinogen
Protamine-corrected clotting times
Normal when clotting time is normal when protamine is added to sample
Used on heparinized patient to detect presence of other inhibitors
Euglobulin lysis times
Normal is 90 minutes to 6 hours
Checks activity of plasma fibrinolytic enzymes
Fibrin/fibrinogen degradation products (FDP)
Normal <10 micrograms/ml
Test for DIC, medication induced, or pathologic fibrinolysis

Modified from Sobel, 1995; values from Pagana & Pagana, 1997.

coagulation. A summary of some commonly available tests is found in Box 3-2. One abnormality that may occur intraoperatively is called **DIC** or **disseminated intravascular coagulation.** DIC is uncontrolled and inappropriate activation of the clotting mechanism with breakdown of fibrinogen and therefore paradoxical bleeding problems. This coagulopathy has many factors and may occur in the presence of extensive surgery or trauma, severe burns, or massive blood transfusion. Intraoperatively the clinical picture is one of generalized oozing from all tissue surfaces. Hypotension, hypothermia, and acidosis contribute to this defect in hemostasis after massive transfusion, 10 to 12 units of blood. DIC is best prevented, but if it occurs, the underlying causes need to be corrected. Heparin may be indicated to prevent the runaway cascade of the hemostatic mechanism that exhausts the available clotting factors (Sobel, 1995) but it is controversial in a bleeding patient (Figure 3-17).

BLOOD CIRCULATION

The body has two basic *arterial* circuits:

- The pulmonary circuit (the right heart pumps blood to the lungs)
- The systemic circuit (the left heart pumps to the rest of the body) (Box 3-3 and Figure 3-18)

The volume in the chambers of the heart is equal, about 60 to 70 milliliters. The major difference is the resistance of the beds they supply. The resistance of the pulmonary bed is much less than the systemic resistance; therefore, the muscle mass is different. The left ventricle needs to be stronger and thus more developed than the right ventricle. The aorta and pulmonary trunk are approximately 30 mm in diameter and as they branch the vessels become smaller and more numerous. Arterioles (0.3 mm in diameter) are just visible to the naked eye. These branch into capillaries that average 0.5 to 1 mm in length with a diameter of 7 microns (0.007 mm), which allows the passage of an RBC (Basmajian & Slonecker, 1989) (Table 3-7).

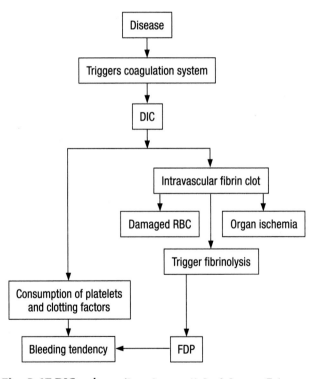

Fig. 3-17 DIC pathway. *(From Pagana, K. D., & Pagana, T. J. [1996]. Mosby's diagnostic and laboratory test reference [3rd ed.]. St. Louis: Mosby.)*

Box 3-3 **Pulmonary and Systemic Circuits**

PULMONARY CIRCUIT
Right atrium—Right ventricle—pulmonary arteries—arterioles—capillaries of lungs—pulmonary venules—pulmonary veins—left atrium

SYSTEMIC CIRCUIT
Left atrium—left ventricle—aorta—arterial branches off aorta to the rest of the body—capillaries—venules—veins—vena cavae (veins)—right atrium

---

Table 3-7 **Average Vessel Pressures**

Vessel	Average Pressure
Aorta	120 mmHg
Arterial end of capillaries	30 mmHg
Venous end of capillaries	12-30 mmHg
Great veins	5 mmHg

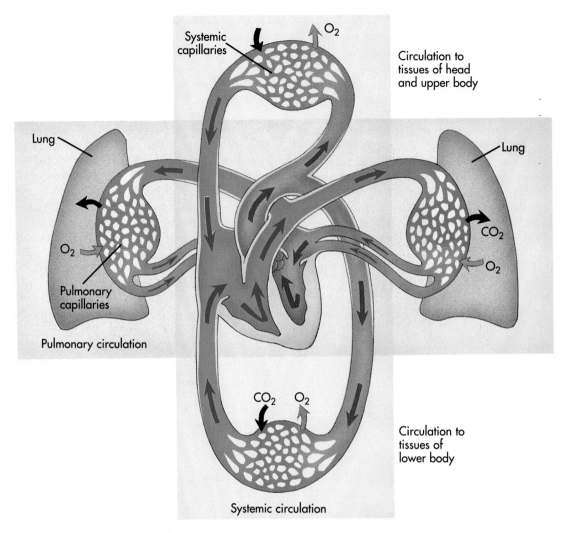

Fig. 3-18 Blood flow through the circulatory system. *(From Thibodeau, G. A., & Patton, K. T. [1996]. Anatomy and physiology [3rd ed.]. St. Louis: Mosby.)*

BLOOD FLOW

Blood flow is a complex process dependent upon many factors (Box 3-4). Blood flow that travels parallel to the vessel wall, relatively undisturbed, is called *laminar.* When an obstruction, stenosis, curve, or bifurcation disrupts flow, the particle motion is called **turbulent.** Turbulence may be evidenced by the presence of a **bruit,** detected by auscultation, or a characteristic Doppler signal. Flow, resistance, and pressure regulate blood flow in the body (Strandness, 1995). Flow is dependent upon blood viscosity, vessel wall resistance, and the peripheral resistance of the arterioles. Pressure and flow are interrelated and governed by **Poiseuille's Law** (Box 3-5). One conclusion of Poiseuille's Law is that a small decrease in the radius results in a big change in pressure (Graham & Ford, 1994). The greater the blood viscosity (thickness) the greater the pressure required to move it. A difference in pressures, or a **pressure gradient,** must exist for blood to flow in the arterial system. The contraction of the left ventricle provides this gradient. In the venous system, it is not the pressure gradient that controls flow so much as the difference in energy levels between one point and another. The left ventricle also provides this energy at rest and in combination with the contraction of the calf muscles (Criado & Johnson, 1991). The negative pressure created by the relaxed right ventricle assists in venous return by creating a suctioning effect and the skeletal and visceral muscles help propel venous return toward the heart. The negative pressures that are created in the abdominal and thoracic cavities by respiration also assist in propelling blood toward the heart. Four factors determine venous flow:

- an unobstructed pathway,
- competent valves,
- blood viscosity,
- and the calf muscle pump or "venous heart" (Jamieson, 1993).

Because two thirds of the volume of blood resides in the venous system, the veins must be able to collapse to accommodate the volume changes. Most of the time, the veins are in a state

---

Box 3-4 **Factors Controlling Circulation**

Three mechanisms of control are exerted by:

- neural
- endocrine
- local factors

AUTONOMIC NERVOUS SYSTEM

Sympathetic nerves release epinephrine (increased heart rate).

Parasympathetic nerves release acetylcholine (slows the heart rate).

Baroreceptors in carotid sinus and aortic arch are activated by stretch or pressure: stimulation causes vasomotor center inhibition and parasympathetic stimulation slows the heart and dilates the vessels (Figure 3-19).

Vasomotor **chemoreceptors** in the carotid body and aortic arch respond to decreased arterial pH and oxygen pressure and increased carbon dioxide pressure.

Vasoconstrictor centers in the medulla are stimulated and cause the arterioles to constrict.

ENDOCRINE CONTROL

Catecholamines released in response to physical activity and stress

Angiotensin

ACTH

Vasopressin

Bradykinin

Prostaglandins

LOCAL FACTORS

pH

oxygen concentration

carbon dioxide concentration

metabolic products

temperature

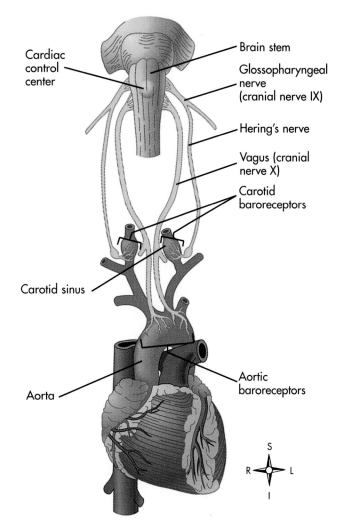

Fig. 3-19 Cardiac baroreceptors and the pressoreflexes. *(From Thibodeau, G. A., & Patton, K. T. [1996]. Anatomy and physiology [3rd ed.]. St. Louis: Mosby.)*

Box 3-5 **Poiseuille's Law**

Poiseuille was a French physician who established the following equation in 1842:

Linear velocity = difference in pressure between the inlet and outlet of a tube × the radius squared divided by the viscosity of the liquid × the tube length × 8 or

$$\text{Linear velocity} = \frac{(P1\text{-}P2)\ r^2}{8nl}$$

P1 = the pressure at the inlet of the tube

P2 = the pressure at the outlet of the tube

r = the radius of the tube

n = the blood viscosity

l = the length of the tube

8 is a constant

Adapted from Jones, 1991.

---

of partial collapse (see Figure 3-12). These mechanisms are used to move blood over long distances. Another mechanism of flow is by diffusion. This works for short distances and is created by concentration gradients (Rhoades & Tanner, 1995).

Blood flow is protected and preserved by the existence of anastomoses and alternate flow pathways. (In surgery, an **anastomosis** is the surgical connection of a vessel to a vessel or graft. In anatomy, the anastomoses, or "collaterals," are natural connections or pathways.) When an artery is damaged or blocked, arterial flow can still deliver oxygen and other nutrients if it can take an alternate pathway through anastomoses. The hands, feet, and brain are protected by anastomoses. The brain has the Circle of Willis as well as dual sources of flow, the right and left carotid arteries and right and left vertebral arteries (see Figures 3-4 and 3-5).

The arterial blood flow is divided into segments according to the resistance to flow. They are described as low, intermediate, and high resistance. The brain, liver, and kidney are low-resistance organs that must have a steady flow of blood in order to function. They do not tolerate periods of ischemia well. The musculoskeletal system and large and small intestines are in the intermediate resistance category. The flow will be regulated depending on the need. For example, during exercise, more flow is diverted to the muscles and less to the intestines. The skin is an organ of high resistance. It will tolerate long periods of low flow without any adverse effect (Strandness, 1995).

NERVES

Efferent fibers of vagal and sympathetic nerves supply the heart. Stimulation of the vagus causes the heart rate to slow; sympathetic stimulation causes the heart rate to accelerate. Increased pressure on the vessel walls (from increased blood pressure) stimulates the **afferent** (sensory) nerve fibers. These include the vagus nerve, cranial nerve X and its branch at the aortic arch (aortic nerve), and the glossopharyngeal, cranial nerve IX, distributed to the internal carotid artery, or carotid sinus (see Chapter 11). This causes a reflex slowing of the heart rate and vasodilation of vessels with a subsequent fall in blood pressure. All vessels are supplied by **efferent** (vasomotor) nerve fibers of the sympathetic nervous system. Stimulation of these nerves causes vasoconstriction and in some areas a parasympathetic vasodilation. Vasoconstriction may vary to allow partial shunting of blood such as shunting to the skin in hot weather and to the digestive tract after ingestion of a meal (Basmajian & Slonecker, 1989).

THE LYMPHATIC CIRCULATION

Proteins, antibodies, and fluids are transferred from arterial blood to the capillaries to the interstitial space to the capillaries of the lymphatic system (see Figure 3-11, *A*). The fluid of the lymph system moves as a result of muscle movement. This system transports fat, protein, and debris to be filtered through the lymph nodes. It then goes through the thoracic duct to the vena cava. The greatest concentration of lymphatic vessels is located in the gastrointestinal tract, the liver, and the skin. The least concentration is in the central nervous system. The capillaries cannot absorb all the fluid that they filter and as a result, plasma and proteins move into the interstitial space by diffusion. One function of the lymphatic vessels is to transport proteins and return them to the plasma. Lymphatic vessels can change diameter readily; they have one-way valves and become progressively larger as they move toward the venous system (Rhoades & Tanner, 1995) (Figure 3-20).

VENOUS DISORDERS

Venous disease is not seen as often in the surgical suite as arterial disease but is more common in the outpatient setting. The surgical interventions that are seen most often for venous problems include excision of varicose veins of the lower extremities (see Chapter 19) and the insertion of vena cava filters (see Chapter 18) to prevent pulmonary embolism caused by lower extremity deep venous thrombosis.

Venous Thrombosis

The most common of the venous disorders is **venous thrombosis.** Three underlying factors contribute to this condition: venous stasis, a hypercoagulable state, and damage to the inti-

mal layer of the vessel. These have been called **Virchow's triad** after the nineteenth century pathologist. Reduced venous flow leads to increased opportunity for platelet aggregation. Trauma such as venipuncture or intravenous drug therapies can cause damage to the intima of the vein. Exposure of the subintimal collagen membrane of the vein sets up the activation of the intrinsic coagulation system, which leads to formation of a thrombus. Hypercoagulable states can be a result of medical disorders such as cancer, excessive use of steroids or estrogens, and some hematologic disorders. When these conditions contribute to venous thrombosis an inflammatory reaction occurs and may eventually result in fibrosis.

Venous thrombosis of the upper extremity is uncommon but the incidence is increasing. This increase may be attributed to chemotherapy, central venous lines, and hyperalimentation catheters. Anatomical abnormalities (e.g., a first rib compression) may contribute to this problem. "Effort thrombosis" is caused by repetitive motion that involves heavy lifting or activity requiring the arms to be over the head. This may lead to compression of the subclavian vein at the level of the thoracic outlet and subsequent thrombosis. Symptoms include sudden onset of arm swelling and complaints of the arm feeling heavy or aching. If ultrasonography confirms venous thrombosis, treatment may be anticoagulation, thrombolysis, thrombectomy, or first rib resection as indicated (Kurgan & Nunnelee, 1995) (see Chapter 4 and Chapter 13).

Venous Stasis Ulcers

Patients with postphlebitic syndrome, also called chronic venous insufficiency, a history of DVT, and incompetent perforating veins may present with leg edema, stasis dermatitis (dark pigmentation around the ankle) and, sometimes, venous leg ulcers. The ulcers are typically found in the "gaiter" area of the lower extremity, pretibial and anteromedial supramalleolar (see Table 5-4). Treatment is focused on prevention of edema with custommade elastic compression stockings, regular exercise, and meticulous skin care to prevent skin injury and further breakdown and promote healing. Leg elevation is most important to promote healing of established ulcers. When conservative treatment fails, stripping of the saphenous veins and ligation of the perforators may be necessary. Local wound debridement and skin grafting are sometimes necessary.

ARTERIAL DISORDERS

Acute

Acute arterial occlusion is due to thrombosis, embolism, and trauma. Thrombi may be from a cardiac origin (atrial fibrillation, prosthetic heart valves, rheumatic heart disease). Acute occlusion may also be due to trauma from compression, shearing, or laceration of a vessel.

Thrombosis

The acute onset of arterial thrombosis is usually related to an atherosclerotic stenosis or thrombosis from an aneurysm (Green & Ouriel, 1993). The most common site of acute arterial thrombosis is at the distal superficial femoral artery. The

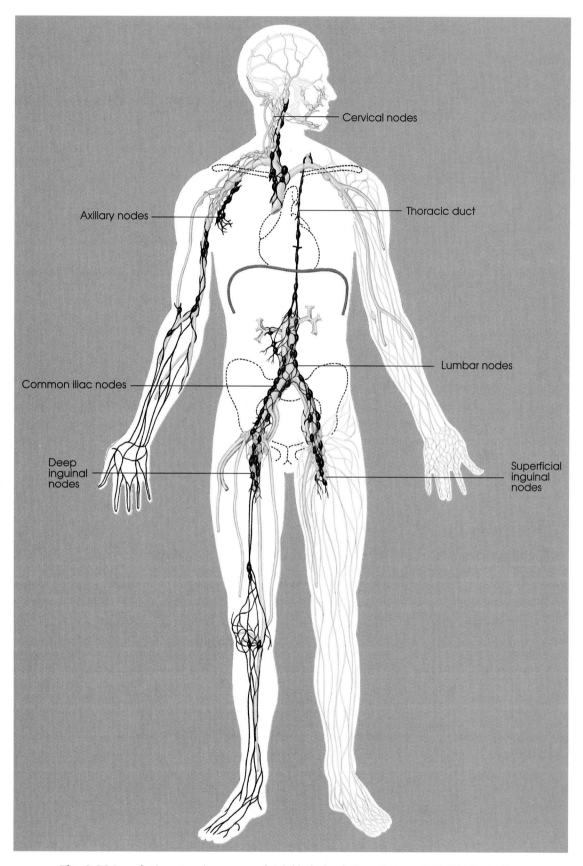

Fig. 3-20 Lymphatic system (*green,* superficial; *black,* deep). *(From Ballinger, P. W. [1995]. Merrill's atlas of radiographic positions and radiologic procedures [8th ed.]. St. Louis: Mosby.)*

initial symptoms are pain, pallor, and pulselessness. The limb may become swollen, waxen looking, and cyanotic. The skin blisters and eventually the limb either becomes infected or mummifies and shrivels if untreated (Pousti, Wilson, & Williams, 1994).

Embolism

Arterial emboli are usually of cardiac origin if they block large vessels (femoral artery). Emboli of the smaller vessels are most often caused by plaque and thrombi of the proximal vessel. (See also Atherogenesis later in this chapter) An embolectomy may be all that is needed to open a vessel if the origin is cardiac. If the occluded vessel is atherosclerotic or aneurysmal, a bypass procedure may be indicated (Green & Ouriel, 1993).

Trauma

Arterial occlusion derived from blunt trauma occurs most often from pressure or injury from a bone fragment or end. The injuries most likely to cause arterial injury are supracondylar fracture of the femur or humerus and dislocation of the shoulder, elbow, or knee. Presenting symptoms, aside from those of the bone injury, resemble those of embolism (Pousti, Wilson, & Williams, 1994).

Chronic

Chronic arterial insufficiency is caused by atherosclerosis, aneurysms, hypertension, hypercoagulable states, or heavy tobacco use (Green & Ouriel, 1993). Acute arterial occlusion may be superimposed upon and a result of chronic disease.

Atherosclerosis and atherogenesis

Atherosclerosis is a disorder of the arteries. The characteristic lesions, called **plaque**, consist of lipid, smooth muscle cells, connective tissue, and calcium. Symptoms are associated with the stenosis of a vessel lumen by the build-up of the plaque. Acute arterial obstruction may occur when blood dissects into or under the plaque (Ross, 1994). The vasa vasorum may also cause acute occlusion by hemorrhaging into the plaque. If an ulceration develops in the plaque, a segment may break off and embolize. As the atherosclerotic process continues, the arterial media degenerates and may result in an aneurysm, a thrombosis, or vessel rupture (Zarins & Glagov, 1994).

Vessel injury and thrombus formation are the basis for the formation of an **atherosclerotic plaque** or lesion. The most accepted hypothesis for this is the "response to injury" view by Ross in 1986 (Green & Ouriel, 1993). Risk factors include diabetes, high blood pressure, hyperlipidemia, smoking, some genetic factors, and lifestyle (Zarins & Glagov, 1994; Ross & Glomset, 1986). This hypothesis has been demonstrated only in nonhuman subjects. Many factors contribute to the formation of atherosclerosis and most likely lipids in the blood, hemodynamics of blood flow, and the arterial wall structure and its complex functions are involved (Haimovici & DePalma, 1996) (Figure 3-21).

One step in the development of atherosclerotic lesions has been described as a normal process detected in children, called the **fatty streak** (Figure 3-22). Fatty streaks are found in populations that do not develop atherosclerosis (Ross, 1994). They

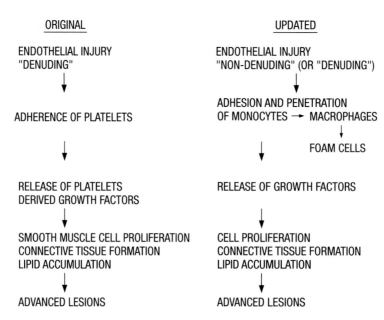

Fig. 3-21 Sequence of events in atherogenesis according to response to injury hypothesis. *(From Clement, D. L., & Shepard, J. T. [1993].* Vascular diseases in the limbs: Mechanisms and principles of treatment. *St. Louis: Mosby.)*

have been seen in arteries at all ages and may be near or part of atherosclerotic lesions. Some fatty streaks are found in areas that are typical of atherosclerotic lesions while other fatty streaks resolve. They apparently do not cause symptoms but their role in atherogenesis has not been clarified. **Fibrous plaques** are found in people in their twenties and typically there is no endothelial involvement. This becomes the most common lesion type in people in their forties. These plaques vary in composition but usually have a connective tissue and smooth muscle cell area under the endothelial cells called the **fibrous cap** (Zarins & Glagov, 1994). These fibrous caps are white and elevated (Ross, 1994). Under this fibrous cap is a central area of lipids, smooth muscle cells, calcium, and other debris called the **necrotic core**. Typically, fibrin accumulates on the lesion, the vasa vasorum penetrate the plaque to nourish it, and the vessel may thin and bulge. Calcification is often found in more advanced lesions and in older patients. Calcification tends to form in the aorta and coronary arteries before other vessels. The extension of the vasa vasorum into

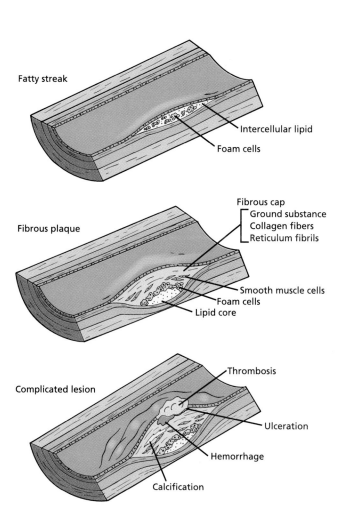

Fig. 3-22 Stages of atherosclerosis.

the plaque is also usually only seen in advanced lesions. This has been implicated in complications of hemorrhage into the plaque, degeneration of the plaque, and a resultant embolization (Zarins & Glagov, 1994). With hemorrhage, there can be the development of a thrombus that may become organized clot and further encroach on the lumen diameter (Ross, 1994).

Atherosclerotic plaque may develop and instead of obstructing the flow of blood, the vessel sometimes accommodates by enlarging. This has been seen in the carotids, the abdominal aorta, and the superficial femoral arteries (Blair, Glagov, & Zarins, 1990). The distribution of atherosclerotic lesions has been the subject of much study. The mesenteric, intercostal, renal, and mammary arteries are less likely to be diseased while the coronary arteries, carotid bifurcation, infrarenal aorta and iliofemoral arteries are the most likely areas of atherosclerosis (Roberts, Moses, & Wilkins, 1959). These patterns have been attributed to different local conditions, vessel wall structure, and blood flow patterns.

Arteriosclerosis

The intima thickens as a part of the aging process (**arteriosclerosis**, often referred to as hardening of the arteries). This tends to be a uniform process throughout the arterial system. This seems to cause no lipid accumulation, stenotic areas, or even a generalized narrowing. The elastic layer of the larger arteries tends to split and exhibit calcium deposition. Aging vessels exhibit the following characteristics: elongation, increased lumen diameter, and tortuosity. It is interesting to note that no connection has been made between these changes and the formation of atherosclerotic lesions (Zarins & Glagov, 1994).

Aneurysmal disease

A **true aneurysm** is the dilation of an artery to one and one half its original diameter with involvement of the entire vessel wall. A **false aneurysm** involves only the adventitial portion of the wall and surrounding tissue. Aneurysms have a variety of causes including infection, trauma, and atherosclerosis. Atherosclerosis has been linked to aneurysm formation but the etiology is not entirely clear. Aneurysms caused by trauma include blunt trauma, as in a motor vehicle accident, and those caused by the trauma of invasive procedures, i.e., arteriograms. Traumatic aneurysms are usually false aneurysms. Arterial anastomoses may lead to the formation of an aneurysm if there is any separation between the graft and artery. A fibrous capsule can develop and become a false aneurysm. Whatever the cause, aneurysms increase in size and may progress to rupture and/or embolization of thrombotic debris.

The abdominal aorta, below the renal arteries and just above the aortic bifurcation, is the most common site for an aneurysm. The iliac arteries are the next most common site. Of the peripheral artery aneurysms, 70% arise in the popliteal artery (Connell & Wilson, 1994) and 33% arise in the femoral artery. Two thirds of patients with a peripheral artery aneurysm have multiple aneurysms (Haimovici, 1996). Green and Ouriel (1993) categorize aneurysms as nonspecific, traumatic, dissecting, anastomotic, mycotic, childhood, and associated with pregnancy. Nonspecific is a term applied to the most common type, generally considered, but unproven, to be due to atherosclerosis.

Trauma-induced aneurysms are usually false aneurysms. In a dissecting aneurysm, the layers of the arterial wall split longitudinally. This is most often associated with hypertension and less often caused by blunt trauma. Mycotic aneurysms or infected aneurysms may arise from an internal or external infection. Until syphilis was controlled, it was the cause of 50% of all aneurysms. This is now rare in the United States. *Salmonella* and *Staphylococcus* are the most common causes of mycotic aneurysms. Anastomotic aneurysms result when the suture line of an arterial anastomosis separates and a fibrous capsule creates a false aneurysm. Childhood aneurysms are rare and usually due to a connective tissue disorder and occasionally to trauma or an arteritis. Aneurysms of pregnancy are also rare, found in the splenic artery or abdominal aorta, and carry a high mortality from rupture.

References

Atkinson, L. J., & Fortunato, N. H. (1996). *Berry & Kohn's operating room technique* (8th ed.). St. Louis: Mosby.

Basmajian, J. V., & Slonecker, C. E. (1989). Cardiovascular and nervous systems and endocrine glands. In J. C. B. Grant, J. V. Basmajian, & C. E. Sloneker (Eds.), *Grants's method of anatomy: A clinical problem solving approach* (11th ed., pp. 25-38). Baltimore: Williams & Wilkins.

Beare, P. G., & Myers, J. L. (1998). *Adult health nursing* (3rd ed.). Nursing assessment of the peripheral vascular system (pp. 404-415). St. Louis: Mosby.

Bishara, R.A., et al. (1986). Deterioration of venous function in normal lower extremities during daily activity. *Journal of Vascular Surgery, 3*(5):700-706.

Blair, J. M., Glagov, S., & Zarins, C. K. (1990). Mechanisms of superficial femoral artery adductor canal stenosis. *Surgical Forum, 41: 359-360.*

Callow, A. D. (1995). The macrocirculation. In A. D. Callow, & C. B. Ernst (Eds.), *Vascular surgery: Theory and practice* (pp. 29-48). Stamford, CT: Applelton & Lange.

Connell, T. P., & Wilson, S. E. (1994). Popliteal artery aneurysms. In F. J. Veith, R. W. Hobson, R. A. Williams, & S. E. Wilson (Eds.). *Vascular surgery: Principle and practice* (2nd ed., pp. 576-579). New York: McGraw-Hill.

Criado, E., & Johnson, G. (1991). Venous disease. *Current Problems in Surgery, 28*(5):339-400.

Graham, L. M., & Ford, M. B. (1994). Arterial disease. In V A. Fahey (Ed.). *Vascular nursing* (pp. 3-20). Philadelphia: W. B. Saunders.

Green, R. M., & Ouriel, K. (1993). Peripheral arterial disease. In S. I. Schwarz, G. T. Shires, & F. C. Spencer (Eds.), *Principles of surgery* (6th ed., pp. 925-987). New York: McGraw-Hill.

Haimovici, H. (1996). Peripheral arterial aneurysms. In H. Haimovici, E. Ascer, L. H. Hollier, D. E. Strandness, & J. B. Towne (Eds.), *Vascular surgery: Principles and techniques* (4th ed., pp. 893-909). Cambridge, MA: Blackwell Science.

Haimovici, H., & DePalma, R. G. (1996). Atherosclerosis: Biologic and surgical considerations. In H. Haimovici, E. Ascer, L. H. Hollier, D. E. Strandness, & J. B. Towne (Eds.), *Vascular surgery: Principles and techniques* (4th ed., pp. 127-157). Cambridge, MA: Blackwell Science.

Jaffe, E. A. (1992). Physiologic functions of normal endothelial cells. In J. Loscalzo, M. A. Creager, & V. J. Dzau (Eds.), *Vascular medicine: A textbook of vascular biology and diseases* (pp. 3-46). Boston: Little, Brown.

Jamieson, W. G. (1993). State of the art of venous investigation and treatment. *Canadian Journal of Surgery, 36*(2): 119-128.

Jones, M. B. (1991). Review of anatomy and physiology: Blood vessels and lymphatics. In M. C. Patrick, S. L. Woods, R. F. Craven, J. S. Rokoky, & P. Bruno (Eds.), *Medical-surgical nursing: Pathophysiological concepts* (2nd ed., pp. 790-801). New York: J. B. Lippincott.

Kurgan, A., & Nunnelee, J. D. (1995). Upper extremity venous thrombosis. *Journal of Vascular Surgery, 13*(1): 21-23.

Linton, R. R. (1938). The communicating veins of the lower leg and the operative technic for their ligation. *Annals of surgery, 107*:582-593.

O'Rourke, S. T., & Vanhoutte, P. M. (1992). Vascular pharmacology. In J. Loscalzo, M. A. Creager, & V. J. Dzau (Eds.), *Vascular medicine: A textbook of vascular biology and diseases* (1st ed.) (pp. 133-155). Boston: Little, Brown.

Pagana, K. D., & Pagana, T. J. (1997). *Mosby's diagnostic and laboratory test reference* (3rd ed.). St. Louis: Mosby.

Pousti, T. J., Wilson, S. E., & Williams, R. A. (1994). Clinical examination of the vascular system. In F. J. Veith, R. W. Hobson, R. A. Williams, & S. E. Wilson (Eds.), *Vascular surgery Principle and practice* (2nd ed.), (pp. 74-89). New York: McGraw-Hill.

Rhoades, R. A., & Tanner, G. A. (1995). An overview of circulation and hemodynamics. In R. A. Rhoades, & G. A. Tanner (Eds.), *Medical physiology* (pp. 230-241). Boston: Little, Brown.

Roberts, J. C. Jr., Moses, C., & Wilkins, R. H. (1959). Autopsy studies in atherosclerosis: I. Distribution and severity of atherosclerosis in patients dying without morphologic evidence of atherosclerotic catastrophe; II. Distribution and severity of atherosclerosis in patients dying with morphologic evidence of atherosclerotic catastrophe. *Circulation, 20*: 511-536.

Ross, R. (1994). Pathophysiology of atherosclerosis. In F. J. Veith, R. W. Hobson, R. A. Williams, & S. E. Wilson (Eds.), *Vascular surgery: Principle and practice* (2nd ed.) (pp. 9-20). New York: McGraw-Hill.

Ross, R., & Glomset, J. A. (1986). The pathogenesis of atherosclerosis-an update. *New England Journal of Medicine, 314*(8):488-500.

Sobel, M. (1995). Hemostatic disorders. In A. D. Callow, & C. B. Ernst (Eds.), *Vascular surgery: Theory and practice* (pp. 797-816). Stamford, CT: Applelton & Lange.

Strandness, Jr., D. E. (1995). Arterial and venous hemodynamics. In K. Ouriel (Ed.) *Lower extremity vascular disease.* (pp. 3-12). Philadelphia: W. B Saunders.

Thibodeau, G. A., & Patton, K. T. (1996). *Anatomy & Physiology* (3rd ed.). St. Louis: Mosby.

Zarins, C. K., & Glagov, S. (1994). Pathophysiology of human atherosclerosis. In F. J. Veith, R. W. Hobson, R. A. Williams, & S. E. Wilson (Eds.), *Vascular surgery: Principle and practice* (2nd ed.) (pp. 21-39). New York: McGraw-Hill.

4 Medications

INTRODUCTION

This text focuses on a fairly small number of medications that are usually utilized in the care of vascular patients. It is appropriate to highlight a few of the basic pharmacologic agents that the perioperative nurse will encounter as she or he elicits a drug history, assesses allergies and sensitivities, and plans care for the surgical patient. Some patients will have visible evidence of previous drug therapy. Some may have had a preoperative course of thrombolytic agents before surgical intervention. It may be useful for the nurse to be able to distinguish bruises caused by heparin therapy from those of other causes. A knowledge of the medical treatment that surgical patients may have had is essential to a complete preoperative assessment. Because the surgical vascular patient may have had medical management of their vascular disease, an overview of the more common medical treatments is covered. (Box 4-1).

Box 4-1 Medication Summary

HEPARIN (ANTICOAGULANT)

Action: (sytemically) direct effect on blood coagulation by blocking conversion of prothrombin to thrombin and fibrinogen to fibrin. As an irrigant: negative charge on tubing wall may mechanically discourage blood adherence and may prevent platelet adherence

Route of administration: IV bolus, continuous IV infusion, SC

May be undiluted or diluted with 0.9% NaCl, dextrose, or Ringer's solution

Irrigation in normal saline or other IV fluid: varies with surgeon's preference, common practice is 1:1 or 500 units/500 cc of saline. Used to irrigate blood vessels and lumens of catheters and tubing

Duration and onset: IV, immediate, peaks in 5 minutes, duration of 2 to 6 hours, half-life of 1.5 hours

SC, onset of 20 to 60 minutes, duration of 8 to 12 hours

Dosages: Prevention of DVT and PE: 5000 units SC q8-12h or PE: 7000 to 10,000 units IVP q4h, then titrate to PTT or ACT

DVT, MI: 5000 to 7000 units IVP q4h initially, titrate to PTT or ACT

Open heart surgery: IV infusion of 150 to 300 units/kg.

Vascular surgery, intraoperatively: just before arterial clamping, usually 5000 to 7000 units IVP and 1000 to 2000 units after the first hour and each hour the clamp remains on or titrated to ACT

Drug Interactions

Because of its high negative charge, it is incompatible with erythromycin, amino glycosides, tetracyclines, phenothiazines, and non-steroidal antiinflammatory drugs (NSAIDs) (Keller & Silver, 1994).

Heparin therapy will decrease the effects of corticosteroids and increase the effects of diazepam.

Heparin's effectiveness is decreased with digitalis, tetracycline, and antihistamines.

Heparin's effectiveness is increased with oral anticoagulants, salicilates, dextran, steroids, and the NSAIDs.

Laboratory test interference:

Triiodothyronine (T3) uptake is increased

Uric acid is decreased

Contraindications

Active or suspected bleeding, e.g., GI, intracranial hemorrhage, or decreased Hct with unknown cause, known coagulation disorders, hemophilia, antithrombin III deficiency, idiopathic thrombocytopenia purpura, use during or after ophthalmic or neurosurgical procedures, endocarditis, threatened abortion, heparin sensitivities, or heparin-induced thrombocytopenia. Caution in the presence of severe liver or kidney disease, open wound, increased capillary fragility, postoperative epidural catheter, alcoholism (see Box 4-2)

Side effects and adverse reactions

Fever and chills, diarrhea, nausea and vomiting, anorexia, hepatitis, abdominal cramps, rash, pruritis, alopecia (reversible), anaphylaxis, hemorrhage, and thrombocytopenia.

ACT, Activated clotting time; *PE,* pulmonary embolism; *PTT,* partial thromboplastin time; *IV,* intravenous; *SC,* subcutaneous.

HEPARIN (HEPARIN SODIUM OR HEPARIN CALCIUM)

Heparin is by far the most commonly used drug in treatment and prophylaxis of thromboembolism. Discovered in 1916, its clinical applicability was not feasible until the 1960s (Nunnelee, 1994). Heparin binds with antithrombin III (or heparin cofactor) to prevent the production of a clot. It binds in a 1:1 ratio, permitting more antithrombin III to bind with thrombin. Heparin prevents the conversion of fibrinogen to fibrin and prothrombin to thrombin (Humphrey & Silver, 1995; Nunnelee, 1994). Heparin is a sulfated polysaccharide with a strong negative charge and is usually extracted from beef lung or pork gut mucosa (Hoch & Silver, 1991). It is a large molecule and this size is an advantage in that it cannot cross the placental barrier and may be used in pregnant woman. It also may be used in lactating women because it does not affect breast milk (Skidmore-Roth, 1995). Other effects of heparin include prolongation of whole blood clotting time, thrombin time, partial thromboplastin time, and prothrombin time. It may also exhibit antiinflammatory and diuretic effects and increase potassium (K+) retention (Govani & Hayes, 1995).

Heparin has many uses. It is used preoperatively to prevent the further extension of thrombus formation (propagation) in acute lower extremity ischemia, crescendo transient ischemic attacks (TIAs), routine prophylaxis of deep venous thrombosis (DVT) in general surgical patients, intraoperatively before vascular clamping, and in acute frostbite (Govani & Hayes, 1995). It is the anticoagulant for cardiopulmonary bypass, renal dialysis, and in blood transfusions. Patients with atrial fibrillation, with the attendant risk of emboli, are treated with heparin initially. It is also used to treat disseminated intravascular coagulation (DIC). It may be instilled into the so-called heparin locks and long-term IV access lines and ports. However, this practice of using heparin in intermittent lines has been studied because of the numerous side effects of heparin and its incompatibility with many other drugs. The studies are showing that instilling saline is effective to maintain patency, presents fewer adverse reactions problems, and is significantly more cost effective in terms of dollars spent on medications, supplies, and decreased nursing time (Goode, et al, 1991). Heparin is used as an irrigant or flush during angiography and endovascular procedures to maintain patency. Its earliest use was in low dosage (minidose) to prevent DVT (Nunnelee, 1994). Research has established that it does in fact decrease the incidence of DVT and fatal pulmonary embolism (PE) in the general surgical patient and remains the drug of choice (Hoch & Silver, 1991).

It is important to understand and teach patients that heparin does not dissolve existing clots but prevents their formation or extension. One disadvantage of heparin is that it must be given parenterally. Intramuscular (IM) injection is contraindicated because its absorption is unpredictable and hematomas form at the site of injection (Govani & Hayes, 1995). IM injection of any other medications in the anticoagulated patient is also discouraged for the same reason. Minidose heparin, for prevention of DVT and PE, is often given subcutaneously (SC) but this is reported to be painful and leaves ecchymotic areas at the injection site. Ice applied to the site of SC injection may help alleviate the discomfort and the bruising. Never aspirate or massage the site when administering SC heparin, but gentle pressure for one minute is recommended (Skidmore-Roth, 1995). The abdomen is the most frequently utilized site for SC administration but the posterior arm, scapular fat pad, and lateral thigh are also cited. Intravenous (IV) heparin via continuous infusion provides steady blood levels but may be inconvenient for the patient because of the presence of the IV line and the potential for bleeding at the IV site (Nunnelee, 1994). Although heparin is metabolized by the liver and excreted in the urine, renal failure and hepatic insufficiency do not affect clearance of the drug (Hoch & Silver, 1991). The elderly may be considered to be at increased risk for hemorrhage (Box 4-2).

Although the adverse effects of heparin are summarized in Box 4-1, two important complications are worthy of discussion: hemorrhage and thrombocytopenia. Bleeding that occurs during minidose heparin is considered a nuisance but poses little risk to the patient (Hoch & Silver, 1991). There has been much research done in the quest for the ideal anticoagulant. Clagett & Reisch (1988) reviewed data from 1600 patients to compare low dose heparin for PE prevention with a combination drug, 5000 units of heparin with 0.5 mg of dihydroergotamine (trade name Embolex). Both regimens were equally effective in preventing fatal PE and the combination drug had significantly fewer major bleeding episodes. Although this appeared promising, the combination drug carried a risk of 0.2% of marked vasoconstriction, which is undesirable in patients with arterial disease. Angina, numbness and tingling of the digits, and lower extremity weakness attributed to vascular ischemia are reported with the use of Embolex (Gever, 1986). Patients who are using other vasoconstrictors, such as nicotine, beta blockers, and dopamine, are particularly at risk (Todd, 1987).

The second important adverse effect of heparin therapy is heparin induced thrombocytopenia (**HIT**), also called **white clot syndrome**, heparin-associated thrombocytopenia and thrombosis (**HATT**), or heparin-induced thrombocytopenia

---

Box 4-2 Conditions That May Increase the Risk of Bleeding

Advanced age
Hypertension
Recent stroke
Recently resuscitated with CPR
Dissecting aneurysm
Any known bleeding tendency
Recent surgery or trauma
Recent GI bleed
Sepsis near the site of the thrombus
Visceral cancer
Collagen disease
Hepatic function impairment
Prolonged dietary insufficiency
Prolonged diarrhea
Prolonged fever
Vitamin C or K deficiency

From Todd, B. (1987). Drugs and the elderly: Use heparin safely. *Geriatric Nursing: The American Journal of Care for the Elderly,* 8(1): 43-44.

syndrome (**HITTS**). This occurs in approximately 2% to 5% of patients on heparin (Hoch & Silver, 1991). When the actual clots are examined in this syndrome, they are not the familiar red clots but are white and composed of fibrin and platelets. The etiology has yet to be elucidated. Bovine-derived heparin has been linked with this reaction more than porcine-derived heparin and again the mechanism is not clear (Kuhar & Hill, 1991). Patients develop antiplatelet antibodies that can cause the complications starting on day 4 to day 15 after treatment. The route and dose do not appear to alter the outcome. Because HIT will occur on the day of reexposure to heparin, a baseline and daily platelet counts are necessary. In addition, a PT and PTT should be routine before the start of anticoagulant therapy (Humphrey & Silver, 1995). Platelet counts can drop dramatically and thrombosis can occur within hours with HIT (Kuhar & Hill, 1991). Though rare, this can be a cause of acute arterial occlusion in the immediate postoperative period. Theories on the cause of HIT suggest that it is an immune response that induces platelet aggregation (Kuc, 1993). Because of the short half-life of heparin, stopping the drug is adequate in mild HIT. Maintaining the heparin is also possible while converting to warfarin and monitoring the patient closely while the oral anticoagulant takes effect, which usually takes 24 to 36 hours. While it makes sense to administer platelets, this is a transient remedy and could exacerbate the existing pathology. Aspirin with dipyridamole and dextran have been used for some patients (Kuc, 1993) (Box 4-3 and Box 4-4). For the patients with HIT, a significant risk of limb loss and even mortality exists. Even with the previously mentioned antiplatelet agents the desired anticoagulation may not be achieved.

ANCROD

Ancrod, derived from the venom of Agkistrodon rhodostoma, the Malayan pit viper, has been used successfully as an anticoagulant in patients who cannot tolerate heparin. Its action is on fibrinogen and produces a fibrin that is incapable of clotting. It has a half-life of 3 to 5 hours. At the same time, platelet function is undisturbed. It has the added advantage of decreasing blood viscosity. The dose for anticoagulation is 1 to 2 units/kg. Like heparin, Ancrod is administered subcutaneously (SC) or by intravenous bolus or push (IVP) with the IV route being more reliable. It has been used for surgery, dialysis, and cardiopulmonary bypass and for thromboembolic prophylaxis. Patients with antithrombin III deficiency, for whom heparin is ineffective, may be treated with ancrod or fresh frozen plasma (FFP) that contains antithrombin III. Side effects from ancrod are minor: fever, minor allergic symptoms, and bleeding. Ancrod can be reversed by administering cryoprecipitate (Humphrey & Silver, 1995; Cole & Bormanis, 1988). Ancrod is not in widespread use in the United States where it is still considered an investigational drug and not approved by the Food and Drug Administration (FDA) (Towne, 1994).

PROTAMINE

Protamine sulfate is the antagonist of heparin (Box 4-5). It appears to bind the heparin, preventing its action with antithrombin (Nunnelee, 1994). It is an anticoagulant itself, but being strongly basic, it combines with the strongly acid heparin to neutralize the effects of both drugs. Its onset of action is 5 minutes and it has a duration of 2 hours (Govani & Hayes, 1995). Because it is derived from fish semen or testes, it has caused allergic reactions in patients allergic to fish. The preoperative assessment of all vascular surgical patients should include a specific question to elicit such a sensitivity. There is also an increased incidence of severe hypersensitivity to protamine in insulin-dependent patients who are taking NPH insulin (Guzzetta & Dossey, 1992). One mg of protamine neutralizes 90 units of heparin from lung tissue or 115 mg of heparin from intestinal mucosa; or more simply, 1 mg neutralizes 100 units of heparin. The dose should be calculated to offset half the last dose of heparin (Clark, Queener, & Karb, 1990). Protamine must be given slowly, at a maximum of 50 mg in 10 minutes, or it may cause dyspnea, flushing, bradycardia, and *severe hypotension.*

Box 4-3 **Drugs That Affect Platelet Function**

ASA
Irreversible, wanes over 5 to 7 days (but DDAVP may be given to significantly shorten bleeding time that is altered by ASA)
NSAIDs
Recovery from platelet inhibition in hours to days
Dextran
Inhibits platelet aggregation, impedes fibrin polymerization, augments clot lysis

---

Box 4-4 **Drugs That Affect Plasma Coagulation**

Heparin
(assess by ACT, PTT, or thrombin time)
Binds antithrombin
Warfarin
Interferes with cofactor activity of vitamin K (vitamin K is needed to synthesize clotting factors II, VII, IX, X)
Starvation, antibiotics, and bowel prep deplete vitamin K

Box 4-5 **Protamine**

Protamine is strongly basic and combines with strongly acid heparin to neutralize the anticoagulant effects of both
Onset is 5 minutes, duration is 2 hours
Adverse reactions: abrupt drop in BP, flush, feeling of warmth, bleeding, N & V, dyspnea, hypersensitivity reaction.
1 mg neutralizes 90 units of heparin from lung tissue or 115 mg of heparin from intestinal mucosa
Monitor blood pressure and pulse
APPT & ACT in 5 to 15 minutes and 2 and 8 hours if desired (Govani & Hayes, 1995)

Another reason for monitoring heparin is that protamine, given in the absence of circulating heparin, acts as an anticoagulant and could delay hemostasis intraoperatively (Baer & Williams, 1996). According to Adkins (1993), a "heparin rebound" can occur by which the heparin stored in the subcutaneous tissue reemerges in the circulation during postoperative reperfusion. This is thought to occur when heparin has been inadequately reversed. Adkins advocates monitoring the activated clotting time (ACT) and partial thromboplastin time (PTT) to gauge adequate reversal and thus prevent rebound. A difference of opinion exists about the need for reversal of heparin. Keller and Silver (1994) claim that reversal is "rarely needed" after intraoperative clamp removal if meticulous attention is given to surgical hemostasis. Others routinely reverse heparin to reduce the incidence of wound hematomas.

HEPARINIZED SALINE IRRIGATION

Heparinized saline solution is used as an irrigant. It may be used to irrigate a blood vessel lumen during surgery, usually after the patient has been systemically heparinized. It is also commonly used to flush the lumen of tubes used to shunt blood. The probable mechanism is twofold: by creating a negative charge on the tubing wall and interfering with platelet adherence (Clark, Queener, & Karb, 1990). The strength of the heparin solution will vary according to the manufacturers' recommendations for certain implant devices or by surgeon preference. A reasonable range is 250 to 1000 units in 250 cc of normal saline.

There are differing ideas on solutions with which to distend, irrigate, or store vein grafts used for bypass procedures. Some surgeons prefer a cold solution to decrease the metabolic demands of the vessel, while others believe this may lead to spasm. Spasm may be of particular concern when working with the small vessels of the distal leg or foot. **Papaverine HCl** may be added to a heparinized saline for its direct antispasmodic effect on the smooth muscle of the vessel wall and its vasodilating properties (Box 4-6) (Govani & Hayes, 1995). A reasonable dose is 120 mg in 250 cc saline. The pressure of a hand-held syringe to distend vein grafts has been viewed as a potential cause of graft failure or graft stenosis because this causes endothelial damage. **Papaverine HCl**, as a smooth muscle relaxant, allows distension at a lower pressure and may decrease the risk of injury (Cunningham, Catinello, Nathan, & Spencer, 1981). Concentrations for infiltration range from 0.05 to 0.6 mg/ml or 12.5 to 150 mg per 250 cc of solution. The literature suggests that more studies are needed to determine whether cold (4° C) or warm storage solutions are better and exactly what constitutes the ideal vein storage solution (Stanley, Sottiurai, Fry, & Fry, 1975). Papaverine is also used intraoperatively to mimic conditions of exercise to establish the location of an arterial blockage. The blood pressure in all vessels should be relatively equal. When a blockage or narrowing of the vessel lumen occurs, as in atherosclerosis, a drop in pressure occurs or what is termed a *pressure gradient*. A direct pressure reading can be obtained by inserting a needle into the artery and connecting it to a monitored transducer, i.e., an arterial monitor (see Chapter 5). The papaverine accentuates the gradient.

> **Box 4-6   Papaverine HCl**
>
> **Action:** Smooth muscle relaxation, vasodilation; direct and immediate
> **Indications:** Prevent or stop vasospasm associated with cerebral or peripheral ischemia
> **Route:** PO as suspension, tablet, or time-release capsule IV or IM
> **Contraindications:** Hypersensitivity or complete heart block

IM, Intramuscular.

WARFARIN SODIUM (COUMADIN)

Warfarin sodium (Coumadin) is the most common oral anticoagulant. It is used for long-term and outpatient anticoagulation. Because it prevents the formation of several clotting factors, it carries the risk of prolonging prothrombin time beyond the desired range. As with any anticoagulant, bleeding is a risk but only 5% of patients will have a serious episode that may require fresh frozen plasma and/or vitamin K to reverse the adverse effects (Harrington & Ansell, 1992). Some more notorious adverse effects include skin necrosis, dermatitis, and blue toe syndrome (Greenfield, 1994). These are probably a result of thrombosed capillaries (Harrington & Ansell, 1992). Warfarin can be given orally or intravenously but is usually given to follow heparin in long-term usage. It cannot be given to pregnant women because it does pass the placental barrier.

ANTIPLATELET AGENTS

Dextran was originally used as a plasma expander in the 1940s. It was considered an inert substance until, in the 1950s, the antithrombotic effects were recognized (Bergqvist, 1983). Its uses are similar to albumin because it expands volume by drawing interstitial fluid to the intravascular space (Skidmore-Roth, 1995). A polysaccharide, it is available in a low molecular weight form, dextran 40, and a high molecular weight form, dextran 70. The plasma expansion seems to improve blood flow and prevent venous stasis. It decreases platelet adhesiveness and platelet aggregation. Its presence also makes fibrin more prone to lysis by plasmin (Hoch & Silver, 1991). The literature varies concerning its efficacy in preventing DVT in surgical patients. It has also been responsible for mild allergic reactions and excessive bleeding but its greatest drawback is that of potential fluid overload (Turpie & Leclerc, 1991). Careful intake and output and vigilant observation for signs and symptoms of circulatory overload is mandatory (Skidmore-Roth, 1995). It is contraindicated in congestive heart failure (CHF) and severe anemia. 500 cc of dextran contain 77mEq of sodium and chloride and must be used with care in patients on low-salt diets. A low specific gravity of urine may be the first sign of inadequate renal clearance in a patient receiving dextran. The hematology laboratory and blood bank should be notified of the administration of dextran because it can interfere with blood typing and cross-matching and Rh factor testing (Govani & Hayes, 1995).

Other antiplatelet agents include aspirin, dipyridamole (Persantine), and NSAIDs (Nunnelee, 1994). Aspirin is commonly used to prevent transient ischemic attacks (TIAs), after myocardial infarctions, and to prevent recurrent myocardial infarctions. Dosage for thromboembolic disorders is 325 to 650 mg once or twice per day; the dosage for TIAs is higher, 325 or 650 mg qid PO. A few points to remember for vascular patients are that the aspirin may need to be discontinued before surgery to prevent bleeding and it may increase the effects of insulin and oral antihypo-glycemics. Aspirin increases the absorption of dipyridamole. Dipyridamole is an antiplatelet agent, antianginal agent, and a vasodilator. It improves coronary blood flow and aids in the generation of collateral coronary vessels. However, it does not have a similar benefit in the peripheral vascular system (Govani & Hayes, 1995). Ticlopidine (Ticlid) is another recent platelet aggregation inhibitor. It inhibits the adenosine diphosphate (ADP) induced effects of platelet aggregation. It is currently being used to prevent thrombotic strokes and is prescribed 250 mg PO twice daily with meals (Skidmore-Roth, 1995). It must be used with caution in patients with renal or liver impairment or other risk factors for bleeding. It is the only antiplatelet drug approved by the FDA in this category (Baer & Williams, 1996). Other drugs in use as antiplatelet agents have other approved uses.

Initially, it may seem reasonable to alleviate symptoms of ischemia with vasodilators for the peripheral vascular patient. However, results of their use for claudication and rest pain have failed. They may cause harm because vessels supplying ischemic tissue may already be fully dilated. Further attempts to dilate the vessels could have the opposite effect by decreasing the systemic blood pressure and thus decreasing perfusion (Nunnelee, 1994). A "steal" phenomenon may also be responsible for this effect, which may be caused by the dilation of normal vessels that diverts flow away from ischemic areas (Green & McNamara, 1988). A steal occurs when an atherosclerotic occlusion to a normal blood flow pattern permits a reversal of flow from the opposite direction. The vessel now supplying this reversed flow is essentially stealing or diverting the full stream from its normal course.

PENTOXIFYLLINE (TRENTAL)

Pentoxifylline is a methyl xanthine derivative. Therefore, the drug is contraindicated in persons intolerant to other drugs in this group, e.g., caffeine, theophylline, and theobromine (Spittell, 1992). Its mechanism of action is still not proven, but it has been prescribed to vascular patients to relieve symptoms of intermittent claudication and improve their walking distance. Classified as a hemorrheologic agent, it appears to decrease blood viscosity, stimulate prostacyclin formation, increase the flexibility of RBCs, decrease platelet aggregation, and decrease fibrinogen concentrations (Skidmore-Roth, 1995). "Hemorrheology is the study of the effects of blood flow on the cellular components of blood and walls of blood vessels" (Mosby's Dictionary, 1995). The theory is that increased blood cell deformability or flexibility allows the cells to move more easily through the microcirculation. Many studies have been undertaken to decide the value of pentoxifylline. In 1984 the FDA approved pentoxifylline as the only medication for treatment of intermittent claudication (Green & McNamara, 1988). While it seems to increase maximum walking distances, careful selection of patients who benefit most is essential (Ingegno & Williams, 1994). AbuRahma & Woodruff (1990), did a study that showed that patients with an ankle/brachial index (**ABI**) of

0.5 or greater responded better to pentoxifylline than did those with more severe disease or an ABI of less than 0.5. Pentoxifylline is rapidly absorbed from the GI tract. Peak plasma levels occur in 2 to 4 hours but the therapeutic effects may take 2 to 4 weeks to be evident, although an 8-week course is suggested before discontinuation. Long-term therapy does not result in tolerance (Govani & Hayes, 1995). The usual dose is 400 mg tid PO. This may be adjusted to 800 mg per day to decrease side effects. Patients on antihypertensive drugs need monitoring and modifications made since pentoxifylline also lowers the blood pressure (Skidmore-Roth, 1995).

DDAVP (DESMOPRESSIN ACETATE)

Desmopressin acetate is classified as a pituitary hormone. It is supplied as a synthetic analog of a human posterior pituitary hormone. According to Adkins (1993), DDAVP enhances platelet function by increasing the levels of factor VIII, von Willebrand factor, and plasminogen activator. The mechanism of action is not clear yet and studies have not shown similar results, especially about its antifibrinolytic effects. The prescribed dosage is 0.3 μg/kg over 20 minutes. Intraoperatively it may be given to renal failure patients who often have a prolonged bleeding time. This prolonged bleeding time has been attributed to the anemia that accompanies renal failure (George & Shattil, 1991). A study by Mannucci, et al, (1983) indicated that DDAVP shortened the bleeding time in both acute and chronic renal failure patients when given preoperatively. The reduced bleeding time lasted at least 4 hours.

TOPICAL HEMOSTATIC AGENTS

Blood coagulation is controlled by intravascular and extravascular (intrinsic and extrinsic) mechanisms. Injury to the endothelium, such as trauma or atherosclerosis, can trigger this mechanism (intrinsic). The extrinsic coagulation mechanism is triggered by the insult of surgery to tissue and vessels, which precipitates exposure of tissue thromboplastin that results in a clot forming (Baer & Williams, 1996). Topical hemostatic agents may be needed. Absorbable hemostatics are effective by creating an environment that promotes the adhesion of platelets (Clark, Queener, & Karb, 1992).

Absorbable Gelatin Sponge (Gelfoam, Gelfilm)

An absorbable gelatin sponge, such as Gelfoam or Gelfilm, may be applied to a bleeding surface to provide a matrix into which clots form. It can absorb many times its weight of whole blood by capillary action (Flynn & Johnston, 1995). It may be applied dry, moistened with saline, or soaked in a topical thrombin/saline solution. 100 to 1000 NIH units of thrombin/cc of saline or blood may be applied to control bleeding. It is recommended that the gelatin sponge be compressed in solution to remove trapped air. It is placed on the site of bleeding, covered with a dry gauze, and left untouched for a minimum of 15 seconds (Govani & Hayes, 1995). It may be applied temporarily until hemostasis is achieved or allowed to remain in the wound. It is completely absorbed in 4 to 6 weeks and is contraindicated in the presence of infection. Thrombin (Thrombinar, Thrombogen, Thrombostat) is usually of bovine origin and therefore contraindicated in patients sensitive to bovine products. Thrombin is part of the normal clotting mechanism and converts fibrinogen to fibrin. The topical thrombin combines with the patient's fibrinogen to create a fibrin-rich plug. The patient may be anticoagulated and this reaction can still occur and assist in local hemostasis (Humphrey & Silver, 1995). It is available in 1000, 5000, 10,000, 20,000 and 50,000 unit vials in powder form (Skidmore-Roth, 1995) that must be refrigerated.

Fibrin Gel

Fibrin gel or "glue" is another topically applied hemostatic agent (Govani & Hayes, 1995). A syringe of saline-reconstituted thrombin and a separate syringe of equal amounts of cryoprecipitate can be sprayed onto a bleeding graft or tissue surface. The fibrinogen in cryoprecipitate is the reagent that combines with topical thrombin to create a dense clot or glue. This preparation can be applied to control diffuse bleeding or augment a vascular anastomoses. A tongue depressor can be used to spread the gel over a larger area or a syringe with a tapered adaptor can be used to place a fine bead of gel to a small area (Pace, 1995). Seifert (1994) describes a batch of fibrin glue made from 20 cc of cryoprecipitate in one syringe and 500 units of thrombin with 20 cc of 10% calcium chloride. Another technique is to reconstitute cryoprecipitate with twice the usual volume and pour it over absorbable or nonabsorbable dressings. In a 20 cc syringe draw up 1000 units of thrombin in 10 cc of saline and 10 cc of calcium chloride (1 g in 10 cc). The dressing is placed over the bleeding area and the contents of the syringe sprayed over it (Flynn & Johnston, 1995).

Microfibrillar Collagen (Avitene)

Microfibrillar collagen (Avitene), a form of bovine collagen, is a powder, or woven web, that induces platelet adhesion. It must be applied with a dry forcep and can be troublesome to contain. It is effective in the anticoagulated patient (Flynn & Johnston, 1995). Avitene may be associated with hematomas and increased risk of wound infection (Skidmore-Roth, 1995). It is important that hemostatic agents not be introduced intravascularly (Govani & Hayes, 1995) nor be suctioned into blood salvaging cannisters (Seifert, 1994).

Oxidized Cellulose (Surgicel, Oxycel, Novocell)

Oxidized cellulose (Surgicel, Oxycel, Novocell) provides a matrix for clot when applied topically. Its action is to absorb blood and create an artificial clot. It is available in knitted fabric, pads, or pledgets. It may be left in place but removing it when hemostasis has been achieved is preferred (Skidmore-Roth, 1995). Removal is best performed with saline irrigation and manual extraction of the cellulose. The low pH of oxidized cellulose destroys thrombin. Therefore, the use of thrombin and Surgicel concurrently is not advised. Topical application of any other hemostatics and antiinfectives is also contraindicated (Govani & Hayes, 1995).

Monoaminocarboxylic Acid (Amicar, Amino Caproic Acid, or Epsilon-Amino Caproic Acid)

Monoaminocarboxylic acid (Amicar, Amino caproic acid, or Epsilon-Amino caproic acid) is available as an injectable or in tablet form. It is used in the presence of hyper fibrinolysis to control hemorrhage. It acts to depress fibrinolysis by inhibiting plasminogen activator substances (Skidmore-Roth, 1995). Extensive tissue damage and vascular inflammation may lead to overactivity of the normal fibrinolysis mechanisms. Amicar can assist in topical hemostasis in these instances (Flynn & Johnston, 1995). It is also administered as an antidote to urokinase or streptokinase toxicity (Govani & Hayes, 1995).

ANTIBIOTIC IRRIGATION

Infections of prosthetic vascular grafts are rare but are extremely serious. Infection may be life-threatening for patients with aortic grafts or limb-threatening in lower extremity procedures. Protecting the prosthetic graft from contact with the skin is essential to prevent bacterial contamination. Prophylactic antibiotic wound irrigation with a Neomycin or Kanamycin and cephalothin solution has resulted in a decreased wound infection rate even in the absence of parenteral antibiotic therapy (Sheng & Busittil, 1991; MacVittie, 1995).

Medications and solutions on the sterile field should always be labeled (MacVittie, 1995). The basic safety practices taught in medication classes must be strictly followed and be practiced by all personnel dispensing medications and irrigation solutions. Check labels when removing a bottle or vial from its storage area, again before drawing it into a syringe or pouring it, and before it is either given to the patient or delivered to the sterile field (Pierson, 1995). Both the circulating nurse and the scrub nurse must concurrently verify the drug or solution, the dosage, and the expiration date. To provide optimal safety, the scrub nurse must verbally identify a drug or irrigation solution *each* time it is passed to a member of the surgical team. This helps decrease the chance of misunderstanding. The majority of solutions may be colorless liquids, e.g., saline, heparinized saline, antibiotic solutions, sterile water, local anesthetics, and x-ray contrast agents. All these are used in the vascular OR in any number of combinations. Relief personnel should be instructed to discard any unlabeled solutions and policies should also reflect this standard. The medications, irrigations, and solutions are documented by the perioperative nurse in the patient record (AORN Standards and Recommended Practices, 1996).

INJECTABLE X-RAY CONTRAST

Invasive diagnostic tests are performed preoperatively and sometimes intraoperatively to identify the extent and location of the patient's peripheral vascular disease. The introduction of contrast media through a catheter into the arterial or venous system facilitates this visualization.

Contrast media for injection have only been around for 100 years but were too toxic for human use until the 1920s. There are three basic categories of radiopaque agents: ionic monomeric, nonionic monomeric (low-osmolar), and ionic dimeric (low-osmolar). Ionic monomeric are triiodobenzoic acid salts. Agents with more sodium are more toxic. The more expensive nonionic monomeric agents do not have the sodium and are half the osmolarity of the first group. The more osmolar, the more toxic and the more adverse local sensations are experienced (pain, burning, flushing). Nausea and vomiting are common side effects and serious allergic reactions can lead to bronchospasm, laryngospasm, and circulatory collapse. There is a 15% chance that a history of an allergic reaction will again result in another. Steroids, Benedryl, and Tagamet may decrease the incidence of these episodes. The contrast agents are removed by the kidneys and nephrotoxicity is a concern to all who utilize it (Lloyd, 1994).

Meticulous technique in injecting contrast can limit side effects. Fader (1986), reminds us that a simple water bath of 37° C to pre-warm the contrast to body temperature significantly decreases the adverse reactions experienced by the patient. Allowing blood to mix in the syringe with contrast may cause clots to form spontaneously in the syringe or on catheters during interventional radiological procedures or angiograms. In the OR the scrub nurse can assist by discarding the blood and contrast mixture.

Nonionic agents have been available in the United States since December 1985. Adverse chemotoxic reactions with these have been reported to be two times less frequent as with ionic agents. The older ionic agents have a moderate anticoagulant effect, compared with the nonionic agents' very slight anticoagulant effect. This indicates a need for caution against allowing the agent to sit in a syringe with blood before injection. Using a stopcock may be helpful in preventing this (Robertson, 1987). The chemotoxic effects of contrast, i.e., pain, vasodilatation, hypervolemia, and endothelial damage, may be due to the fact that they are hyperosmolar. The volume injected is directly related to the severity of the results. The allergic type of reactions, i.e., urticaria, respiratory arrest, and vasomotor collapse, may occur with any volume administered. The nonionic agents reportedly cause fewer of both types of reactions, as well as being less nephrotoxic (Malott & Fodor, 1984).

Nephrotoxicity of ionic versus nonionic contrast agents was studied in a randomized trial of almost 2000 patients. Adequate hydration was considered imperative for all subjects. The conclusion was that patients at risk for acute contrast reactions were those with preexisting renal insufficiency, especially diabetics. Patients receiving ionic contrast were 3.3 times more likely to develop nephrotoxicity (Rudnick et al, 1995).

THROMBOLYTICS

Thrombolytic therapy and thrombolytic agents are the subjects of much interest. None of the anticoagulants or antiplatelet drugs will rid the body of existing clots. The three most commonly used agents are urokinase, streptokinase, and tissue-type plasminogen activator (t-PA). The body maintains a balance of the creation and dissolution of clots as needed. When an area of vessel wall integrity is disrupted or any other tissue injury triggers the creation of the relatively insoluble fibrin plug, a counter measure is triggered to remove the plug when it is no longer needed. This fibrinolysis is a proteolytic process. When abnormal or pathologic thrombosis occurs, external agents may be useful as well as lifesaving.

Streptokinase

Streptokinase is one of the first clinically useful agents. It acts by facilitating the transformation of plasminogen to plasmin, which lyses clot. Streptokinase is indicated for DVT, PE, arterial thrombosis, and failed A-V fistulae. It has not been useful for thrombi that are a week old or more (Skidmore-Roth, 1995).

This is used in emergency rooms throughout the United States to open acutely blocked coronary arteries. It is produced from Lancefield group C beta hemolytic streptococci. Because most people have had a streptococcal infection, they are likely to have also produced an antibody that can render the streptokinase inactive. The body views this as a foreign antigen and responds accordingly with 2% of patients exhibiting an anaphylactic reaction. Some of these reactions can be prevented with steroids or antihistamines (Rubin, 1995).

Streptokinase indirectly induces the activation of plasminogen, whereas urokinase is a direct plasminogen activator. Streptokinase binds with plasminogen and causes adjacent plasminogen molecules to convert to plasmin, which then breaks down fibrinogen and fibrin (Harrington & Ansell, 1992). The onset is immediate and may last for 12 hours, with a half-life of 20 minutes. If it needs to be reversed, cryoprecipitate or fresh frozen plasma may be administered. A 0.8 micrometer filter is recommended when infusing streptokinase (Skidmore-Roth, 1995). Streptokinase doses are expressed in international units (IU). One IU activates enough blood plasminogen to lyse a standard fibrin clot in 10 minutes under standard conditions (Govani & Hayes, 1995).

Urokinase

Urokinase was named for the original study that described the fibrin lysing activities of human urine. It is currently obtained from urine and tissue cultures of fetal kidney cells (Verstraete, 1995). It was first discovered by Williams in 1951 in a quest for a fibrinolytic agent that did not cause the febrile reactions of streptokinase. 1500 liters of urine are needed to obtain a single dose of urokinase. Using recombinant DNA methods on E. coli may be the source of the future (Bell, 1995). One important point is that urokinase must be reconstituted with sterile water for injection and not bacteriostatic water (Skidmore-Roth, 1995).

Thrombolysis may be achieved by placing a catheter directly into a clot. This may be done in an x-ray or operating suite. Regional therapy with streptokinase or urokinase has been used to open both occluded grafts and native vessels (Box 4-7 and Box 4-8). Perloff and Berkowitz (1994) describe a method of

---

Box 4-7 **Thrombolysis of Occluded Grafts**

A small study of 31 patients (33 grafts) was analyzed to determine the value of thrombolysis in occluded popliteal and tibial bypass grafts. The conclusion was that thrombolysis, having been achieved in 92% of the attempts, was effective for rapid patency. Grafts that failed in the first year should be replaced. Thrombolytic therapy appears to be best when used to open grafts older than one year. It was also noted that synthetic grafts have a longer patency rate after thrombosis than vein grafts.

From Hye, et al. (1994). Is thrombolysis of occluded popliteal and tibial bypass grafts worthwhile? *Journal of Vascular Surgery, 20*(4): 588-596.

**Box 4-8 Tourniquet Use During
Intraoperative Thrombolysis**

Goodman, et al (1993) reported their technique of using a limb tourniquet intraoperatively to more effectively lyse clots during surgical embolectomy. Urokinase or streptokinase was infused into the limb in high doses. The use of the tourniquet permitted the infusion of higher than usual doses and limitation of the drug that entered the general circulation. Five of the six limbs were salvaged. None of the patients experienced any complications despite the fact that two patients had major surgery within the week. Variations of this technique may be promising for the treatment of acutely thrombosed limbs.

Adapted from Goodman, G. R., Tersigni, S., Li, K., & Lawrence, P. F. (1993). Thrombolytic therapy in an isolated limb. *Annals of Vascular Surgery*, 7(6): 512-520.

"lacing" a clot with a fibrinolytic agent via an angiography catheter. A guidewire is run through a clot and 250,000 units of urokinase is placed throughout the clot. Urokinase is continued at a rate of 4000 units per minute for 1 to 2 hours. If the vessel is opened by this procedure, 1000 to 2000 units per minute are continued until the clot is completely removed. An alternate method of using a large bolus of the drug at the top of the clot (5000 to 8000 units per minute of streptokinase or 20,000 to 60,000 units of urokinase) has also been reported (Perloff & Berkowitz, 1994).

Tissue-Type Plasminogen Activator (t-PA)

A third fibrinolytic agent used clinically is t-PA or tissue-type plasminogen activator. It acts both directly and indirectly on plasminogen. Endothelial cells synthesize and secrete t-PA naturally. Considered a relatively new drug, limited trials and bleeding complications have not been encouraging and it has not gained widespread use (Perloff & Berkowitz, 1995).

Thrombolytic therapy may be most helpful for patients who undergo concomitant surgical embolectomy. However, not all thrombi are accessible by balloon catheter access. The catheter cannot be introduced into small, collateral vessels, multiple passes of the catheter can cause damage to the intima or may even perforate a vessel wall. Use of embolectomy in conjunction with thrombolysis in selected patients is proving to be effective. The cost must be weighed and in some instances, Fogarty embolectomy remains the treatment of choice. Patients with acute vessel or graft occlusion of less than 72 hours are found to have better long-term results from thrombolysis than those with chronic occlusions caused by atherosclerosis (Garcia, et al, 1990).

Patients at risk for bleeding complication, such as those receiving anticoagulant or thrombolytic therapy, need to have special precautions taken on their behalf. Patients who are elderly, have uncontrolled hypertension, and are thin are at greatest risk for bleeding. Assess patients thoroughly for other risk factors. Intravenous lines should be started before drug therapy and should not be discontinued unnecessarily until 24

hours after thrombolysis. Careful, gentle handling and moving of patients is mandatory. Any unnecessary movement should be avoided to minimize tissue trauma. Urine, stool, and emesis should be tested for occult blood. It may be useful to place a sign above the patient's bed to remind all personnel that the patient is on bleeding precautions (Magee, 1989). Although probably not needed in the operating room, a means to alert the next nursing unit, PACU or ICU, may be advisable.

References

AbuRahma, A. F., & Woodruff, B. A. (1990). Effects and limitations of pentoxyfilline therapy in various stages of peripheral vascular disease of the lower extremity. *American Journal of Surgery, 160*:266-270.

Adkins, P. J. (1993). Postoperative coagulopathies. In K. A. Gould (Ed.), *Critical care nursing clinics of North America: Coagulopathy and hematology* (pp. 459-473). Philadelphia: W. B. Saunders.

AORN Standards and Recommended Practices (1996). Denver: The Association of Operating Room Nurses.

Baer, C. L., & Williams, B. B. (1996). *Clinical pharmacology and nursing* (3rd ed.). Springhouse, PA.

Bell, W. R. (1995). Current thrombolytic agents: Comparative analysis. In A. J. Comerata (Ed.), *Thrombolytic therapy for peripheral vascular disease* (pp. 143-160). Philadelphia: J. B. Lippincott.

Bergquvist, D. (1983). Dextran. *Post-operative thrombo-embolism: Frequency, etiology, prophylaxis* (pp. 129-139). New York: Springer-Verlag.

Clark, J. B., Queener, S. F., & Karb, V. B. (1990). *Pharmacological basis of nursing practice* (3rd ed.). St. Louis: Mosby.

Clagett, G. P., & Reisch, J. S. (1988). Prevention of venous thromboembolism in general surgical patients. *Annals of Surgery, 208*:227-240.

Cole, C. W., & Bormanis, J. (1988). Ancrod: A practical alternative to heparin. *Journal of Vascular Surgery,* (8)59-63.

Fader, M. I. (1986). Preheated contrastmedia: The advantage of intravenous injection. *Radiologic Technology, 58*(2): 117-119.

Flynn, M. F. X., & Johnston, K. W. (1995). In R. B. Rutherford (Ed.), *Vascular Surgery* (4th ed., pp. 552-571). Philadelphia: W. B. Saunders.

Garcia, R., Saroyan, R. M., Senkowsky, J., Smith, F., & Kerstein, M. (1990). Intraoperative intra-arterial urokinase infusion as an adjunct to fogarty catheter embolectomy in acute arterial occlusion. *Surgery, Gynocology & Obstetrics, 171*: 201-205.

Gever, L. N. (1986). Embolex: To prevent a double postop danger. *Nursing 86.*

George, J. N., & Shattil, S. J. (1991). The clinical importance of acquired abnormalities of platelet function. *The New England Journal of Medicine, 324*(1): 27-39.

Goode, C. J. et al. (1991). A meta-analysis of effects of heparin flush and saline flush: Quality and cost implications. *Nursing Research, 40*(6): 324-330.

Goodman, G. R., Tersigni, S., Li, K., & Lawrence, P. F. (1993). Thrombolytic therapy in an isolated limb. *Annals of Vascular Surgery, 7*(6): 512-520.

Govani, L. E. (1985). *Drugs and Nursing Implications (5th ed.).* Norwalk, CT: Appleton-Century-Crofts.

Green, R. M., & McNamara, J. (1988). The effects of pentoxifylline on patients with intermittent claudication. *Journal of Vascular Surgery, 7*(2): 356-362.

Greenfield, L. (1994). Deep venous thrombosis: Prevention and management. In F. J Veith, R. W. Hobson, R. A. Williams, & S. E. Wilson (Eds.), *Vascular surgery: Principles and practice* (2nd ed., pp. 852-864). New York: McGraw-Hill.

Guzzetta, C. E., & Dossey, B. M. (1992). *Cardiovascular nursing: Holistic practice.* St. Louis: Mosby.

Harrington, R., & Ansell, J. E. (1992). Trends in antithrombotic therapy. *Journal of the Academay of Physicians Assistants, 5*(2): 131-141.

Hoch, J. R., & Silver, D. (1991). Hematologic factors, anticoagulation, and anticoagulant complications in venous thromboembolism. In J. J. Bergan, & S. T. Yao (Eds.), *Venous disorders* (pp. 19-35). Philadelphia: W. B. Saunders.

Humphrey, P. W., & Silver, D. (1995). In R. B. Rutherford (Ed.), *Vascular surgery* (4th ed., pp. 311-323). Philadelphia: W. B. Saunders.

Hye, R. J., et al. (1994). Is thrombolysis of occluded popliteal and tibial bypass grafts worthwhile? *Journal of Vascular Surgery, 20*(4): 588-596.

Ingegno, M. D., & Williams, R. A. (1994). Pentoxyfilline, vasodilators, and metabolic agents. In F. J Veith, R. W. Hobson, R. A. Williams, & S. E. Wilson (Eds.), *Vascular surgery: Principles and practice (2nd ed.)* (pp. 242-245). New York: McGraw-Hill.

Keller, M. P. & Silver, D. (1994). Anticoagulants: Heparin and warfarin. In F. J Veith, R. W. Hobson, R. A. Williams, & S. E. Wilson (Eds.), *Vascular surgery: Principles and practice* (2nd ed., pp. 219-228). New York: McGraw-Hill.

Kuc, J. (1993). When heparin causes clots. *RN, 56*(3): 34-38.

Kuhar, P. A., & Hill, K. M. (1991). White clot syndrome: When heparin goes haywire. *American Journal of Nursing, 91*(3): 59-60.

Lloyd, K. (1994). Ionic vs. non-ionic contrast media. *Radiologic Technology, 66*(1): 57-59.

MacVittie, B. A. (1995). Vascular surgery. In M. H. Meeker, & J. C. Rothrock (Eds.). *Alexander's care of the patient in surgery* (10th ed., pp. 1032-1057). St. Louis: Mosby.

Magee, M. (1989). Nursing care of the patient receiving thrombolytic therapy. *Journal of Emergency Nursing, 15*(2): 165-173.

Malott, J. C., & Fodor, J. (1984). Advantages of non-ionic contrast media in vascular applications. *Radiologic Technology, 56*(2): 95-98.

Mosby's Medical, nursing, & allied health dictionary (4th ed.) (1994). St. Louis: Mosby.

Mannucci, P. M., et al. (1991). Deamino-8-D-Arginine vasopressin shortens the bleeding time in uremia. *The New England Journal of Medicine, 308*(1): 8-12.

Nunnelee, J. D. (1994). Medications used in vascular patients. In V. A. Fahey (Ed.), *Vascular nursing* (2nd ed., pp. 219-234). Philadelphia: W. B. Saunders.

Pace, R. M. (1995). Intraoperative preparation of autologous fibrin gel. *AORN Journal, 62*(4): 604-607.

Perloff, L. J., & Berkowitz, H. D. (1994). Throbolytic therapy. In F. J Veith, R. W. Hobson, R. A. Williams, & S. E. Wilson (Eds.), *Vascular surgery: Principles and practice* (2nd ed., pp. 229-236). New York: McGraw-Hill.

Pierson, M. A. (1995). Patient and environmental safety. In M. H. Meeker, & J. C. Rothrock (Eds.), *Alexander's care of the patient in surgery* (10th ed., pp. 19-34). St. Louis: Mosby.

Robertson, H. J. F. (1987). Blood clot formation in angiographic syringes containing non-ionic contrast media. *Radiology, 162*(3): 621-622.

Rubin, R. N. (1995). Streptokinase. In A. J. Comerata (Ed.), *Thrombolytic therapy for peripheral vascular disease* (pp. 87-97). Philadelphia: J. B. Lippincott.

Rudnick, M. R. et al. (1995). Nephrotoxicity of ionic and nonionic contrast media in 1196 patients: A randomized trial. The Iohexol Cooperative Study. *Kidney Int., 47*(1): 254-256.

Seifert, P. C. (1994). *Cardiac surgery.* St. Louis: Mosby.

Sheng, F. C., & Busuttil, R. W. (1991). Antibiotics in vascular surgery. In W. S. Moore (Ed.), *Vascular surgery: A comprehensive review* (pp. 262-274). Philadelphia: W. B. Saunders.

Skidmore-Roth, L. (1995). *Mosby's nursing drug reference.* St. Louis: Mosby.

Spittell, J. A. Jr. (1992). Conservative management of occlusive peripheral arterial disease. In J. A. Spittell, Jr. (Ed.), *Contemporary issues in peripheral vascular disease* (pp. 209-215). Philadelphia: F. A. Davis.

Stanley, J. C., Sottiurai, V., Fry, R. E., & Fry, W. J. (1975). Comparative evolution of vein graft preparation media: Electron and microscopic studies. *Journal of Surgical Research, 18*(3), 235-246.

Szilagyi, D. E., Elliott, J. P., Guzzetta, C. E., & Dossey, B. M. (1992). *Cardiovascular nursing: Holistic practice.* St. Louis: Mosby.

Todd, B. (1987). Drugs and the elderly: Use heparin safely. *Geriatric Nursing: The American Journal of Care for the Elderly, 8*(1): 43-44.

Towne, J. B. (1994). Hyperthrombotic states in vascular surgery. In F. J Veith, R. W. Hobson, R. A. Williams, & S. E. Wilson (Eds.), *Vascular surgery: Principles and practice* (2nd ed., pp. 209-218). New York: McGraw-Hill.

Turpie, A. G. G., & Leclerc, J. R. (1991). Prophylaxis of venous thromboembolism. In J. R. Leclerc (Ed.), *Venous thromboembolic disorders* (pp. 303-345). Philadelphia: Lea & Febiger

Verstraete, M. (1995). Urokinase. In A. J. Comerata (Ed.), *Thrombolytic therapy for peripheral vascular disease* (pp. 99-114). Philadelphia: J. B. Lippincott.

Preoperative Patient Assessment

THE VASCULAR PATIENT PROFILE

The majority of patients who present with vascular disease, particularly arterial disease, are elderly, diabetics, smokers, or a combination of these. These are very complex patients and may have a variety of medical problems related to or in addition to their vascular disease. In assessing these patients the nurse must have an understanding of the special considerations necessary for conducting a reasonable interview, evaluating the data collected, and planning for special needs in the perioperative period. The elderly and diabetic patient is considered first, followed by information about the smoking patient. Surprisingly little actual hard data exists to prove the deleterious effects of smoking in the vascular patient. Advanced age, a history of smoking, and diabetes are risk factors associated with impaired wound healing. Patients with cancer, malnutrition (including obesity or cachexia), and cardiovascular disease are also at risk, and the elderly have an increased chance of having these comorbidity factors (Feistritzer, 1995).

Burnside (1988) suggests the following basic five guidelines for working with elderly patients:

- do not hurry an elderly person
- explain procedures before requesting cooperation
- speak as if expecting comprehension
- treat with dignity and respect (i.e., do not call them "honey" or "pops")
- encourage self-care (also, to decrease disorientation address the person by name and title, speak slowly, do not agree with confused ideas, and do not argue or insist on correction).

Confusion is often the first symptom of a problem, i.e., pain, myocardial infarction (MI), or urinary tract infection (UTI). Orientation to time, place, and person are lost in that order. Something as simple and seemingly benign as a sleep disturbance may lead to periods of confusion. Reasons for sleep disturbances include overstimulation, understimulation, uremia, congestive heart failure, respiratory insufficiency, need to void at night, and leg pain from peripheral vascular disease (Burnside, 1988). Confusion is not normal nor is it an inevitable consequence of aging. Sensory changes result in a slowing of the person's responses that can affect their safety, socialization, and self esteem and can sometimes result in a patient being labeled as confused because they have misinterpreted sensory cues.

Sensory Changes (Vision, Hearing, Touch)

Sensory changes are reviewed first because they are the first consideration when meeting and talking with an elderly client. Sensory changes have multiple effects upon the elderly. Visual changes are a result of lens opacity that may scatter light and cause a glare, while simultaneously the older patient needs more light to see. The elderly have been estimated to need about three times the amount of light that a 20-year-old needs. Loss of lens elasticity results in a decreased ability for accommodation that leads to a loss of near vision first and finally a diminished ability to adjust from near to far and to changes in lighting. Ciliary muscles become weaker and more relaxed, lenses become more opaque, and the corneas flatten. This muscle weakening leads to **presbyopia** (farsightedness) and diminished peripheral vision. The iris atrophies and is not able to respond quickly to light changes. Rigidity of the iris diminishes pupillary size and inhibits light from reaching the retina. Color perception alters as a result of cataracts and lens yellowing that often results in loss of blues and violets. The lens yellowing is caused by alterations in proteins. This also leads to a loss of corneal luster and the appearance of rainbows around lights. Reduced blood supply leads to macular deterioration. The ability to respond to changes in lighting declines causing lessened acuity, night blindness, halos around lights, diminished recovery from a glare, and adds to the already present difficulties with depth perception. An increase in orbital fat, fatty tissue in the lacrimal apparatus, and diminished lid elasticity result in "crows' feet," pouches under the eyes, and dry eyes. Arcus senilis or visible yellow lipid deposits in the margin of the cornea are a benign change (Burggraf & Donlon, 1985; Ebersole & Hess, 1994).

Hearing loss is also a normal result of aging. The reduction of blood flow to the cochlea leads to deterioration of the cochlea, the hair cells, and the neurons. The eardrum itself thickens, which leads to a decrease in the transmission of sound. This loss is usually a gradual process. The ability to hear high frequency tones is lost first. This is called **presbycusis.** High frequency tones are the consonants f, g, s, sk, sh, t, and z. A male voice may be easier for a patient to hear than a female voice. Many causes have been suggested for presbycusis, including nutrition, noise, hypertension (HTN), stress, and arteriosclerosis (Mhoon, 1990). The second most frequent hearing problem is the inability to detect volume intensity (see the Nursing Care Plan on p. 51).

Mental Status

The second most basic consideration before gaining cooperation and providing explanations should be a mental status check. Another complex area of assessment is that of cognitive function and changes in mental status. Patients may present with an acute confused state, dementia, or generalized cognitive impairment or disturbed thinking related to an emotional or psychiatric problem. A variety of physiologic problems can cause acute confusion in the elderly (Box 5-1). Basic to a mental

Nursing Diagnosis: Alteration in Sensory/Perceptual Function: Hearing

NURSING OUTCOMES	NURSING INTERVENTIONS
Patient is able to hear conversation	Speak in a tone of voice that does not include shouting (shouting increases the pitch of the voice) Face the patient when speaking Speak slowly and distinctly Use touch to get the patient's attention if standing behind him or her Use simple sentences Lower the pitch of the voice Be aware of nonverbal communication (e.g., facial expression) Speak toward the better or aided ear from a distance of 2 to 3 feet Use nonverbal cues to alert the person to a change in topic Speech should be slow and clear with more pauses than normal If the person does not understand, paraphrase instead of repeating Keep your face visible; do not eat, chew gum, or cover your mouth

Data from Gallman, R. L. (1995). The sensory system and its problems in the elderly. In M. Stanley & P. G. Beare (Eds.), *Gerontological nursing* (pp. 134-147). Philadelphia: F. A. Davis; and Mhoon, E. (1990). Otology. In C. K. Cassel, D .E. Riesenberg, L. B. Sorensen, & J. R. Walsh (Eds.), *Geriatric medicine (2nd Ed.)* (pp. 405-419). New York: Springer-Verlag.

Box 5-1 **Causes of Acute Confusion in the Elderly**

Myocardial infarction	Dehydration
Gastrointestinal bleeding	Pneumonia
Urinary tract infection	Drug intoxication
Heart failure	Ischemia
Electrolyte imbalance	Pulmonary embolism
Alcohol withdrawal	Occult malignancy
Fecal impaction	

status examination is ensuring that the patient has heard the questions and that sensory impairment is not mistaken for confusion.

Treatment of any medical problem that may be contributing to altered mental status should be managed with reassurance for both the patient and family members (Reichel & Rabins, 1995). The disoriented patient may be acutely distressed and fearful and very much aware that they are not able to think clearly. Never agree with confused or disoriented persons but also do not insist on corrections. Gently reorient and treat the patient as if expecting comprehension. Acknowledge their fears and explain corrective interventions.

A variety of screening tools are in use to evaluate cognition and mental status. While no perfect, universal tool exists, it is imperative that data for a baseline assessment be gathered. For quick assessment, level of consciousness and orientation to person, place, and time may be helpful. However, do not assume that cognitive functioning has been assessed. McDougall (1990) reviewed 11 popular screening instruments and charted the parameters measured by each. He advised that the tools are only one aspect of evaluation and not a substitute for a thorough examination. The Mini-Mental State Exam (MMSE) has been widely used since 1975 (Folstein, Folstein & McHugh, 1975). The test is short and easy to administer (Table 5-1). It has the endorsement of the National Institute of Neurological and Communicative Disorders and Stroke and the Alzheimer's Disease and Related Disorders Association work group. A second short and practical tool is the Mental Status Questionnaire (MSQ). It consists of 10 questions (Box 5-2). Both have been described as allowing mildly affected patients to be labeled as having dementia. Nevertheless, if used properly, this should not be a problem (McDougall, 1990). Although this may seem very formal and time consuming, the perioperative nurse may find it extremely important. More patients are experiencing same day surgery. Assessment must be efficient. However, it is imperative to decide whether a patient can understand and retain basic instructions, is able to give informed consent, that there is a baseline mental status documented, and that a determination of any change from a recent office or telephone interaction is made.

REVIEW OF SYSTEMS

Neurologic

Multiple, widespread alterations affect the neurologic system in the elderly patient. The blood flow and subsequent oxygen supply to the brain decrease and neurons decrease in number as they die and are not replaced. This leads to a diminished pain response that should be distinguished from diabetic neuropathy. Motor neuron conduction lessens as a result of myelin sheath

---

Box 5-2 **Mental Status Questionnaire**

1. What is the name of this place?
2. Where is it located?
3. What is today's date?
4. What is the month?
5. What is the year?
6. How old are you?
7. What month were you born?
8. What year were you born?
9. Who is the president now?
10. Who was the president before him?

   Each answer is worth one point. Zero to two errors means no or minimal mental dysfunction; 3-8 is moderate mental dysfunction; 9-10 errors indicate severe dysfunction. This may need to be modified for those in institutions for whom time may be less relevant.

Adapted from Kahn, R. L., Goldfarb, A. I., Pollack, M., & Peck, A. (1960). Brief objective measures for the determination of mental status in the aged. *American Journal of Psychiatry*, 326-329.

Table 5-1 **Mini-Mental State Examination (MMS)**

MAXIMUM SCORE	SCORE	
		Orientation
5	( )	1. What is the (year) (season) (date) (day) (month)?
5	( )	2. Where are we: (state) (country) (town) (hospital) (floor)?
		Registration
3	( )	3. Name 3 objects: 1 second to say each. Then ask the patient all 3 after you have said them.
		Give 1 point for each correct answer. Then repeat them until he learns all 3. Count trials and record.
		TRIALS
		Attention and calculation
5	( )	4. Serial 7s. 1 point for each correct. Stop after 5 answers. Alternatively, spell "world" backwards, if cannot subtract.
		Recall
3	( )	5. Ask for 3 objects repeated above. Give 1 point for each correct.
		Language
9	( )	6. Name a pencil, and watch (2 points) 7. Repeat the following: "No ifs, ands, or buts" (1 point) 8. Follow a 3-stage command: "Take a paper in your right hand, fold it in half, and put it on the floor." (3 points) 9. Read and obey the following: "Close your eyes" (1 point) 10. Write a sentence. (1 point) 11. Copy design. (1 point)

_____
TOTAL SCORE

1. 1 point for each correct answer.
2. 1 point for each correct answer.
3. 1 point for each of the 3 object names that is correctly repeated the first time. Then repeat them until all 3 are repeated but give no further points.
4. 1 point for each correct subtraction. If the patient does not or cannot make any subtractions have him spell the word "world" backwards. If an attempted subtraction is made this is the preferred task.
5. 1 point for each object.
6. 1 point for each correctly named object. Give no points if an approximate but incorrect word is used.
7. 1 point if completely and correctly completed.
8. 1 point for each command followed.
9. 1 point only if the patient carries out the activity. No points if the sentence is read correctly but the act is not done.
10. Sentence should be grammatically correct and have subject, verb, and predicate.
11. 1 point if each figure has 5 sides and the overlap is correct.

Modified from Folstein MF, Folstein SE, McHugh PR. Mini-Mental State: A practical method for grading the cognitive state of patients for the clinician. *J Psychiatr Res 12*:189, 1975. Copyright 1975, Pergamon Journals, Ltd. Courtesy of Dr. Marshal Folstein.
The highest possible score is 30; 21 or less may indicate dementia, schizophrenia, delirium, or an affective disorder. The part of the test that requires reading and writing may be difficult for visually impaired or illiterate patients.

degeneration, which results in slowed reaction times and slowed reflexes. Sweat glands diminish in number and, combined with a slowed autonomic nervous system response, the elderly are much more susceptible to heat stroke. Slowed autonomic responses are also responsible for orthostatic hypotension.

Musculoskeletal

Intervertebral discs become dehydrated and narrow with the resultant loss in height and increased risk of back pain and fractures. Cartilage erodes, synovial membranes become fibrotic, and synovial fluid thickens. This causes joint swelling, stiffness, and decreased range of motion. Muscle cells dwindle in size and number as protein synthesis decreases, causing muscle atrophy. Decreased muscle mass also results in decreased glycogen stores with a diminished response to exercise. Extracellular water, Na, and Cl levels increase and intracellular K levels decrease, resulting in leg cramps at night.

Genitourinary

Bladder capacity drops from an average of 500 cc to 250 cc. The ureters, bladder, and urethra lose muscle tone and elasticity. Combine this with delayed sensation and the outcome may be urinary frequency, urgency and nocturia. Nocturia may also be caused by lower extremity edema resorption from the legs being elevated. Pelvic floor relaxation is associated with estrogen deficiency in women and contributes to stress incontinence. In men, prostate enlargement and uninhibited bladder contractions may occur, leading to stress incontinence and dribbling. Cystoceles or benign prostatic hypertrophy (BPH) can cause urinary retention. Lowered cardiac output (CO) decreases renal blood flow, glomerular filtration rate, and tubular resorption, placing the elderly at risk for altered acid-base balance and drug toxicity.

Cardiovascular

Multiple anatomical changes occur that compromise the elderly patient's ability to respond to changes in the cardiovascular system (Box 5-3). The cardiac output drops as a result of fibrosis and sclerosis in the endocardium, the left ventricular wall thickens, increased fat infiltration is found in the right atrium and left ventricle, and stroke volume lessens. Decreased renal flow (caused by decreased CO) may lead to Na and water retention

---

Box 5-3 Anatomic Changes of the Heart

Increase in collagen leads to:
- stiffness
- decreased compliance
- altered electrical conduction

Increased fat deposition

Fibrosis of and decrease of myofibers

Decreased number of cells in sinus node

Decreased number of mitochondria cells for energy production

Data from Moss A. J. (1995). Diagnosis and management of heart disease in the elderly. In Reichel, W., et al., *Care of the elderly: Clinical aspects of aging* (4th ed). Baltimore: Williams & Wilkins.

and peripheral edema. The baroreceptor response decreases as the arterial wall stiffens and is less able to stretch and respond to blood pressure changes. Mitral and aortic valves calcify and fibrose, resulting in systolic murmurs. Nerve transmission decreases in speed and strength. Nerve impulses through the SA and AV nodes decrease and the excitation-relaxation cycles take longer. The slowed bundle branches result in a slowed pulse rate, palpitations, atrial arrhythmias, and extra systoles. The elderly have a higher incidence of bundle branch block, SA node disorders, and increased ventricular filling pressures (Burggraf & Donlon, 1985; Ebersole & Hess, 1994).

Moss (1995) reminds us that the important concept to recall is that the elderly have an altered response to stress. Symptoms of MI are not the same in the elderly patient as in younger patients. While the classic picture of an acute myocardial infarction is substernal pain, the elderly patient will present with "dyspnea, syncope, stroke or GI symptoms." Laboratory testing and blood work have not been as diagnostic for the elderly because of the lack of a norm for the older age groups, the wide variation in patients, and the confounding factors of normal aging changes. Changes that occur are normal for aging but they take place at very different rates and may be profoundly influenced by stressors and environmental factors.

As the intimal layer of the arteries thicken and fibrose, vascular resistance increases. Arteries become rigid as the elastin content of the wall thins. This leads to hypertension (HTN). Vessel wall alterations also occur in the veins. Veins thicken, dilate, fibrose, and stretch, which can result in varicosities and venous stasis (Ebersole & Hess, 1994).

Pulmonary

Respiratory muscles atrophy, resulting in an increased A-P diameter. The loss of lung elasticity leads to a reduced vital capacity. Pulmonary wall thickening impedes oxygen diffusion. O_2-CO_2 exchange is less efficient because of the increase in residual volume. Fewer capillaries and thickening of alveoli lead to a decline in PaO_2 levels and the frequent result is the complaint of fatigue. Maximum breathing capacity has a linear decline with age. The epithelial cells that line the alveoli atrophy and this reduces ciliary movement that slows cough reflex. Atrophy and weakness of respiratory muscles lead to thoracic wall rigidity, which means coughing becomes less effective and the risk of pneumonia and influenza increases.

Gastrointestinal

The beginning of the GI tract, the mouth, has a large impact on comfort and nutrition. With age saliva declines in amount and is more alkaline, causing halitosis and dry mouth. Dentures add to these problems. The capillary blood supply to the gums lessens, making the gums appear pale. Bone resorption increases and vitamin absorption decreases, which contributes to loose or missing teeth. The teeth appear to darken as a result of wear and tear and the dark dentin of the tooth is more exposed. The appearance of tooth elongation is due to migration of gingiva toward the gums ("long in the tooth").

Hydrochloric acid (HCl) secretion decreases, resulting in impaired absorption of vitamins and minerals. The decrease in saliva production slows starch breakdown and has been implicated in malnutrition and a resultant increased risk of infection. This combines with the decreased number of taste buds (decreased appetite, increased use of salt). Smooth muscle tone loss leads to delayed gastric and esophageal emptying. The diaphragm is then displaced upward and symptoms of heartburn, nausea and vomiting, and dysphagia are common. Peristalsis slows, abdominal muscles lose their elasticity, secretion of mucus reduces lubrication, and the elderly have more real problems with constipation. The diminished flow to the liver (related to decreased cardiac output) means less drug detoxification. This fact coupled with decreased gastric motility and thus increased drug absorption places the elderly at significant risk for drug toxicity.

Skin

A general loss of body water content is reflected in the dryness of the skin and the thinning of the epidermis. Nerve endings decrease in number, especially in the fingers. Touch is a multifaceted area of stimulation but safety is again a major issue. The decreased ability to respond to pressure, heat, or cold has serious implications for the elderly patient, especially when superimposed upon vascular disease (Gallman, 1995). Touch can impart many social and therapeutic messages and responses. Stimulation of the skin may cause the production of endorphins, which block the sensation of pain. Gentle massage or stroking can stimulate improved circulation and relaxation that may result in a decreased need for medications. The cultural aspects of touch must be considered individually. Touching by males or females, the type of touch, and the timing of touch may be interpreted positively or negatively. The nurse must assess the response to touch with each patient. Offering a hand to hold during a procedure may be the first way to determine the patient's response (Weiss, 1992).

Cell mitosis slows, resulting in increased vascular fragility. Capillaries become fragile and contribute to the formation of liver spots or senile lentigo, senile purpura; this capillary fragility increases the risk of pressure sores. Reduced vascularity may also contribute to delayed wound healing. The connective tissue thickens and the result is seen as seborrhea keratosis (yellow-brown warts) and skin tags. Collagen, subcutaneous fat, and the number of sweat glands diminish, leading to wrinkles and the appearance of dry, leathery skin. The facial pallor so typical of the frail elderly is attributed to the decrease in capillaries and melanocytes (Burggraf & Donlon, 1985). Changes caused by decreased body water content and altered connective tissue alter the way that skin turgor is assessed. On a younger patient, it is checked on the forehead, wrist, or clavicular area. In an elderly patient, using the abdomen to check hydration is better because of the above described alterations. Fat distribution is found less on arms and legs and more on the trunk. There is often a decreased growth of nails, compounded by decreased blood flow. Hair thins, and men generally have a decrease in facial hair while women have an increase (Ebersole & Hess, 1994).

DRUGS IN THE ELDERLY

Because so many physical changes of aging decrease the ability of the elderly to metabolize and detoxify medications, a drug history is critical to their overall assessment. Those patients who do not have a regular health care provider, those on a fixed income, and those with chronic symptoms may be at risk for excessive over-the-counter (OTC) drug use. Most people believe that if the drug does not need a prescription, it must be benign. As a result, many people inappropriately use them with prescription drugs. Patients often fail to mention OTC drugs and many health care providers neglect to specifically elicit this important information. The following is a brief look at a few very common OTC drugs that can have potentially lethal effects in combination with prescription drugs.

Acetaminophen potentiates anticoagulants and may increase hepatotoxicity of alcohol. Chronic aspirin use may lead to renal disease. Laxatives have been linked to malabsorption syndromes, hypokalemia, and hypocalcemia. Cold remedies with anticholinergic or antihistamines could cause sedation, toxic psychosis, urinary retention, and worsened glaucoma. The many factors that contribute to constipation in the elderly can result in long-term antacid use. Those preparations with magnesium, calcium, or aluminum content can cause serious harm. Aluminum may cause dementia-like symptoms with impaired renal function. Hypermagnesium can cause nausea and vomiting and central nervous system (CNS) depression (Kofoed, 1985). The elderly are at risk for problems caused by increased sensitivity and diminished reserve. The two most common reasons for falls in the elderly are surgery and drugs.

PAIN ASSESSMENT

Awareness of age-related changes is necessary to accurately interpret physical findings and laboratory data. Many elderly patients neglect to report pain and other symptoms because they may believe these to be normal for their advanced age. Unfortunately, these misconceptions may be considered the norm by family members and health care providers.

Pain is a complex topic that has serious implications for the elderly patient. They are at increased risk for pain because their longevity increases the likelihood that they have developed a chronic condition. Because of their lessened reserves for responding to alterations in physiologic and other stressors, they appear to respond atypically. Their responses are atypical only when veiled in the narrow confines of "normal" being based on descriptions for healthy young males. Pain sensation may be diminished in the elderly because of the previously described changes of aging. Older people may also believe that pain is expected or cannot be relieved and thus report it less. Pain may be manifested in very subtle ways such as sleep or eating disturbances or altered mental status. The support systems available to older patients may be severely diminished as well. This may also decrease their emotional reserve to manage pain and distress. Many elderly are adjusting to the multiple losses that occur with deaths of spouses and friends. They mourn the loss of many of their roles in life, such as that of the breadwinner, caregiver, and advisor. Added to this are the physical changes that may diminish their ability to manage self-care or be independent, e.g., driving, shopping, cooking, and remaining in their home. Grief and depression can have a profound impact on a person's ability to learn and make appropriate decisions and it may interfere with the healing process. An added challenge exists in elucidating the pain of patients who are either nonverbal or cognitively impaired.

Pain assessment must include consideration for the patients' spiritual and cultural beliefs and practices. Some patients may believe that pain has a punitive aspect for mistakes they have made in their past. Others express their discomfort in an exaggerated manner because it is their custom. It has been estimated that 50% of surgical patients do not obtain pain relief (Ebersole & Hess, 1994). The U.S. Department of Health and Human Services published guidelines to address this problem in 1992: *Clinical Practice Guidelines: Acute Pain Management.* These guidelines essentially promote an interdisciplinary approach to pain control individualized and developed before surgery. Assessment and reassessment must be performed and interventions instituted to prevent and relieve pain. Institutions bear the responsibility for establishing a formal approach to pain management with policies established for accountability.

VITAL SIGNS AND LABORATORY TESTS IN THE ELDERLY

Vital signs in the old-old patient (over age 85) may differ from younger patients. Multiple factors contribute to a baseline temperature lower than the 98.6° F (37° C) standard. Obtaining a baseline for each individual is critical. The tympanic membrane thermometer is considered the most accurate tool. The average temperature for an adult is 97.6° F, but for those above 85 years it is 94 to 96° F. If a mercury thermometer is used, it must be shaken down to 94° before use. Older people are less able to regulate their body heat, have less insulation, and are more susceptible to inadvertent perioperative hypothermia. A temperature of 37.5° C may be a fever in an elderly patient and failure to recognize this contributes to morbidity and mortality in the frail elderly. The pulse rate remains fairly stable throughout life although it may decrease in the old-old to 50 to 55 beats per minute without medication or pathology. Respiratory rate usually increases to compensate for the decrease in depth. The most accurate method to assess respirations is to place a hand on the abdomen rather than the chest. Blood pressure is the same for all adults, i.e., 140/90 as the upper range. Pulse pressure varies and increases in the elderly from the 30 to 50 norm of the average adult to 50 to 100 in the old-old (Hogstel, 1994) (Boxes 5-4 and 5-5).

The elderly population generally has a diminished flow of blood to the brain compared with the flow in their younger days and the feedback mechanisms that regulate blood flow and blood pressure are less efficient and slower to adjust. Vasoconstriction and dilation of blood to the brain are not as automatic as in younger patients. As a result, the elderly are predisposed to orthostatic hypotension. Anything that alters blood flow to the brain may contribute to stroke. Some of these factors are cardiac arrhythmias, dehydration, atherosclerosis, and hypertension. Atrial fibrillation is a cause of atrial thrombi that may travel to the brain and cause an infarct. The most common cause of a stroke is infarction (80%); of these, thrombosis is the most likely event. Hemorrhagic stroke (15%) is primarily caused by hypertension and less often (5%) by trauma, tumor, or cerebral aneurysm. After a cerebral infarct, there is a period called the **hyperemic phase** (vascular dilation) that is a result of the lack of autoregulation. This defect in the autoregulatory mechanism persists for many days after a stroke. Hyperemia and altered metabolic processes cause more damage to the neurons and other adjacent

> *Box 5-4* **Laboratory Values That Remain Unchanged in the Elderly**
>
> - Hematocrit
> - Hemoglobin
> - Platelet count
> - Electrolytes (Na, Ca, Cl, K, bicarbonate)
> - Blood urea nitrogen
> - Liver function tests (transaminases, bilirubin, prothrombin time)
> - Free thyroxine index
> - Thyroid-stimulating hormone
> - Calcium
> - Phosphorus
>
> When the above values are outside of normal ranges, the patient should be referred for further workup.

cells in addition to those already damaged from the initial event. Free-radical damage has been proposed as one mechanism of cellular injury (Kyriazis, 1994).

There are many complications from a stroke that the nurse must consider in caring for a vascular surgical patient. Depending on the area of the brain affected, emotional lability may be present. As a result, the patient may respond inappropriately at times and cry in response to a seemingly benign question or statement. Remain sensitive to the possibility that the response was very appropriate but do not become startled and overreact or withdraw in the face of emotional lability. Projecting an attitude of acceptance goes far to calm and reassure a patient. Depression may also complicate interactions. Be wary of labeling a patient as disoriented if depression makes them reluctant or slow to answer. Another complication of stroke is paralysis. These patients are at greater risk for alterations in skin integrity because of limited mobility and sensation. The initial flaccidity that occurs after a stroke is followed by spasticity and hyperactive reflexes. Assess patients for their ability to transfer and ask them for the best way to help them. Be extremely careful in moving weakened limbs to prevent spasms and the resultant pain that can occur with sudden movements. Patients' shoulders are particularly at risk for injuries that may seriously impede their rehabilitation. The flaccid arm may be responsible for causing shoulder dislocation (Cochran, et al, 1994). If the patient's arm needs to be abducted to position it on an armrest, do so slowly and with the patient awake.

Paralysis on the left side of the body indicates a right brain stroke and vice-versa. Right brain damage often results in the patient being unable to concentrate and becoming very impulsive. Because of a short attention span, they need tasks and requests explained repeatedly and just before requesting cooperation. Patients with left hemiparesis are frequently unaware of the affected side of their body. With right-sided hemiparesis, the patients may have no sensation and altered visual fields but are aware of the affected side. The patient with speech problems can be challenging. A number of terms are used to express the different problems. Dysarthria is altered speech caused by muscle weakness. Aphasia is impaired speech, not impaired intellect.

Box 5-5 **Laboratory Values Commonly Found to Be Abnormal in the Elderly**

Sedimentation rate
10 to 20 mm elevation may be age-related change.

Glucose
Glucose tolerance decreases.

Creatinine
Because lean body mass and daily endogenous creatinine production decline, high-normal and minimally elevated values may indicate substantially reduced renal function.

Albumin
Average values decline (<0.5 g/ml) with age, especially in hospitalized elderly patients, but generally indicate undernutrition.

Alkaline phosphatase
Mild elevation is common in asymptomatic elderly patients; liver and Paget's disease should be considered if moderately elevated.

Serum iron and iron-binding capacity
Decreased values are not an aging change and usually indicate undernutrition and/or GI blood loss.

Prostate specific antigen
May be elevated in patients with benign prostatic hypertrophy. Marked elevation or increasing values when followed over time should prompt further investigation.

Chest radiographs
Interstitial changes are a common age-related finding; diffusely diminished bone density should generally indicate advanced osteoporosis.

ECG
ST-segment and T-wave changes, atrial and ventricular arrhythmias, and various blocks are common in asymptomatic elderly patients and may not need specific evaluation or treatment.

Mellillo (1993) emphasizes the need to consider the BUN and creatinine in older patients as inaccurate despite the normal laboratory values. They do not measure the true renal function. The decline in serum creatinine production is coupled with a decline in lean body mass to give a false idea of its clearance. This can lead to drug overdose from faulty calculations.

$$\text{Creatinine clearance} = \frac{(40 - \text{age}) \times \text{body wt (kg)}}{72 \times \text{serum creatinine}}$$

This formula is for men; multiply the number by 0.85 for females. BUN and creatinine levels that are in the upper limits of a standard normal range or are slightly elevated must be considered to be indicative of significantly compromised kidney function.

Adapted from Kane, 1994.

These patients may not be able to read or write but they understand. Expressive aphasia is altered sentence structure and the patient exerts great effort with limited results. Receptive aphasia is normal articulation with the use of jargon, such as repetitive use of one word for many meanings or the use of meaningless phrases. Global aphasia is a combination of any of these different types of aphasia. This person may use only a few words repeatedly (Cochran, et al, 1994).

Some basic guidelines will help the nurse to care for the stroke patient. Maintain the patient's dignity by assuming comprehension on their part. Maintaining eye contact will acknowledge the patient as your focus and help keep their attention. Just as raising your voice with a person who does not speak your language is ineffective, shouting at a stroke patient is demeaning unless they also have a severe hearing deficit. When you do not understand the patient be honest. Do not nod and pretend comprehension. Acknowledge their frustration and suggest that a pause or rest may permit more success with a subsequent attempt. Use silence and pauses generously. All elderly need extra time and stroke patients need even more. Rushing a patient just adds to their stress level making it more difficult for them to respond (Cochran, et al, 1994). Although verbal skills may be impaired, the patient may respond to pantomime or demonstration of what is wanted. Patting the bed to show that the patient should move to it may be more useful than words.

THE DIABETIC PATIENT

The risk of having diabetes mellitus increases dramatically with age to more than 10% for those age 60 and older (Wilson, Anderson, & Kannel, 1986). It is prevalent at a rate of 3% to 5% in ages 30 to 50 and up to 20% by age 80. An additional 20% of the elderly population has hyperglycemia. Some researchers believe that diabetes may be a form of accelerated aging. This may partially account for the accelerated atherosclerosis in the diabetic. Older patients who develop diabetes tend to have a more insidious onset and milder progression than younger patients. (Lipson, 1986a). The presence of diabetes leads to more coronary artery disease, peripheral arterial occlusive disease, neuropathies, and retinopathy. Control of blood sugar is important in preventing the complications of the disease but overtreatment that leads to hypoglycemia is a danger in the elderly. Hypoglycemia can cause tissue damage to the organs (Lipson, 1986b).

The patient with diabetes is at increased risk for many problems that lead them to the vascular surgeon. They are particularly susceptible to lower extremity complications because of diabetic neuropathy, infection, and peripheral arterial disease. Bilateral neuropathy expresses itself as a loss of vibratory sensation, then a diminished reflex of the Achilles tendon, and loss of pinprick sensation in the distal extremities. Patients report symptoms of numbness, tingling, and itching. Controlling blood sugar seems to help in pain relief (Bell, 1991).

There is increased vascular disease in the diabetic patient of any age. The vascular changes in the lower extremity of the diabetic tend to be diffuse and bilateral. The disease progresses more rapidly and involves the small vessels and collateral circulation. Arterial occlusive disease occurs more frequently below the knee in the tibial and peroneal arteries (Bell, 1991). Arteries may be noncompressible, making some tests such as the ankle-brachial index unreliable.

Because regulation of blood glucose levels in both insulin-dependent and non–insulin-dependent diabetics is best controlled by established patterns of caloric intake and activity levels, surgery will affect that control. Diabetic patients do best if their surgery is scheduled as early in the day as possible to minimize the disruption of their routines. Diabetic patients, like elderly patients, are at increased risk for infection, altered skin integrity, delayed wound healing, and fluid and electrolyte imbalance (Atkinson, 1992).

SMOKING

The first noted observation that cigarette smoking could be linked to cardiovascular disease was in 1934. A sharp rise in the number of smokers coincided with World War II. However, it was not until 1958 that a formal study made a connection between smoking and cardiovascular disease. The Framingham study contributed more data to implicate smoking as a major risk factor with HTN, elevated blood cholesterol, diabetes, and glucose intolerance in cardiovascular disease. Of all patients with atherosclerosis, 70% are smokers. **Thromboangiitis obliterans** is similar to occlusive disease but is usually seen in males aged 30 to 49. It only occurs in smokers and the disease progress is halted when the patient quits smoking (Lakier, 1992).

Smoking causes vasospasm that aggravates diminished blood flow to the patient's feet (Nunnelee, 1994). Vascular disease occurs three times more frequently in smokers versus nonsmokers. Smokers are 15 times more likely to experience lower extremity claudication. They are at a significant risk for limb amputation, aortic aneurysm, stroke, and MI. Studies have shown that quitting smoking reduces the risk (Green & Ouriel, 1994). Nicotine is known to lead to arterial constriction by direct stimulation of the sympathetic nervous system and may expedite platelet aggregation (Emma, 1992). The diabetic patient who smokes is four to five times more likely to have cardiovascular disease (Maryniuk, 1993). Rimm, et al (1993) prospectively studied the relationship between non–insulin-dependent diabetes and cigarette smoking. They collected data on more than 114,000 female nurses since 1976 who had no cardiovascular disease, cancer, or diabetes. There was a significant increased risk of non–insulin-dependent diabetes in women who smoked. The study demonstrated a dose-related trend. This is an area that has received little attention. Their conclusion was that smoking may be an independent risk factor in the development of diabetes in women.

Lesmes (1992), in summarizing the conclusions of a symposium on smoking and health effects, stated that "perhaps no single intervention has more potential to combat the skyrocketing costs of health care than smoking cessation" (p. 55S). He concluded that smoking cessation is more important than controlling blood lipids. Smoking not only acts directly on the vessel walls but increases the negative effects of the other major risk factors such as HTN, hypercholesterolemia, and diabetes. More attention needs to be paid to the impact of smoking on wound healing. No large scale studies have been done to prove the causal relationship between smoking and wound healing delays. However, the effects of cigarette smoking are also the known factors in delayed wound healing: vasoconstriction, platelet adherence, and decreased oxygen transport.

No formal study of peripheral vascular disease and cigarette smoking has been done in North America in 20 years. Consequently, Cole, et al (1993) studied a group of patients (men) with claudication compared with a control group. Their conclusion was that after factoring out confounding factors, 76% of the claudication was attributable to smoking. Studying the effects of cigarette smoking has been difficult for many reasons, one being the existence of 4000 constituents in the smoke (Hoffman & Wynder, 1986). Research is in progress to explain the exact mechanism of injury by cigarettes. One study showed that smoking led to a significant increase of monocyte adherence to vessel endothelium. The process of foam cell production (see Chapter 3) is initiated by monocyte adherence. These steps are considered basic to the development of atherosclerosis. Interestingly, nicotine did not seem responsible for this process (Kalra, et al, 1994). Muluk, et al (1994) compared two groups of patients, those above and below the cutoff of 60 years of age. An abdominal aortic aneurysm (AAA) is uncommon before age 60. These researchers concluded that besides a genetic factor, the greatest risk factor for the development of AAA in patients less than 60 years old is smoking. Their aneurysms were larger by 1 cm and they had more symptoms.

While the physical effects remain to be explained, the physical dependence is clear. Nicotine is an extremely addictive substance. Cessation usually results in withdrawal symptoms that occur within 24 hours and last several weeks. The *Diagnostic and Statistical Manual of Mental Disorders* (1995) lists the following signs of withdrawal:

- nicotine craving
- irritability, frustration, or anger
- anxiety
- difficulty concentrating
- restlessness
- decreased heart rate
- increased appetite

Four of these symptoms are usually in evidence. Nicotine is a psychoactive substance that has neuroregulatory effects on the central nervous system. Epinephrine and norepinephrine levels rise with the rise of nicotine in the blood. There are a number of other neurotransmitters affected and that have an immediate effect on mood and the ability to think and concentrate. As a result, the smoker has an immediate reward that reinforces continued smoking. All the environmental and physiologic effects have not been fully demonstrated. Other sources of nicotine, such as gum, do not have the immediate effect that smoking does and may be less effective as a result. If these substitutes are to be most effective in smoking cessation efforts, they must be tailored to produce an equal dose of nicotine. Successful interventions must include the behavioral cues that are part of the response to smoking (Pomerlau, 1992).

Nurses must be involved in helping patients to stop, or at least decrease, smoking as a part of health promotion. Smoking is the number one preventable health risk in the United States. Smoking doubles the risk of death from heart disease. It is a factor in cancer, strokes, amputations, and respiratory disease. Rice et al (1994) reviewed the literature for factors affecting smoking cessation. These factors include age, race, sex, marital status, income, smoking history, medical diagnosis, exposure to other smokers, a perceived threat to health status, and the desire to quit. Results vary with age; some studies found older people were more likely to quit, while others found no difference. Whites quit more readily than other races and women less readily than men. Those who are single, have a low income, and less formal education are less likely to be amenable to smoking interventions. Married white males in higher income brackets seem to have the best success rates. The longer someone smokes, the more difficult it is to stop. Fear may be a motivator for quitting for those who feel a greater threat to their health. Rice, et al (1994) did a study to examine three presentations of smoking cessation programs with adults in the hospital. Nurse-client intervention was more effective than just written material but the most successful group was the group that had no intervention. This result may have been because the patients were post coronary artery bypass surgery. More studies need to be done to determine the most effective time and manner to help patients in their smoking cessation efforts.

When a patient is facing surgery for a smoking-related illness, they may be more amenable to interventions. Most people are aware that smoking is hazardous to their health; it is written on cigarette packages. A nationwide campaign started in the 1970s to focus on the rights of nonsmokers. Smoke-free workplaces, restaurants, and other public buildings have become commonplace. Some progress has been made as seen in the decline of per capita adult smoking that has correlated with public health messages in the media (Couch, 1986). However, a strong component of denial exists in the smoker as with any addict. Nurses should include a smoking assessment in their nursing history and determine strategies to encourage cessation. Use the available community resources. The American Cancer Society and the American Lung Association have a variety of printed materials and audiovisual aides (Wewers, et al, 1994). Check with the local libraries for free information. Refer patients to the free smoking clinics available in many communities. Support groups may be helpful for some (Box 5-6).

PATIENT TESTING

Invasive and noninvasive testing is done to assess the presence of disease, the extent of disease, and for follow-up to detect the progression of the problem or the resolution as in postoperative assessment. Vascular testing can both document and quantify abnormalities. Hundreds of tests exist and may vary with physician preference and the availability (because of cost) of sophisticated machinery. This chapter is limited to those tests that are widely accepted as standard and relevant to the surgical procedures described in Part Two. The vascular laboratory, devoted to noninvasive patient studies, has become a necessity for the

---

Box 5-6 **Position Statement: Tobacco Abuse**

The Society for Vascular Nursing (SVN) is an international specialty organization dedicated to promoting excellence in the compassionate and comprehensive treatment for persons with vascular disease. The mission is accomplished in the following ways:
- Assuming the leadership role in defining the vascular component of fundamental nursing education
- Establish and implement research-based standards of practice for vascular nursing
- Collaborate with other professions to address the unique needs of the patient with vascular disease

In turn, SVN believes that nurses caring for these individuals require a specialized body of knowledge and skills to deliver the highest standard of care. As advocates for persons with vascular disease and quality care delivery, SVN is taking an active role in support of tobacco abuse health care issues.

SVN identifies the following areas of concern with regard to tobacco abuse:
- Tobacco abuse is defined as smoking cigarettes, pipes, and cigars or use of tobacco in oral form
- Tobacco use can be both psychologically and physically addictive
- Smoking is a major contributing factor in development and progression of disease of the vascular system (peripheral arterial disease)
- Although detrimental effects of second-hand smoke are not yet completely understood, it is a major contributor to morbidity and death

Furthermore there are additional areas of concern:
- Increased use of tobacco in school-age children
- Increased use of tobacco among women
- Detrimental effect of second-hand smoke
- Glamorization of smoking in the media and entertainment field
- Advertising targeted to school-age children
- Continued use of tobacco products by public figures in sports

SVN would like to mount a collaborative effort with other professional organizations to do the following:
- Assess individual use of tobacco
- Educate individuals on systemic effects of smoking
- Promote ongoing school-based programs on awareness prevention, and cessation of smoking at elementary, middle, junior, and senior levels
- Facilitate public awareness of smoking cessation materials, devices, and kits available
- Develop and implement educational materials as needed
- Support policies created by government, industry, and institutions to provide nonsmoking environments
- Support research related to prevention, treatments, cessation, and effects of tobacco abuse

SVN's main focus is "managing wellness" as the driving force in meeting the unique challenges to effectively address tobacco abuse issues to reduce the incidence of vascular disease.

Adapted from The Society of Vascular Nursing, Position statement: Tobacco abuse (1995). *Journal of Vascular Nursing, 13*(3):93.

diagnosis of peripheral vascular disease. Anatomical tests provide information on the location or physical aspects of the vascular lesion. Imaging studies fall in this category (CT or MRI scans, segmental pressure studies, and Doppler). Segmental pressure measurements give partial **anatomic** information in that they assist in locating lesions. **Hemodynamic** tests provide information on the flow of blood, such as to the brain or an extremity, and the effects on flow caused by a vascular lesion (segmental pressures, CW Doppler, plethysmography) (Rooke, 1992).

Ultrasonography

Ultrasonography is done to obtain information about structures through the emission of high frequency sound waves. These sound waves are reflected or bounced back to the probe, or transducer, that emits them and they are electronically transformed into an image.

Doppler

The Doppler effect, initially described by Christian Johann Doppler (1803-1953), is the *change in the frequency* of echo signals that occurs whenever there is a *change in the distance* between the source of a sound and the receiving object (McGraw & Rubin, 1995). The probe, or transducer, is aimed toward the blood vessel at an angle of 45 to 60 degrees. This directs an ultrasound beam that is reflected back to the probe by moving RBCs. The velocity of the flow of cells is converted into an audible signal heard through a speaker. The signal is described as a **swishing** sound (Pagana & Pagana, 1995). The sound is called a **signal** not a pulse. The tip of the probe is made of an element called a ceramic piezoelectric crystal. This can send, receive, and convert signals when an electric current is applied. The element becomes thicker and thinner, thus resulting in a pressure wave converted to an audible signal (McGraw & Rubin, 1995). The simplest form is the **continuous wave (CW) Doppler.** It has two elements; one sends a high frequency wave and the other receives it. In a **pulsed Doppler,** the same element sends and receives signals. The pulsed Doppler has the advantage of being able to differentiate between vessels of different depths. A normal arterial Doppler signal is either biphasic or triphasic. The first sound corresponds to systolic flow and is forward moving and high velocity. The second sound is related to early diastole and has a lesser reversal of flow. The third is later diastole and is smaller, forward flowing, and of a lower velocity. The pitch is described as rising quickly in systole and dropping quickly in early diastole. An abnormal signal, indicating stenosis or occlusion, is heard as low pitched and monophasic. These abnormal arterial signals may sound like venous signals (Zierler & Sumner, 1995). The Doppler can provide information in three forms: the audible signal, a visible graph printout similar to an ECG tracing, and a spectral analysis that appears on a screen and may be recorded on paper as well (Blackburn & Peterson-Kennedy, 1994). The Doppler is the most widely used instrument for vascular study. It has the advantages of being readily available, inexpensive, and easy to use. A small, portable battery unit is durable and can be transported and stored easily (see Chapter 8, Figure 8-29). When used on intact skin, a water-soluble gel is needed to conduct a signal. Probes can be used directly on a vessel intraoperatively (Box 5-7). The probes are heat sensitive and must be sterilized accordingly to be used

intraoperatively on the sterile field or they may be inserted into a sterile sleeve or probe cover. If they are handled gently, the probes have a reasonable life span. Care must be taken to protect the sensitive tip from being dropped or crushed. The biggest drawback of the Doppler is a negative finding in the presence of a stenotic lesion pronounced enough to produce a flow disturbance that results in an altered signal. A **bruit** is a sound disturbance that is sometimes described as a low-pitched blowing sound. It can be heard through a stethoscope over an area of blood flow turbulence that occurs at points of vessel stenoses. Bruits do not provide information on the extent of a lesion, only that an abnormal flow may exist. They occur at points of significant stenosis and are not heard when severe flow restriction or total flow occlusion occurs (Zierler & Sumner, 1995). The Doppler is noninvasive and painless for patients.

The interpretation of the Doppler signal provides important information to the surgeon but is very subjective. The recording that looks like an ECG tracing, called the **zero-crossing output,** gives immediate information on the wave contour but is potentially inaccurate (Figure 5-1). Spectral analysis is the preferred method (Zierler & Sumner, 1995). Spectral analysis provides a tracing of the frequency and amplitude of a Doppler signal. Amplitude is displayed by the brightness of the tracing that appears on the screen.

B-mode ultrasonography

B-mode is brightness modulation, a technique in ultrasound imaging that projects a two-dimensional image on an oscilloscope screen. The image appears as dots from the echoes of the signal. The strength of the echo is shown by the intensity and brightness of the dots on the screen (Anderson, 1994).

Duplex ultrasonography

A duplex ultrasound machine is a combination of the pulsed Doppler image and the so-called "real-time" B-mode image ultrasound. Real time simply refers to the image projecting the current, undelayed information. B-mode image is best when the probe is perpendicular to the vessel but the Doppler does not pick up signals at a perpendicular angle. Some manipulation of the probe angle is required to obtain the best results (McGraw & Rubin, 1995). Color duplex imaging converts the detected signals caused by blood flow into a color depending on the direction of flow. Flow toward the probe may be displayed as red, away from the probe as blue, and turbulence as multiple colors. This imaging provides both hemodynamic and anatomical information (Blackburn & Peterson-Kennedy, 1994). This technology is used in transesophageal echocardigraphy (Table 5-2).

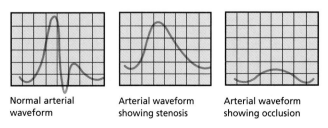

| Normal arterial waveform | Arterial waveform showing stenosis | Arterial waveform showing occlusion |

Fig. 5-1 Doppler printout and spectral analysis.

Table 5-2 **Summary of Common Vascular Tests**

TEST	PURPOSE	ADVANTAGES	DISADVANTAGES
NONINVASIVE **Arterial studies**			
Continuous wave Doppler	Diagnose occlusive disease; General assessment of severity; Assist in localizing occlusions	Inexpensive; Portable; Multiple applications	Operator dependent; Limited ability to quantify disease severity; Inaccurate in assessing collateral flow
Duplex scanning	Provides anatomic and hemodynamic information on arteries (extracranial carotid, aorta, upper and lower extremity lesions, and for following aneurysms, locating A-V fistulas; some usefulness in assessing renal and mesenteric lesions)	Correlates well with arteriography (may replace arteriography); Highly accurate; Provides anatomic and dynamic information simultaneously	Very expensive; Requires high level of operator skill and interpretation
Segmental pressures (ankle-brachial index [ABI], toe pressures, and penile pressures included in this category)	Diagnose and document occlusive disease; Assess severity; Localize lesion to specific vessel segment; Penile pressures may rule out vascular disease as cause of impotence and provides information on pudental artery (off the iliac)	Least expensive; Fastest; Easiest; Most accurate; Most reproducible	Does not work with incompressible vessels (diabetic); Useful only at or below midthigh; Difficult to assess small collateral vessels
Oculoplethysmography (OPG)	Assess cerebral perfusion pressure by measuring ocular arterial pressure	Accurate indicator of cerebral perfusion	Contraindicated in patients with ocular lens implants; Insensitive to severe stenosis of carotid when collateralization is well developed
Pulse volume recording (PVR) or sequential volume plethysmography (A **plethysmograph** measures and records the changes in the sizes and volumes in extremities by measuring the blood volumes; methods include electrical impedance, mercury in Silastic strain gauges, air or fluid displacement, and others)	Determine the location of arterial lesion; Estimate the severity of the disease	More accurate than segmental pressure measurements	Need for careful limb positioning and patient cooperation; Artifacts are possible; Inability to estimate blood flow to specific tissue (bone, muscle)
Computed tomography scan (CT) measures attenuation of an x-ray beam	Accurate staging of AAA; Assessment of graft occlusion; Assessment of graft infection, hemorrhage, or abscess	Superior to arteriography for visualizing vessel walls and other structures; Fast, good in emergency situations	If contrast is injected, it carries the same complications as arteriography; Equipment is expensive; Exposure to x-rays (a three-dimensional computer-generated reconstruction may be helpful for visualizing the aortic cuff and renal arteries)

Test	Purpose/Use	Advantages	Disadvantages
Magnetic resonance imaging (MRI) measures behavior of atoms in strong magnetic field	Provides detailed and three-dimensional image of anatomy for evaluation of carotid, aortic, and lower extremity disease	Provides more detail than ultrasonography or CT scan Avoids complications of contrast injection No exposure to x-ray Superior to CT scan for cerebral and spinal disease	Contraindicated in patients with pacemakers or metal cerebral aneurysm clips; vena cava filters may cause large image artifacts Less accurate in obese patients Very expensive Very time consuming; may not be useful in emergency
Venous Doppler	Continuous wave (CW) Doppler can identify presence and location of venous obstruction and assess the severity Good screening tool	Quick, easy, inexpensive	Significant number of false positives and false negatives Cannot differentiate between veins of different depths
Impedance or air plethysmography	Used to quantify venous outflow from the extremity, which is decreased in presence of venous thrombosis Tests for valve function Negative study is good predictor of low risk for pulmonary embolism (PE)	Low cost Good predictive value Accurate in detecting thrombosis	False positive rate is high (old DVT, CHF, and external compression) Poor for DVT below the popliteal artery; may miss partially blocking thrombosis Poor positioning or patient discomfort may cause artifact
Phleborheography (PRG) (a type of air plethysmograph)	Used to assess DVT, venous outflow obstruction, gross valvular incompetence, and efficacy of venous thrombolytic therapy	Most accurate method to assess DVT; provides objective hard copy of results	Cost estimated at $10,000 Time-consuming Requires very cooperative patient Bulky machine Does not pick up small thrombi in calf, obstruction of deep femoral or internal iliac veins Time and expense for its use (therefore, not a screening tool)
Venous duplex imaging	Most often used to identify DVT Locate and assess diameter of veins before harvest for arterial bypass procedures Identify function of specific valves	Almost 100% specificity and sensitivity for detection of proximal DVT	
INVASIVE Arteriography	Provides information on arterial anatomy, location of stenotic or occluded vessels, assists surgeon in planning bypass procedures Documentation of surgical outcome (completion angiogram)	Detailed anatomic information	May be uncomfortable for patient; pain with injection, flushing Multiple complications from mechanical trauma*: hemorrhage, dissection of vessel walls, false aneurysm, A-V fistula, thrombosis Multiple complications of injection of contrast: seizure, stroke, allergic reactions, laryngeal spasm or edema, cardiovascular collapse, renal failure; patients at increased risk include those with known allergy to iodine, with previous reactions, and alcoholics
CT scan			Considered invasive whenever contrast is injected Carries same complications as arteriography
Venogram (contrast venography)	Show venous abnormalities in extremities, vena cava, hepatic or renal systems **Ascending venography** can differentiate between acute and chronic thrombosis and define anatomy **Descending venography** assesses valve competence of lower extremity	Accurate	Complications include thrombophlebitis Contrast may leak into tissue and cause tissue necrosis (rare) Hypersensitivity to contrast media

Data from Zierler & Sumner, 1995; Rooke, 1992; Green & Ouriel, 1994.
*May require surgical correction.

Box 5-7 **Intraoperative Uses of Doppler**

- Assess and document patency of vascular graft or vessel (e.g., after thrombectomy or arterial bypass surgery)
- Locate areas of stenosis in vessel or graft
- Detect presence of blood flow to intestines after placement of aortic or mesenteric graft
- During carotid endarterectomy verify blood flow through a shunt
- Locating an arteriovenous fistula
- Locating a branch of a vein graft (in situ)

INTRAOPERATIVE DUPLEX SCANNER (DOPPLER AND ULTRASOUND)

- Transesophageal echocardiography; monitor and detect early cardiac ischemia

---

PATIENT HISTORY AND PHYSICAL

The history and physical may be performed by a variety of health care team members (see Chapter 2). The information should be readily available to all health care providers involved in the patient's care. The perioperative nurse should review it (if another team member gathered the data) and clarify and expand on the information needed to provide care.

The following should be considered for vascular patients:

- History
- Chief complaint or presenting problem
- Medical history

  Angina, myocardial infarction, congestive heart failure (CHF), renal disease, chronic obstructive pulmonary disease (COPD), hypertension (HTN), diabetes (Type I or II), pain, deep venous thrombosis (DVT), intermittent claudication

  Injuries, trauma, nonhealing wounds, back pain, arthritis

  Medications: both prescription and nonprescription

  Allergies: drugs, topicals, seafood, or fish products

  Previous vascular surgeries, orthopedic (implants), scars
  Family history

- Health/lifestyle habits, health-promoting activities, foot care in diabetics
- Psychosocial

  Recent stressors or significant life change

  Marital status/significant other

  Composition of family and support system

  Educational and occupational history

  Understanding of illness and surgery

  Response to pain

  Alcohol, tobacco, and diet (recent weight gain or loss, current weight)

  Activities of daily living (ADLs), exercise, functional status

  Coping strategies, e.g., religion, hobbies, activities

  Mental status

  Knowledge deficits related to surgery or health care

- Physical assessment
- Inspection

Skin assessment: color (pallor, cyanosis), turgor, temperature, and moisture

Nails: color, shape, symmetry, thickness, clubbing

Extremities: color, hair distribution, skin abnormalities (atrophy, ulcers, thickening, varicosities, swelling, discoloration, hair distribution, nails)

Abdomen: aortic pulsations

- Auscultation

  Bruits (check carotid arteries, iliac arteries, femoral)

  Palpation (pulses, Doppler signal) (Figure 5-2 and Figure 5-3)

  Palpation provides information on temperature, texture, edema, pulses, capillary refill, and pain

- Trendelenburg test
- Perthes test

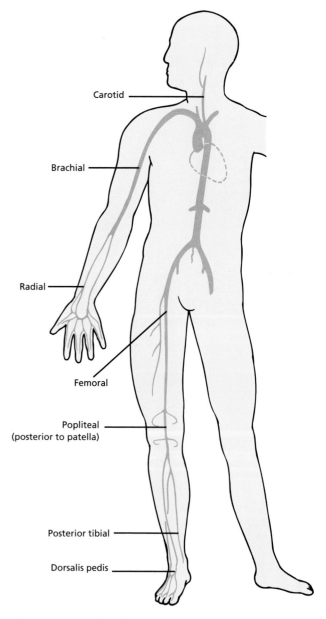

Fig. 5-2 Arteries for taking pulses. *(From Canobbio M. M. [1990]. Cardiovascular disorders. St. Louis: Mosby.)*

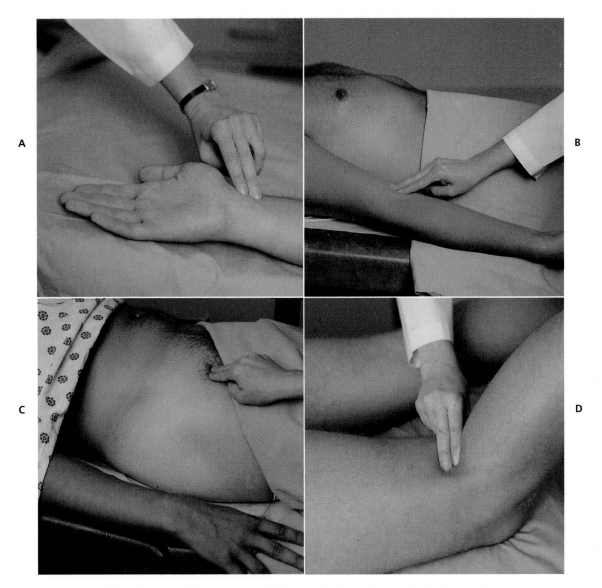

Fig. 5-3 **A,** Radial pulse. **B,** Brachial pulse. **C,** Femoral pulse. **D,** Popliteal pulse.

The **Trendelenburg** test can be done in an office setting. The patient is requested to lie down and the leg is elevated. Pressure is applied to the saphenofemoral junction with a tourniquet or using manual pressure. Instruct the patient to stand while the rate of varicose vein filling is observed. Release the pressure on the vein. When the perforating veins have competent valves, the refilling occurs gradually. When the valves are incompetent, the refilling occurs rapidly. Competence of the saphenofemoral valve can be determined in the same manner.

The **Perthes** test is performed by placing a tourniquet on the upper leg. Observe the patient ambulating. When varicose veins disappear, the deep venous valves are patent. If the patient complains of pain, this is an indication that the deep veins are not patent and the superficial system is functioning as the main conduit (Greenfield, 1994).

The **Allen test** may be used to assess the patency of the ulnar artery distal to the wrist. This is done before the insertion of an arterial monitoring line into the wrist. Manually occlude the radial artery, have the patient clench his or her fist to cause blanching, then relax the fist. The ulnar artery is patent if color returns immediately while the radial artery remains compressed (Wild, Craven, & Cunningham, 1991).

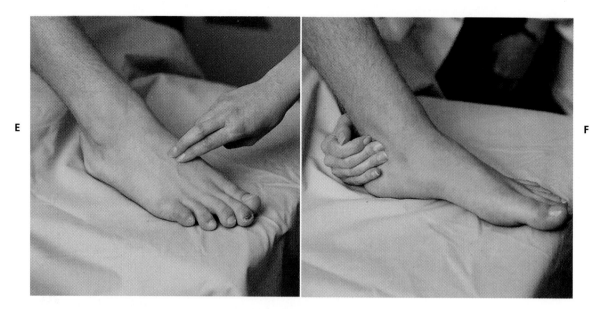

Fig. 5-3, cont'd E, Dorsalis pedis pulse. F, Posterior tibial pulse. *(From Potter P. A., & Perry, A. G. [1995]. Basic nursing [3rd ed.]. St. Louis: Mosby.)*

PHYSICAL ASSESSMENT

Inspection

Physical assessment should be done in an orderly fashion. However, some information will be obtained by observation during the interview and some through palpation. Assessment of the skin is often an ongoing process. Color variations should be noted. Pallor or cyanosis is more difficult to detect in dark-skinned patients. Nail beds, lips, and gums may have a bluish coloration in some black-skinned individuals that is normal. Inspect the patients' palms, conjunctiva, and buccal mucosa. Pallor may be due to superficial vasoconstriction if the patient is nervous or cold and may not be indicative of pathology. Pallor from a disease state may be caused by a low concentration of oxyhemoglobin. Cyanosis is due to an increase in deoxygenated hemoglobin (Canobbio, 1990). With the patient supine, elevate the patient's leg at about 45 degrees and inspect for color changes. Pallor within 30 seconds of elevation indicates a lack of adequate arterial circulation when working against gravity. Healthy limbs maintain their color. Lower the patient's legs below the examination table level. Again, healthy limbs maintain their color. Patients with arterial disease will have what is called **dependent rubor** that is a deep red color. Capillary refill is assessed by pressing on the tip of a toe or the heel and timing how long it takes to change from white to pink (Fahey & White, 1994). Another method of assessing capillary refill is to blanch a nail bed. Normal refill time is from a fraction of a second to 3 seconds. Capillary refill checks peripheral perfusion and cardiac output (Wild, Craven, & Cunningham, 1991). Blue toes or areas of darkened skin on one or more toes may be due to microemboli blocking small vessels. This is often referred to as **"blue toe syndrome."** Note any muscle atrophy, varicosities, and scars from either injuries or previous surgeries. Note all skin changes or abnormalities, especially ulcers. Venous and arterial causes of ulcers and skin changes often have typical characteristics that help in diagnosis (Table 5-3).

Auscultation

Auscultate with the bell of a stethoscope. If a bruit is heard in the neck, a carotid bruit should be distinguished from a vertebral artery bruit (Callow, 1995). Ask the patient to hold his or her breath. Listen by starting at the base of the neck and moving upward. If a bruit is heard, it is usually from the carotid artery if it is loudest in the upper third of the neck and cardiac in origin (or subclavian) if it gets louder toward the clavicle (Fahey & White, 1994). The vertebral artery is heard by placing the stethoscope posterior to the sternocleidomastoid muscle. A murmur from the aortic valve may be heard in all four vessels of the neck as equal. Abdominal bruits are a common finding in middle-aged patients. They may be detected over the aorta, iliac arteries, and other major branches of the aorta. Bruits from the renal arteries may be heard by listening at the flank or back (Callow, 1995). When the vibration of a blood disturbance is palpated, it is called a **thrill.** When referring to a thrill, be sure to inform the patient of the medical interpretation of the term. The detection of a bruit may indicate the need for further study. This must be determined within the context of the location and the entire patient presentation.

Palpation

Palpation provides information on skin temperature, skin texture, edema, pulses, capillary refill, and pain. Palpation is used *after* inspection and auscultation. Use care in palpating the carotid bifurcation. Causing embolic material to break off is possible and massage of the carotid sinus can cause a sudden drop in BP from the bradycardia reflex. Pulses are taken at the

Table 5-3 **Common Characteristics of Arterial versus Venous Disease**

	ARTERIAL	VENOUS
Pain	Intermittent claudication	Possible relief with exercise
	Rest pain	Mild to none, feeling of heaviness or fatigue
	Acute, severe	
Hair	Decreased	Normal
Nails	Thick, brittle	Normal
Skin color	Pallor, cyanosis, mottling, pigmentation	Brawny (red-brown) pigmentation
Skin temperature	Decreased to cold	Normal or increased with inflammation
Pulses	Decreased	Normal
	Absent	
Edema	None to mild	Typically calf to foot, worse at end of day
		Relieved with elevation
Sensation	Decreased, numbness, tingling, paresthesia	Normal
Ulcers	Very painful	Medial distal third of leg ("gaiter" area), pretibial area
	Found on or between toes, heel, dorsum of foot, above lateral malleolus	Uneven edges
	Surrounding skin is atrophic, possibly black and necrotic, defined edges	Shallow, moist
	Deep	

Data from Wild, Craven, & Cunningham (1991); Fahey & White (1994); and Bright & Georgi (1992).

carotid, brachial, radial, femoral, popliteal, posterior tibial, and dorsalis pedis arteries (see Figures 5-2 and 5-3). Document the rate, rhythm, and amplitude at each point separately and simultaneously to detect differences. An exception to this is in palpating the carotid arteries. The carotids should be palpated separately to prevent decreasing cerebral blood flow (Canobbio, 1990). Asymmetry may indicate occlusive disease. Using your index and second fingers is best (avoid using your thumb because you may feel your own pulse). Marking the site of a pulse when it is difficult to detect is sometimes helpful. This saves time in subsequent assessments, especially those done by different personnel. The location of the dorsalis pedis pulse is especially variable in individuals. In describing a pulse, use a scale accepted by the health care setting. One scale is written as 0+ for no pulse, 1+ for diminished, 2+ for normal, 3+ for full volume, and 4+ for bounding, hyperkinetic (Box 5-8). Obesity may interfere with the ability to detect a palpable pulse. The Doppler may be used for detection of arterial flow when pulses are not palpable. Edema is also described by a scale (determined by setting) or may be simply noted by the depth in millimeters (Canobbio, 1990). Edema may be caused by venous disease or congestive heart failure (CHF). Edema should be assessed and documented (Figure 5-4).

Blood Pressure

The blood pressure should be taken in both arms, at three levels of the legs, and with the patient standing, seated, and lying down. The blood pressure cuff should be the correct size for the limb. A brachial pressure above 140/90 is considered elevated. The dominant arm usually reads 10 mmHg higher than the other arm and the legs are normally higher than the arms. The diastolic pressure tends to be more stable and less dependent on external stimuli and is therefore the number used in

diagnosing HTN. Diastolic pressures of 90 to 104 are considered mild, 105 to 114 is moderate, and 115 and above is severe. Hypotension is generally considered to be 95/60 and benign unless accompanied by other symptoms. Patients who are taking antihypertensive medications should be assessed for **orthostatic hypotension** (Canobbio, 1990) as should all elderly patients. In a normal, healthy person, diastolic blood

---

Box 5-8 **Scales for Grading Pulses**

EXAMPLE 1
4 = bounding
3 = full, increased
2 = expected
1 = diminished, barely palpable
0 = absent, not palpable

EXAMPLE 2
3+ = bounding
2+ = normal
1+ = weak, thready
 0 = absent

EXAMPLE 3
4+ = normal
3+ = mildly impaired
2+ = moderately impaired
1+ = markedly impaired
 0 = absent

From Beare P.G., & Myers, J. L. (1998). *Adult health nursing* (3rd ed.). St. Louis: Mosby.

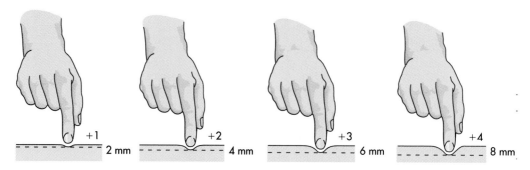

Fig. 5-4 Grading of edema. *(From Beare P. G., & Myers J. L. [1998]. Adult health nursing [3rd ed.].
St. Louis: Mosby.)*

pressure will drop about 10 mmHg and systolic BP rises 5 mmHg when the person alters their position from supine to sitting. Heart rate increases about 5 to 10 beats. A systolic BP drop of more than 15 mmHg, any drop in diastolic BP, and symptoms such as dizziness or visual changes indicate orthostatic hypotension. The patient should have been supine for 10 minutes before checking the BP and allowed to remain about 1 to 3 minutes in subsequent positions (Wild, Craven, & Cunningham, 1991). Blood pressures in the legs should be assessed from distal to proximal. A lower pressure distally as compared with proximally may indicate an arterial stenosis between the two locations.

ANKLE-BRACHIAL INDEX (ABI)

A widely used measurement in the assessment of lower extremity arterial perfusion is the **ankle-brachial index (ABI)**. A cuff is placed just above the malleolus and the diastolic pressure obtained using a Doppler probe on the dorsalis pedis pulse. The ankle systolic pressure divided by the arm (brachial) systolic pressure equals a number called the index. A normal ABI is equal to 1 or more. The patient will often have intermittent claudication when the ABI is 0.3 to 0.8, and rest pain with impending tissue loss at 0.3 or below (Fahey & White, 1994). According to Strandness (1995), an ABI of 0.95 is recommended as the dividing point between normal versus abnormal readings. A normal ABI does not mean that no disease is present. This is especially true of diabetics because of the nature of their disease. Diabetic vessels are calcified and may be incompressible resulting in false ABIs. Strandness suggests some guidelines for reading the ABI of 0.50 or above to indicate single segment disease and less than 0.50 to indicate multisegment disease.

COMPUTED AXIAL TOMOGRAPHY (CT SCAN)

The CAT or CT scan is a noninvasive test or invasive if IV contrast is injected to enhance the image. It is useful and accurate for diagnosing abdominal tumors, aneurysms, abscesses, or bleeding. It is also helpful to the surgeon in planning a surgical interventional. Images are achieved by using x-rays to pass through the body at various angles. The tissues and organs vary in their density and allow an image to be generated by a computer. Each tissue density is assigned a density value called the density coefficient, which is converted to dots on a screen in shades of gray. The images generated are like slices taken at

frequent intervals. When looking at a CT scan, the x-ray film is placed on a lighted view box like any other x-ray. The viewer sees the sliced image as from below, looking upward toward the patient's head. Bone is very dense and appears white. Locating familiar bony structures helps orient the viewer to other structures (Figure 5-5). An alternative image that can be generated from the CT scan is a three-dimensional projection. This image may be helpful in showing the relationship of various structures more clearly (Figure 5-6).

X-RAY

For the typical elderly patient, a current chest x-ray is usually required before the consideration of an anesthetic. A great deal of information can be obtained from a chest film and an abdominal flat plate x-ray. Having a working knowledge of a normal film to recognize any abnormal findings is helpful (Figure 5-7). Nurses should be able to select the best view of an x-ray study and any other anatomic views that may be requested intraoperatively. The image projected from an x-ray is influenced by the density or absorptive capacity of the material. The four basic densities are exhibited by metal, fluid, fat, and air. Metal shows up as the most dense or white image; bone is next, followed by blood vessels (their density is due to the water content), then fat, and air, which appears black (Dettenmeier, 1995).

Angiography

An **angiogram** is a series of x-rays taken to follow the flow of an injected contrast material. Contrast injection may also be followed by viewing the image using an image intensifier. These may be either intravenous or intraarterial injections. These images give an approximation of the size and shape of the vessels, any obstructions, and irregularities. Because the image is two dimensional, it is possible to see an erroneous impression of a vessel that appears patent. An atherosclerotic plaque may not be pictured depending on the angle of the view. Digital subtraction is a computer-generated image by which the dense bony structures are subtracted out to permit easier visualization of the blood vessels. An image of the anatomy before the subtraction is often found next to the subtracted image (Figure 5-8). This is helpful in orienting the viewer to the location. Any time a contrast agent is injected there are increased risks of discomfort and allergic reactions (see Chapter 4).

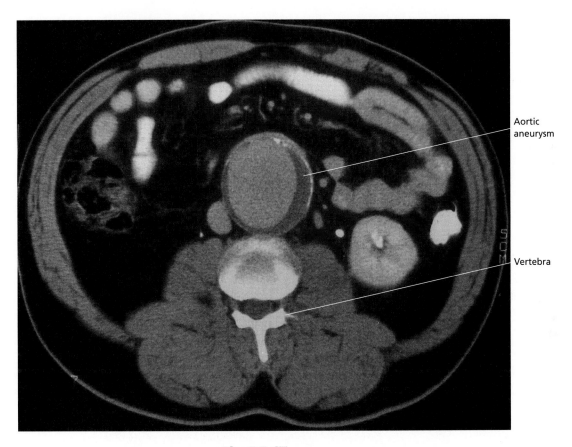

Aortic
aneurysm

Vertebra

Fig. 5-5 CT scan.

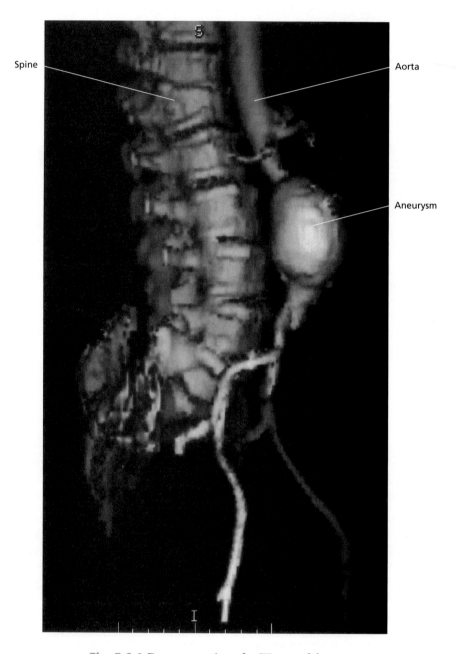

Fig. 5-6 3-D reconstruction of a CT scan of the aorta.

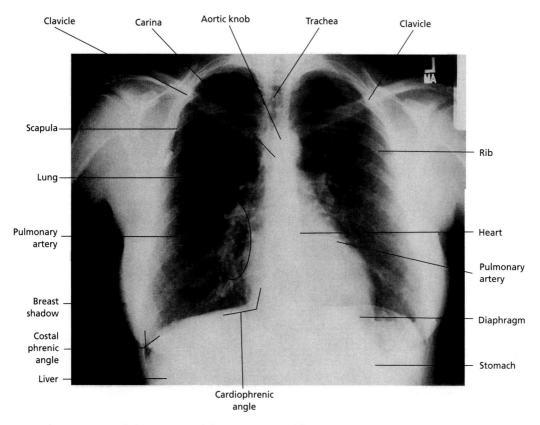

Fig. 5-7 Normal chest x-ray and the structures visible. *(From Dettenmeir P. A. [1995].* Radiographic assessment for nurses. *St. Louis: Mosby.)*

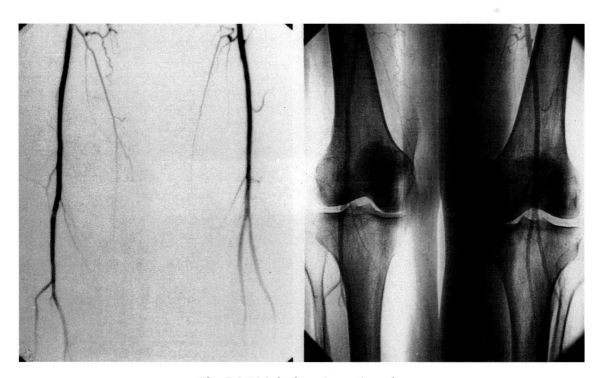

Fig. 5-8 Digital subtraction angiography.

VENTILATION-PERFUSION SCAN

Patients who are suspected of having a pulmonary embolism (PE) may have a ventilation-perfusion scan, also known as a V/Q scan. To study these two parameters, ventilation and perfusion, the patient inhales a radioactive gas to allow scanning of the ventilation. They also are given a radioisotope intravenously to allow scanning of the pulmonary circulation, or perfusion. Normal scans have equal ventilation to perfusion or are said to "match." Mismatched scans indicate a probable PE (Figure 5-9). A negative scan can rule out a pulmonary embolism. However, concurrent pulmonary pathology (e.g., pneumonia, congestive heart failure) may interfere with the results (Fahey, 1994). The next test performed when a V/Q scan is inconclusive is the pulmonary angiogram, considered the "gold standard" or most conclusive for diagnosing a PE (Dettenmeier, 1995; Fahey, 1994).

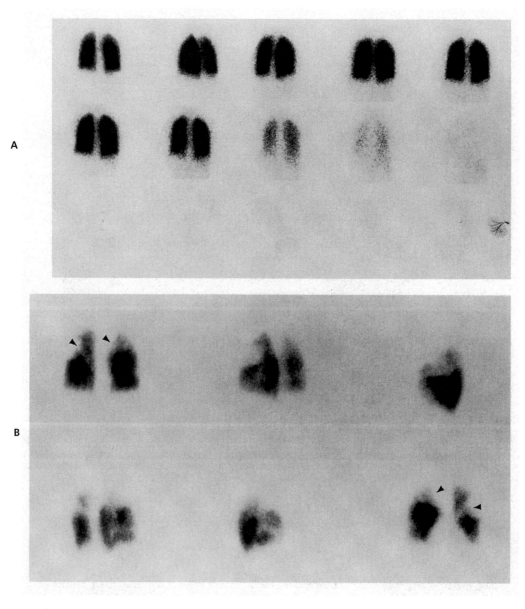

Fig. 5-9 Ventilation-perfusion (V/Q) scan. *(From Dettenmeir P. A. [1995]. Radiographic assessment for nurses. St. Louis: Mosby.)*

MAGNETIC RESONANCE IMAGING (MRI)

MRI is a type of imaging that uses a magnetic field to transmit radio waves through the patient to a computer. Like CT imaging, the image projected is determined by the tissue density. Unlike CT scans, no x-rays are used. This may produce better imaging for soft tissue than other methods (Thibodeau & Patton, 1996).

RENAL VEIN RENIN ASSAYS

Patients who are suspected of having renal hypertension may require a renal vein assay test. This is an invasive procedure, performed under fluoroscopy. Radiopaque contrast is injected into the inferior vena cava to visualize the renal veins. A catheter is inserted to withdraw a blood sample from each renal vein. The renin level is equal in a normal study. If the patient has renal hypertension as a result of a renal artery stenosis, the renin level in the affected kidney is 1.4 times greater than the other kidney (Pagana & Pagana, 1995).

References

Anderson, K.N. (ed.) (1994). *Mosby's medical, nursing, & allied health dictionary* (4th ed.). St. Louis: Mosby.

Atkinson, L.J. (1992). The patient: The reason for your existence. In *Berry & Kohn's Operating Room Technique* (7th ed., pp. 46-64). St. Louis: Mosby.

Barnes, R.W., & Vitti, M.J. (1996). Noninvasive diagnosis of venous disease. In H. Haimovici (Ed.), *Haimovici's vascular surgery* (4th ed., pp. 1149-1165). Cambridge, MA: Blackwell Science.

Bell, D.S.H. (1991). Lower limb problems in diabetic patients. *Postgraduate Medicine, 89*(8):237-244.

Blackburn, D.R., & Peterson-Kennedy, L. (1994). Noninvasive vascular testing. In V.A. Fahey (Ed.), *Vascular nursing* (2nd ed., pp. 73-103). Philadelphia: W.B. Saunders.

Bright, L.D., & Georgi. S. (1992). Peripheral vascular disease: Is it arterial or venous? *American Journal of Nursing, 92*(9): 34-43.

Burggraf, V., & Donlon, B. (1985). Assessing the elderly: System by system: Part I *American Journal of Nursing, 85*(9): 974-984.

Burnside, I.M. (1988). Communication. In I.M. Burnside (Ed.), *Nursing and the aged: A self-care approach* (3rd ed., pp. 193-213). New York: McGraw-Hill.

Callow, A.D. (1995). Clinical assessment of the peripheral circulation. In A.D. Callow & C.B. Ernst (Eds.), *Vascular surgery: Theory and practice* (pp. 181-199). Stamford, CT: Appleton & Lange.

Canobbio, M.M. (1990). Assessment. In M.M. Canobbio (Ed.), *Cardiovascular disorders* (pp. 17-40). St. Louis: Mosby.

Cochran, I., et al (1994). Stroke care. *Nursing 94, 24*(6): 34-41.

Cole, C. W., et al (1993). Cigarette smoking and peripheral arterial occlusive disease. *Surgery, 114*(4): 753-756.

Couch, N. P. (1986). On the arterial consequences of smoking. *Journal of Vascular Surgery, 3*(5): 807-812.

Dettenmeier, P.A. (1995). *Radiographic assessment for nurses.* St. Louis: Mosby.

Diagnostic and statistical manual of mental disorders: Primary care version (4th ed.) (1995). American Psychiatric Association. Washington, D. C.

Ebersole, P., & Hess, P. (1994). Age-related changes. In *Toward healthy aging: Human needs and nursing response* (4th ed., pp. 69-108). St. Louis: Mosby.

Emma, L.A. (1992). Chronic arterial occlusive disease. *Journal of Cardiovascular Nursing, 7*(1): 14-24.

Fahey, V.A., & White, S.A. (1994). Physical assessment of the vascular system. In V.A. Fahey (Ed.), *Vascular nursing* (2nd ed., pp. 53-72). Philadelphia: W.B. Saunders.

Feistritzer, N.R. (1995). Wound healing, dressing, and drains. In M.H. Meeker, & J.C. Rothrock (Eds.), *Alexander's care of the patient in surgery* (10th ed., pp. 182-191). St. Louis: Mosby.

Folstein, M.F., Folstein, S.E., & McHugh, P.R. (1975). "Mini-Mental State": A practical method for grading the cognitive state of patients for the clinician. *Journal of Psychiatric Research, 12*:189-198.

Gallman, R.L. (1995). The sensory system and its problems in the elderly. In M Stanley, & P.G. Beare (Eds.), *Gerontological nursing* (pp. 134-147). Philadelphia: F.A. Davis.

Green, R.M., & Ouriel, K. (1994). Peripheral arterial disease. In S.I. Schwarz, G.T. Shires, & F.C. Spencer (Eds.), *Principles of surgery* (pp. 925-987). New York: McGraw-Hill.

Greenfield, L.J. (1994). Venous and lymphatic disease. In S.I. Schwarz, G.T. Shires, & F.C. Spencer (Eds.), *Principles of surgery* (pp. 989-1014). New York: McGraw-Hill.

Hoffman, D., & Wynder, E. L. (1986). Chemical constituents and bioactivity of tobacco smoke. In D. R. Zaridge, & R. Peto (Eds.), *Tobacco, a major international health hazard*. International Agency for Research on Cancer, WHO. London: Oxford Press.

Hogstel, M.O. (1994). Vital signs are really vital in the old-old. *Geriatric Nursing, 15*:252-255.

Kalra, V. K., et al (1994). Mechanism of cigarette smoke condensate induced adhesion of human monocytes to cultured endothelial cells. *Journal of Cellular Physiology, 160*(1): 154-162.

Kane, R.L., Ouslander, J.G., & Abrass, I.B. (Eds.) (1994). Evaluating the elderly patients. In *Essentials of clinical geriatrics* (3rd ed., pp. 44-79). New York: McGraw-Hill.

Kofoed, L.L. (1985). OTC drug use in the elderly: What to watch for. *Geriatrics, 40*(10): 55-60.

Kyriazis, M. (1994). Developments in the treatment of stroke patients. *Nursing Times, 20*(90): 30-32.

Lakier, J. B. (1992). Smoking and cardiovascular disease. *American Journal of Medicine, 93*(1A): 85-125.

Lesmes, G. R. (1992). Smoking and cardiovascular disease: Summary and conclusion. *American Journal of Medicine, 93*(1A): 55s-56s.

Lipson, L.G. (1986a). Diabetes in the elderly: A multifaceted problem. *American Journal of Medicine, 80*(suppl 5A): 1-2.

Lipson, L.G. (1986b). Diabetes in the elderly: Diagnosis, pathogenesis, and therapy. *American Journal of Medicine, 80*(suppl 5A): 10-21.

Maryniuk, M.D. (1993). Lipid-lowering diets: Putting guidelines into parctice. *Diabetes Educator, 19*(5): 440-441.

McDougall, G.J. (1990). A review of screening instruments for assessing cognition and mental status in older adults. *Nurse Practitioner, 15*(11):18-28.

McGraw, D.J., & Rubin, B.G. (1995). The Doppler principle and sonographic imaging: applications in the noninvasive vascular laboratory. In A.D. Callow, & C.B. Ernst (Eds.), *Vascular surgery: Theory and practice* (pp. 309-317). Stemford, CT: Appleton & Lange.

Mellillo, K. D. (1993). Interpretation of laboratory values in older adults: Part II. Journal of Gerontological Nursing, *19*(2): 35-40.

Mhoon, E. (1990) Otology, In C.K. Cassel, D.E. Riesenberg, L.B. Sorensen, & J.R. Walsh (Eds.), *Geriatric medicine* (2nd ed., pp. 405-419). New York: Springer-Verlag.

Moss, A.J. (1995). Diagnosis and management of heart disease in the elderly. In W. Reichel, J.J. Gallo, J. Busby-Whitehead, & J.B. Murphy (Eds.). *Care of the elderly: Clinical aspects of aging* (4th ed., pp. 69-86). Baltimore: Williams & Wilkins.

Muluk, S. C., et al (1994). Presentation and patterns of aortic aneurysms in young patients. *Journal of Vascular Surgery, 20*(6): 880-886.

Nunnelee, J.D. (1994). Patient education: Hospital to home. In V.A. Fahey (Ed.), *Vascular Nursing* (2nd ed., pp 206-218). Philadelphia: W.B. Saunders.

Pagana, K.D., & Pagana, T.J. (1995). *Mosby's diagnostic and laboratory test reference* (2nd ed.). St. Louis: Mosby.

Pomerlau, O. F. (1992). Nicotine and the central nervous system: biobehavioral effects of cigarette smoking. *American Journal of Medicine, 93*(1A): 2s-7s.

Reichel, W., & Rabins, P.V. (1995). Evaluation and management of the confused, disoriented, or demented elderly patient. In W. Reichel, J.J. Gallo, J. Busby-Whitehead, & J.B. Murphy (Eds.). *Care of the elderly: Clinical aspects of aging* (4th ed., pp. 142-154). Baltimore: Williams & Wilkins.

Rice, V.H., Lepczyk, M., & Templin, T. (1994). A comparison of nursing interventions for smoking cessation in adults with cardiovascular health problems. *Heart Lung, 23:* 473-486.

Rimm, E. B., et al (1993). Cigarette smoking and the risk of diabetes in women. *American Journal of Public Health, 83*(2): 211-214.

Rooke, T.W. (1992). The noninvasive vascular laboratory. *Cardiovascular Clinics, Comtemporary Issues in Peripheral Vascular Disease, 22*(3):27-44.

The Society of Vascular Nursing (1995). Position statement: Tobacco abuse. *Journal of Vascular Nursing, 13*(3); 93.

Strandness, Jr., D.E. (1995). Arterial and venous hemodynamics. In K. Ouriel (Ed.), *Lower extremity vascular disease* (pp. 3-12). Philadelphia: W.B. Saunders.

Thibodeau, G.A., & Patton, K.T. (1996). Organization of the body. In G.A. Thibodeau, & K.T. Patton (Eds.), *Anatomy & physiology* (3rd ed.). St. Louis: Mosby.

Weiss, S. (1992). Measurement of the sensory qualities in tactile interaction. *Nursing Research, 41:*82-86.

Weiss, S. (1992). Measurement of the sensory qualities in tactile interaction. *Nursing Research, 41:*82-86.

Wewers, M., Bowen, J., Stanislaw, A., & Desimone, V. (1994). A nurse delivered smoking cessation intervention among hospitalized postoperative patients—influence of a smoking related diagnosis: A pilot study. *Heart Lung, 23:*151-156.

Wild, L.R., Craven, R.F., & Cunningham, S.L. (1991). Assessment of vascular function. In M.C. Patrick, S.L. Woods, R.F. Craven, J.S., Rokoky, & P. Bruno (Eds.), *Medical-surgical nursing: Pathophysiological concepts* (2nd ed., pp. 802-811). New York: J.B. Lippincott.

Wilson, P.F., Anderson, K.M., & Kannel, W.B. (1986). Epidemiology of diabetes mellitus in the elderly: The Framingham study. *American Journal of Medicine, 80*(Suppl. 5A);3-9.

Zierler, R.E., & Sumner, D.S. (1995). Physiologic assessment of peripheral occlusive disease. In R.B. Rutherford (Ed.), *Vascular surgery* (4th ed., pp. 65-117). Philadelphia: W.B. Saunders.

6 Nursing Diagnoses for the Vascular Patient

AORNs Recommended Practices for Documentation of Perioperative Nursing Care (1996), provides guidelines for charting the **nursing process**. Assessment, diagnosis, planning, implementation, evaluation, and expected outcome are the accepted steps in this process. Chapter 5 covers the medical and nursing assessments for this population. After the initial patient assessment, the planning phase is initiated with the formulation of nursing diagnoses that lead to desired patient outcomes. Since nursing diagnoses are driven by these patient outcomes, diagnoses and outcomes are discussed together. The professional judgement that is necessary to carry out these steps falls within the jurisdiction of the professional Registered Nurse. The professional nurse is responsible for the care but may delegate aspects of the implementation phase to assistive personnel. Abbott (1994) describes components of "embedded nursing judgement" as based on environmental cues, changes in patient responses, anticipation of surgical events, and assessment of resources, both material and human. She further predicts that as the patient acuity increases in the current uncertain health care environment, the ability to control and predict patient outcomes decreases.

A systematic description of the process of defining and collecting patient data (nursing diagnosis) to direct care planning has been growing since the 1950s. The North American Nursing Diagnosis Association (**NANDA**) develops and approves this evolving list of accepted nursing diagnoses. Documentation of the nursing process must reflect the continual assessment of the patient, the interventions that are implemented, and the actual or pending **outcomes**. Standardized forms that reflect the nursing process ideally minimize the time spent on charting but should reflect the care uniquely tailored for the individual patient (Ladden, 1995). Perioperative nurses who care for the patient in the intraoperative phase have a unique perspective of the patient experience. The patient is at his or her most vulnerable and the nurse must ensure that this phase of the patient's care is accurately communicated so that care is continuous and outcomes are achieved. Many outcomes cannot be measured in the intraoperative phase and must be assessed in the recovery to discharge periods. Patient outcome standards such as freedom from infection, preserved skin integrity, and freedom from injuries caused by intraoperative positioning or equipment may be assessed on an ongoing basis (Box 6-1). An initial assessment is performed and documented by the nurse in the operating room but achievement of the desired outcomes occurs at different points in the recovery process. Many aspects of intraoperative care are totally unique and unfortunately unknown to other nursing colleagues. Written and verbal communication is important to ensure that any patient problems that may arise from intraoperative care (or lack of care) are understood and appropriate interventions instituted.

NANDA NURSING DIAGNOSES HEADINGS

In 1973 nursing diagnoses began the evolution process of acceptance and usage. NANDA has categorized nursing diagnoses under nine headings. These headings are patterns of human response and include the following:

- Exchanging
- Communicating
- Relating
- Valuing
- Choosing
- Moving
- Perceiving
- Knowing
- Feeling (Carpenito, 1992)

The terminology for expressing patient problems has become more specific and complex. All surgical patients are at

---

Box 6-1 **Patient Outcomes: Standards of Perioperative Care**

Standard I
The patient demonstrates knowledge of the physiologic and psychologic responses to surgical intervention.
Standard II
The patient is free from infection.
Standard III
The patient's skin integrity is maintained.
Standard IV
The patient is free from injury related to positioning, extraneous objects, and chemical, physical, and electrical hazards.
Standard V
The patient's fluid and electrolyte balance is maintained.
Standard VI
The patient participated in the rehabilitation process.

Adapted from AORN, 1996.

some risk for infection but this is not a useful nursing diagnosis for every patient because not all patients are at *risk for infection*. The elderly diabetic patient is at high risk for infection because of the many physiologic changes wrought by both attributes. *Possible* nursing diagnoses are different from the former *potential*. Possible has been likened to the medical term *rule-out*. It focuses attention on the need to continue investigation into an area to decide if it is problematic for the patient (Carpenito, 1992).

HUMAN RESPONSE PATTERNS AND NURSING DIAGNOSES

Communicating

Impaired ability to communicate may be a subtle or obvious problem in dealings with the average vascular patient. Because most are elderly, they may have various degrees of hearing loss, limited visual acuity, or have suffered a stroke that has left them with a form of aphasia (see Chapter 5). Many people are aware of their limitations and are embarrassed to admit them. As a result they may fabricate responses to cover up hearing deficits and end up seeming confused or inappropriate. Pain, anxiety, and depression may prevent the patient from listening and comprehending instructions or requests.

Perceiving

Perceptual alterations usually refer to changes related to physiologic factors, e.g., pain, sleep deprivation, immobility, and a general decrease of the usual environmental stimuli. These patients may have an electrolyte imbalance, low blood sugar, or may be sedated.

Feeling

Feelings of anxiety are common to most patients who expect to undergo a surgical procedure. However, the vascular patient who faces a carotid endarterectomy may be particularly fearful of the surgical outcome. Although the incidence of a stroke is low (1% to 2%), it can produce great anxiety for the patient and family. The patient who presents with a leaking or "ruptured" abdominal aortic aneurysm (AAA) is at risk for death or prolonged residence in an intensive care unit (ICU). Patients with lower extremity arterial occlusive disease, especially diabetics, fear amputation.

Knowing

Knowledge deficits are common in the vascular surgery patient. Many people do not understand even the basic anatomy enough to differentiate between arteries and veins. These patients may be in denial over the poor health habits that place them at risk, such as smoking and high fat diets. It may be challenging to teach these patients about their disease, the surgical procedures, and the desired outcomes and recommended lifestyle changes.

Moving

The vascular patient population is prone to impaired physical mobility. Patients with venous disorders such as severe varicose veins or lower extremity phlebitis may need to elevate their legs for long periods. Elderly patients may be limited by musculoskeletal problems such as arthritis or poor cardiac function.

This can have a major impact on discharge planning because of the limitations for safety and self care. The amputation patient will have many of these same needs with the additional need to teach functional adaptation to a prosthesis or wheelchair.

Exchanging

The human response patterns that fall under exchanging encompass many physiologic concerns of intraoperative care planning. Circulation is a focus because of the nature of venous and arterial disease. Cardiac status is affected and many patients must be evaluated thoroughly for cardiac status before any surgical intervention. These patients are at risk for impaired skin integrity, skin injury, and impaired tissue perfusion. Very elderly, cachectic, obese, and diabetic patients need special protection in the operating room to prevent pressure injuries to their already compromised tissue. Elderly and diabetic patients are at risk for infection because of their altered immune response. Any breach in sterile technique or less than optimal skin preparation (e.g., shaving versus clipping) or skin protection should be taken seriously and corrective measures instituted immediately. A fluid volume deficit (bleeding) or fluid volume excess (fluid overload in the cardiac patient) are other risk areas. Inadvertent hypothermia is a risk area for elderly patients, those undergoing long surgeries, and those with a potential for prolonged exposure of a major body cavity.

Relating

Vascular disease can have a profound impact on many of the patient's usual roles. They may be so limited by the inability to walk long distances that their employment is affected, they may become unable to carry out the necessary activities of daily living, and they become increasingly isolated. Pain, such as night rest pain, can lead to sleep deprivation and chronic fatigue that have consequences for the quality of family interactions. Aortoiliac occlusive disease may affect sexual performance in men.

Valuing

The chronicity of vascular disease can lead to feelings of hopelessness and spiritual distress. Spiritual beliefs may be the key for many patients' ability to cope with changes and loss. Spiritual practices may help the patient to handle acute situations. A brief spiritual assessment may unlock many areas of relief for the patient and family.

Choosing

Problems may be encountered as the patient makes choices for lifestyle changes. They must be assisted to obtain the information they need to make informed choices. Patients go through stages of grieving when faced with the need to alter lifelong patterns of coping no matter how maladaptive the coping mechanisms may seem to the health care professional. Acceptance is important to allow the patient the requisite time to advance rather than regress or deny in the face of demands made upon them. It is important to make sure that the plans and interventions are based on the patient's wishes so that they are realistic. It would be unrealistic to map out a plan that a patient does not agree with (choose) and would not follow.

SELECTED NURSING DIAGNOSES FOR THE VASCULAR PATIENT

As the perioperative nurse assesses the vascular patient, he or she prioritizes the appropriate nursing diagnoses for focusing and individualizing the plan of care. The nursing diagnoses selected for incorporation into the care rendered utilize the ultimate goal or patient outcome as a guide. The outcomes are ideal goals and may not be achievable. They are modified over time to be realistic for the patient. Some outcomes may be influenced by the nurse but may not be entirely within his or her control.

1. **Nursing diagnosis:** A knowledge deficit related to the anatomy and physiology of vascular disease, pending surgical procedure, and the immediate postoperative events.

Patient outcomes: The patient verbalizes acceptance and understanding of the surgical procedure, its purpose, and the impact it will have on health and functioning. The patient verbalizes expected events in the immediate postoperative period.

2. **Nursing diagnosis:** Alteration in sensory/perceptual function: hearing deficits related to aging changes.

Nursing outcome: The patient can hear the conversation and respond appropriately.

3. **Nursing diagnosis:** Anxiety related to the surgical procedure and/or perioperative events.

Nursing outcome: The patient exhibits a decrease in the manifestations of anxiety as evidenced by the reduction or absence of crying, verbal expressions of fear, poor attention, or agitation.

4. **Nursing diagnosis:** Risk for injury related to the surgical position.

Nursing outcome: The patient is free from injury related to the surgical position as evidenced by the absence of neuromuscular impairment or tissue necrosis.

5. **Nursing diagnosis:** Risk for injury related to retained foreign objects.

Nursing outcome: The patient is free from retained foreign objects as evidenced by correct counts of surgical supplies and instrumentation or an x-ray film read as having no retained object when a count is in question.

6. **Nursing diagnosis:** Risk for injury related to chemical, physical, or electrical hazards.

Nursing outcome: The patient is free from injury related to chemical, physical, or electrical hazards as evidenced by the absence of allergic reactions, skin reactions to prep solutions, adhesives, or the return electrode of the electrocautery.

7. **Nursing diagnosis:** Risk for infection related to physiologic changes of aging and compromised immunology as a result of diabetes mellitus, prosthetic implant, or groin incision.

Nursing outcome: The patient remains free of infection in the immediate postoperative phase as evidenced by stable baseline vital signs and absence of wound symptoms.

8. **Nursing diagnosis:** Risk for impaired wound healing related to peripheral vascular disease, advanced age, diabetes mellitus, malnutrition, or surgical clamping.

Nursing outcomes: The patient will participate in the plan to promote optimal wound healing. Surgical incisions show progressive healing.

9. **Nursing diagnosis:** Risk for altered body heat regulation: inadvertent hypothermia related to advanced age (decreased basal metabolism and loss of adipose tissue), operating room suite temperature, exposure of body surface and body cavities during surgery, unheated fluid infusions, and anesthetics.

Nursing outcome: The patient will remain normothermic, based upon baseline body temperature, throughout the surgical procedure and during the immediate postoperative period.

10. **Nursing diagnosis:** Risk for impaired skin integrity related to advanced age, diabetes mellitus, history of smoking, lengthy surgical procedure (immobility), peripheral vascular disease, and surgical clamping.

Nursing outcome: The patient's skin integrity will be maintained as evidenced by the absence of bruises, discoloration, skin breakdown, or excoriation during the perioperative period.

11. **Nursing diagnosis:** Risk for a fluid volume deficit related to blood loss from a ruptured aneurysm or surgical intervention.

Nursing outcome: The patient's fluid volume will be maintained as evidenced by hematocrit, blood pressure, urinary output, arterial blood gases, and electrolytes within normal limits.

12. **Nursing diagnosis:** Risk for altered participation in the rehabilitation process related to physical barriers, functional barriers, or lack of information.

Nursing outcome: The patient participates in his or her own care depending on the physical and psychologic status by identifying problems related to the surgical experience and performing activities related to care (AORN Standards & Recommended Practices, 1996).

References

Abbott, C.A. (1994). Intraoperative nursing activities performed by surgical technologists. *AORN Journal, 60*(3): 382-393.

Association of Operating Room Nurses: Standards and Recommended Practices (1996). *Patient outcomes: Standards of perioperative care.* Denver: AORN.

Association of Operating Room Nurses: Standards and Recommended Practices (1996). *Recommended practices for documentation of perioperative nursing care.* Denver: AORN.

Carpenito, L.J. (1992). *Nursing diagnosis: Application to clinical practice* (4th ed.). Philadelphia: J.B. Lippincott.

Ladden, C.S. (1995). Concepts basic to perioperative nursing. In M.H. Meeker, & J.C. Rothrock (Eds.), *Alexander's care of the patient in surgery* (10th ed., pp 3-18). St. Louis: Mosby.

Perioperative Nursing Care

Perioperative nursing care encompasses a wide variety of practice settings and job responsibilities. Perioperative care is provided from the time that the patient becomes a candidate for surgery either electively or emergently through the postoperative period. Practice settings and requirements will vary depending on the patient, proposed procedure, physician preferences and scope of practice, institution, reimbursement policies, and region of the country. The nursing care and teaching will also vary and depend on the patient's needs and the team members roles (see Chapter 2). Nursing care planning is individualized to the patient and must be based on expected outcomes. Teaching is done to prevent complications, maximize the patient's self-care potential, and plan for discharge from the onset. More patients are being admitted for surgery to minimize the length of hospital stay. Patient days are predicted to continue to decline by a third by 1999 (Declining hospital, 1995). Patients who do not necessarily require the availability of complex hospital care and resources are entering ambulatory surgical settings for procedures such as varicose vein excision and ligation. Hospital admission on the day of surgery is becoming the norm. Patients have preoperative tests, histories, and physicals before the day of surgery. This eliminates an unnecessary night in the hospital. Most patients prefer to remain home as long as possible, thereby promoting patient and family comfort as well as reducing medical costs. This may also prevent a surgical cancellation if tests or other assessments indicate a need for further work-up or a lack of indications for surgery.

The trend toward same-day admission decreases the opportunities for patient-staff interaction. Patients need time for questions to be answered and instructions to be assimilated. Teaching must be streamlined and tools refined to allow the maximum patient benefit. The time immediately preceding surgery may be very stressful for the patient and may not be the best time to give new information. Reinforcement of information is appropriate at this time but the teaching is best done during the preadmission interview. Patients prefer preadmission teaching (Brumfield et al, 1996). This may be done primarily by a nurse practitioner, RNFA, or the inpatient unit nurse. Some places use a team approach to utilize nurses from the OR, ICU, and PACU who have developed skill in effective interviewing.

CHART REVIEW

The perioperative nurse must be able to efficiently assess the patient and his or her specific needs. This includes time to perform an adequate chart review (Box 7-1). The first sight of the patient may give much information but must be confirmed by thorough assessment to avoid mistaken assumptions. The patient must be greeted by name and identification confirmed by the patient when possible and by a name band and the medical record. Comfort should be the next most important assessment before continuing any interview. This is caring and will promote the establishment of a nurse-patient rapport and facilitate obtaining accurate and complete information. Patient acuity will also affect the prioritizing of the assessments and interactions. Safety is always uppermost. The surgical procedure must be confirmed and the patient's understanding assessed. Informed consent is not a piece of paper with a signature. Informed consent written requirements vary from region to institution. The nurse must necessarily follow the policies of the institution, but his or her role as advocate mandates that he or she determine that the patient comprehend the pending intervention to the best of his or her ability. Inaccuracies or misconceptions must be clarified before proceeding with surgery. The Patient's Bill of Rights specifies that the patient has the right to receive information about treatment that is pertinent, up-to-date, and clear to them (Atkinson & Fortunato, 1996). The surgeon is responsible for providing this information. Written documentation may be in the form of a narrative description by the physician or a preprinted form that the patient or legal alternate signs. A consent is designed to protect the patient by allowing clarification in

---

Box 7-1 **Chart Review**

The nurse will review the surgical patient's chart for the following items:

- Correct and current chart
- Surgical consent
- History and physical examination
- Baseline vital signs (include height and weight)
- Mental status
- Medications
- Allergies or adverse reactions to drugs, topical agents, or other substances
- Skin tone and integrity
- Physical limitations
- Laboratory data (blood work, ECG report, urinalysis, ultrasound or x-ray studies, or other pertinent tests)
- Religious preferences
- Nursing plan of care or other notations from transferring nurse
- Presence or disposition of prosthetic devices (hearing aides, dentures, glasses, etc.)

Modified from Pierson, 1995; Atkinson & Fortunato, 1996.

writing of the proposed procedure. It is not legal proof that the patient is truly informed; however, it does lend support that the patient gave permission. Consents that are valid, obtained freely, and from a competent person remain in effect for as long as the person still agrees to the surgery or procedure. This may vary by institutional modification (Atkinson & Fortunato, 1996). Complex decision making and the availability of new technologies may make informed consent difficult. The American College of Obstetricians and Gynecologists have developed a computer program for an interactive informed consent. It requires the patient to touch the computer screen to answer questions and then creates a summary for the health care provider to review teaching needs (Workplace, 1995).

LIVING WILLS, HEALTH CARE PROXIES, DNR

Passage of the Patient Self-Determination Act in 1991 permits patients to provide specific instructions about their choices if they become incapacitated. The health care institution must ensure that all adults have been given written information on these rights but it falls to the nurse to check that the patient has been given this opportunity. The law does not require a patient to have an advanced directive but to have the option to make a choice. Advance directives such as living wills, durable powers of attorney, health care proxies, and anatomic gifts must be considered when in place. The legality and terminology varies from state to state. For example, an advanced directive made in one state may not be accepted in another (Pokalo, 1992). Forms may vary but the intent is important. The issue of organ donation may be less relevant for the aged population that comprises the majority of the vascular patients, but DNR (do not resuscitate) orders may be very relevant. The public is very aware of the potential for prolonging life beyond the point that they or their families deem desirable. Health care providers must be knowledgeable about their state law and hospital policies. Although these plans should have been well thought out, discussed, and documented, the stress of impending surgery often elicits last minute conversations and patients need reassurance that their wishes will be respected.

The DNR orders should be addressed in institution policy. They must be explicitly written if the institution is accredited by JCAHO (Cohen & Cohen, 1991). However, this tends to be an area of concern when patients are brought to the operating room. One of the major problems is the difficulty in defining DNR. What it means to the patient, health care provider, family, and the courts is not clear. Patient autonomy is considered a basic right. The patient determines what may or may not be done for them. The health care arena ethically centers on not doing harm and instead doing good. Institutions have tried to limit their operative mortalities in their medical model framework and quest to preserve life. The anesthetists must tailor their actions to optimize care to the *individual*. The administration of anesthetics makes it difficult to determine whether the drugs lead to a cardiac or respiratory arrest or whether this is a natural outcome of the patient's underlying health status. Discussion with the patient, family, and experts in the field of ethical decision making provides a sound basis for making critical decisions before entry into the OR (Clark, Lucas & Stephens, 1994). Nurses must be involved in this dialogue and

policy development as part of their patient advocacy responsibilities. The nurse in the PACU is directly involved by virtue of the fact that he or she is responsible for the patient as they emerge from the effects of anesthesia. Some institutions include a paragraph on DNR in their surgical consent form. This at least opens up the opportunity for discussion (Golanowski, 1995). It becomes an ethical dilemma for many because the anesthesia providers must treat any reactions that may have been caused by the administration of anesthetics. It may be an unwritten rule to err on the legally safe side and treat a cardiac or respiratory arrest in the OR. Patients may elect to undergo surgery to provide relief of pain or otherwise improve the quality of their life. The ethically sound practice is to be sure that the patients are aware that DNR orders are suspended in the OR if such is the case.

DNR aside, the ethical concerns for CPR in the elderly population must be considered. CPR was developed in 1960 as closed chest massage to treat cardiac arrest from anesthetics or MI. It has been widely taught to hospital workers, emergency personnel, and lay persons. While it has saved many lives, its use in every situation is being questioned. Age is a factor in the likelihood of impending death and studies have indicated that more harm than good may result for elderly persons. Survival rates for the elderly after CPR are low. A number of legal issues have arisen as a result of questioning the wisdom of CPR in all situations. Age is a factor in the patient's situation but age alone does not diminish their worth as an individual. Withholding care based on age alone would be unethical and illegal. Physicians are not mandated to provide care and treatment that is futile. The care should benefit the patient. The patient's best interests remain the legal basis for accountability. Although medical care is aimed at preserving life, the physician is not legally required to do so at all costs (Carton & Brown, 1993).

PREOPERATIVE PREPARATIONS

Before the patient's entry into the OR, certain preparations may be needed. These may be performed in the same-day admission area or holding room, depending on space and privacy. The holding room nurse may be the one to perform a chart review and patient assessment. The intraoperative nurse may perform these or complete the assessment process. This is the place where any errors or omissions may be corrected, e.g., removal of dentures or constricting jewelry. If hair removal is needed, it is done here with clippers or wet razor. Insertion of intravenous lines, arterial, or other invasive monitoring devices may be completed. With monitoring as needed, some institutions insert regional blocks in a holding area. Preoperative sedation may be given. It is important that the patient be given the opportunity to speak with the surgeon, anesthesiologist, and nurse before sedation to allow them to have their questions and concerns addressed (Atkinson & Fortunato, 1996).

ENTRY INTO THE OPERATING ROOM

The patient enters the operating room after all the requirements of the chart review have been met to prevent delays and ensure patient safety and optimal care. The nurse has completed his or her initial assessment and prepared the operating room for the specific patient and procedural needs. Preparation about the sights, sounds, and other environmental features of the OR as appropriate will assist in making the patient comfortable. The room should be warm while the patient is aware, and comfort measures such as warm blankets and pillows provided without the patient having to request these. The room should be quiet. The patient must remain the focus of attention. Patients' hearing is acute from sedatives and during the initial phase of the induction of general anesthesia. Loud music and conversations about other patients are inappropriate. Patients can misconstrue overheard information to pertain to them and this may elicit unnecessary fear or anxiety. The patient must be supervised and protected from falls or other injuries by having the appropriate number of personnel during any patient transfers. Tell the patient what you plan to do and request their assistance. If the patient is able to transfer himself, the stretcher and OR bed must be locked and a person standing on either side. If the patient must be lifted, at least four people are needed. Body alignment must be maintained at all times to prevent injury or discomfort.

ANESTHETIC CONSIDERATIONS

The anesthetic options for vascular procedures include local anesthesia, local anesthesia with monitored anesthesia care, regional, general, and combinations of the above. A few minor procedures lend themselves to straight local anesthesia. These may include ligation of a single arteriovenous AV fistula after arterial leg bypass, creation of an AV fistula or other vascular access device for dialysis, or insertion of a vena cava filter. The condition of the patient, basic competency training of the staff, surgeon preference, and potential for complications necessarily guide the surgeon in requesting the appropriate provider of care. Institutional policy must clearly designate the patient acuity level for local anesthesia cases monitored by a nurse. The nurse monitoring a local patient must have no other duties that will interrupt this. The minimum monitoring includes BP, pulse, heart rate and rhythm, oxygen saturation, skin condition, and mental state (AORN Recommended Practices for Monitoring the Patient Receiving Local Anesthesia, 1996).

The surgeon generally initiates a preference for local anesthesia or the services of the anesthesia team at the time the surgery is scheduled. The final choice of anesthetic is determined by the anesthetist with the informed consent of the patient. This choice will be based primarily on patient safety. The patient's emotional and mental status are considered. A patient's fear of a particular type of anesthetic may determine the choice made. The surgical site, length and invasiveness of procedure, and patient position are considered. Patient acuity and coexisting disease will heavily influence the choice. A regional anesthetic may be chosen in patients with severe cardiac disease. An epidural anesthetic may be used alone, in conjunction with general anesthesia, or for those patients needing postoperative pain control (Hoffer, 1995). Epidural catheter placement has the advantage over a spinal in that it can be augmented to increase the length of time of anesthesia for a surgical procedure that lasts longer than anticipated. Spinal anesthesia has an almost immediate onset while epidurals can take 10 to 20 minutes before surgical care can commence. The induction of anesthesia is a critical time for the patient. The circulating nurse should suspend all other duties to be in

attendance at the patient's side. The nurse should provide comfort and support by his or her presence and touch as appropriate by offering a hand to hold. The nurse is available to assist as needed such as by applying cricoid pressure (Sellick's maneuver) during intubation as requested by the anesthetist. This reduces the risk of regurgitation and aspiration by occluding the esophagus. Cricoid pressure may be applied before induction and maintained until the endotracheal tube cuff is inflated and the anesthetist is satisfied with the airway (Atkinson & Fortunato, 1996). Some anesthesiologists may elect to apply cricoid pressure for the induction and intubation of all diabetics because these patients have delayed stomach emptying under normal circumstances (Chlebowski, 1996). The nurse also remains available and alert to assist in any other way and whenever emergency measures are needed. The same vigilance applies to extubation and emergence from anesthesia.

In the role of patient advocate and manager and coordinator of intraoperative care, the circulating nurse must ensure that the patient's dignity and privacy are maintained. The patient must remain covered for these reasons as well as to maintain normal body temperature. Patient awareness during anesthesia is not always predictable. The last sensation to diminish during general anesthesia is hearing. In a literature review, Eldor and Frankel (1991) found the smallest percentage of cases with patient's reporting awareness during surgery were those who had light anesthesia because they were unstable at a serious point of the operation. Patients have recalled conversations during anesthesia and some have had lasting psychologic sequelae from subconscious hearing of negative events and sounds. Hypnosis has been used and patients have repeated things said during surgery using anesthetic techniques and assessments that presumed recall was impossible that they could not consciously recall (Eldor & Frankel, 1991). No anesthetic technique can be considered completely free of the possibility of patient awareness. It has been suggested that the possibility of awareness be explained to patients as a minor risk of anesthesia. As public awareness increases, so does litigation. Patients have been awarded claims for recall and resultant posttraumatic stress syndrome. Many patients fear they will wake up during anesthesia. Their fears may be based on previous experience and should be discussed with sympathy. Anesthetic techniques of balanced anesthesia, widely used in the 1970s and 1980s, contributed to this problem. Positive suggestions during general anesthesia have reportedly contributed to favorable surgical outcomes and decreased lengths of stay. Adverse situations could trigger adverse outcomes (Heneghan, 1993). Any unnecessary stimulation must be avoided during induction, but especially noise. The scrub nurse must be aware of this and avoid the sounds produced by the enthusiastic handling of metal instruments. OR doors must be kept closed to prevent noise from the halls, for adequate air exchange for asepsis, and for privacy.

INTRAOPERATIVE MONITORING

The American Society of Anesthesiologists (ASA) has developed standards for patient monitoring. These include the presence of qualified personnel and the documentation and assessment of the patient's oxygenation, ventilation, circulation, and temperature. The perioperative nurse must be aware of the basic standards for patient monitoring (Box 7-2). Two significant advances in monitoring include the use of a pulse oximeter (SpO_2) to measure the percentage of oxygen in the blood and a means to measure the end tidal carbon dioxide ($ETCO_2$). Different types of monitors exist but basically they allow an approximation of alveolar function and arterial CO_2 (Hoffer, 1995).

Intraoperative monitoring for vascular patients consists of the basic ECG, pulse oximeter, and blood pressure cuff ($ETCO_2$ for general anesthesia). For patients undergoing saphenous vein stripping or amputation these are usually adequate. For lengthy procedures, as in arterial bypass or reconstruction, an arterial line is usually placed percutaneously in the radial artery. This is kept open by a heparin drip attached to a transducer, and a waveform monitor reads out the systolic and diastolic pressures. The monitor also calculates the mean arterial pressure (MAP, 70 to 105 mmHg), which aids in the evaluation of the perfusion of systemic and cardiac circulation. This arterial line also allows easy access for collecting specimens for arterial blood gas analysis. The electrocardiogram and direct arterial lines are used for monitoring and assessment. Continuous assessment of the patient's arterial pressure is a critical part of the surgical procedure. Pulmonary capillary wedge pressure as an index of left atrial pressure (LAP) and left ventricular end diastolic pressure (LVEDP) may be monitored depending on the patient's physiologic status. Because many patients undergoing vascular surgery have generalized atherosclerotic disease, the nurse should be constantly alert for cardiac arrhythmias and blood pressure changes. Acid-base balance and pulmonary gas exchange may be assessed from the blood gas analysis (Atkinson & Fortunato, 1996) (Tables 7-1 and 7-2).

A central venous pressure catheter (CVP) or various types of pulmonary artery (PA) catheters may be inserted via the right internal jugular (RIJ) vein. The CVP line allows assessment of blood volume and vascular tone in a patient with a normal heart. The more sophisticated PA catheters (e.g., the Swan-Ganz) can monitor cardiac output, fluid balance, and the cardiac response to drugs (Guzzetta & Dossey, 1992). These would be used for aortic surgery or patients with cardiac disease (MacVittie, 1995).

The carotid endarterectomy patient can be monitored with electroencephalography (EEG). This allows immediate observation of slowing of the brain waves caused by cerebral ischemia or reduced perfusion. The surgeon may elect to place a temporary shunt in the artery if this occurs when she or he clamps. This could reduce the chance of perioperative stroke.

Table 7-1 **Normal Blood Chemistry Laboratory Values**

PARAMETER	NORMAL VALUES FOR ADULTS
Base excess of blood	0 ± 2 mmol/L
Bicarbonate (HCO_3)	22-26 mEq/L
Bilirubin (total)	0.1-1.0 mg/dl
Blood urea nitrogen (BUN)	5-20 mg/dl
Calcium (Ca)	9.0-10.5 mg/dl
Carbon dioxide (CO_2) in serum	23-30 mEq/L
Chloride (Cl)	90-110 mEq/L
Creatinine	0.7-1.5 mg/dl
Creatinine phosphokinase (CPK)	12-80 U/L
Glucose	70-115 mg/dl
Magnesium (Mg)	1.6-3.0 mEq/L
pH of serum	7.35-7.45
Phosphate (P)	2.5-4.5 mg/dl
Potassium (K)	3.5-5.0 mEq/L
Sodium (Na)	136-145 mEq/L
Serum glutamic oxaloacetic transaminase (SGOT)	5-40 IU/L
Serum glutamic pyruvic transaminase (SGPT)	5-35 IU/L

From Atkinson L. J., & Fortunato N. H. (1996). *Operating room technique* (8th ed.). St. Louis: Mosby.

Table 7-2 **Normal Values for Arterial Blood Gases and Abnormal Values in Uncompensated Acid-Base Disturbances**

ACID-BASE DISTURBANCES	pH	Pco_2 (MMHG)	HCO_3^- (MEQ/L)	COMMON CAUSE
None (normal values)	7.35-7.45	35-45	22-26	
Respiratory acidosis	↓	↑	Normal	Respiratory depression (drugs, central nervous system trauma) Pulmonary disease (pneumonia, chronic obstructive pulmonary disease, respiratory underventilation)
Respiratory alkalosis	↑	↓	Normal	Hyperventilation (emotions, pain, respirator overventilation)
Metabolic acidosis	↓	Normal	↓	Diabetes, shock, renal failure, intestinal fistula
Metabolic alkalosis	↑	Normal	↑	Sodium bicarbonate overdose, prolonged vomiting, nasogastric drainage

Pagana K. D., & Pagana J. (1997). *Mosby's diagnostic and laboratory test reference* (3rd ed.). St. Louis: Mosby.

Box 7-2 **Standards for Basic Anesthetic Monitoring**

STANDARD I

Qualified anesthesia personnel shall be present in the room throughout the conduct of all general anesthetics, regional anesthetics and monitored anesthesia care.

OBJECTIVE

Because of the rapid changes in patient status during anesthesia, qualified anesthesia personnel shall be continuously present to monitor the patient and provide anesthesia care. In the event there is a direct known hazard, e.g., radiation, to the anesthesia personnel which might require intermittent remote observation of the patient, some provision for monitoring the patient must be made. In the event that an emergency requires the temporary absence of the person primarily responsible for the anesthetic, the best judgment of the anesthesiologist will be exercised in comparing the emergency with the anesthetized patient's condition and in the selection of the person left responsible for the anesthetic during the temporary absence.

STANDARD II

During all anesthetics, the patient's oxygenation, ventilation, circulation and temperature shall be continually evaluated.

OXYGENATION

Objective

To ensure adequate oxygen concentration in the inspired gas and the blood during all anesthetics.

Methods

1) Inspired gas: During every administration of general anesthesia using an anesthesia machine, the concentration of oxygen in the patient breathing system shall be measured by an oxygen analyzer with a low oxygen concentration limit alarm in use.
2) Blood oxygenation: During all anesthetics, a quantitative method of assessing oxygenation such as pulse oximetry shall be employed. Adequate illumination and exposure of the patient are necessary to assess color.

VENTILATION

Objective

To ensure adequate ventilation of the patient during all anesthetics.

Methods

1) Every patient receiving general anesthesia shall have the adequacy of ventilation continually evaluated. While qualitative clinical signs such as chest excursion, observation of the reservoir breathing bag and auscultation of breath sounds may be useful, quantitative monitoring of the carbon dioxide content and/or volume of expired gas is strongly encouraged.
2) When an endotracheal tube is inserted, its presence in the trachea must be verified by clinical assessment and by identification of carbon dioxide in the expired gas. Continual end-tidal carbon dioxide analysis, in the use from the time of endotracheal tube placement, until extubation or initiating transfer to a postoperative care location, shall be performed using a quantitative method such as capnography, capnometry or mass spectroscopy.
3) When ventilation is controlled by a mechanical ventilator, there shall be in continuous use a device that is capable of detecting disconnection of components of the breathing system. The device must give an audible signal when its alarm threshold is exceeded.
4) During regional anesthesia and monitored anesthesia care, the adequacy of ventilation shall be evaluated, at least, by continual observation of qualitative clinical signs.

CIRCULATION

Objective

To ensure the adequacy of the patient's circulatory function during all anesthetics.

Methods

1) Every patient receiving anesthesia shall have the electrocardiogram continuously displayed from the beginning of anesthesia until preparing to leave the anesthetizing location.
2) Every patient receiving anesthesia shall have arterial blood pressure and heart rate determined and evaluated at least every five minutes.
3) Every patient receiving general anesthesia shall have, in addition to the above, circulatory function continually evaluated by at least one of the following: palpation of a pulse, auscultation of heart sounds, monitoring of a tracing of intra-arterial pressure, ultrasound peripheral pulse monitoring, or pulse plethysmography or oximetry.

BODY TEMPERATURE

Objective

To aid in the maintenance of appropriate body temperature during all anesthetics.

Methods

There shall be readily available a means to continuously measure the patient's temperature. When changes in body temperature are intended, anticipated or suspected, the temperature shall be measured.

Adapted from Standards for Basic Anesthetic Monitoring, as amended 1995, of the American Society of Anesthesiologists. A copy of the full text can be obtained from ASA, 520 N. Northwest Highway, Park Ridge, Il, 60068-2573

Transesophageal echocardiography may be used to noninvasively monitor the heart during aortic surgery. The device looks similar to a bronchoscope and can be passed down the esophagus to provide an ultrasonic image. The cardiac structures, blood flow, wall motion, and great vessels can be observed (Canobbio, 1990). The equipment is very expensive and requires highly skilled personnel and thus may not be available in many settings. However, it can detect cardiac changes of impending MI before other monitoring modalities (Docker, Muthasamy, Balasundaramy, & Duran, 1992) and could be important to evaluate the effect of aortic cross-clamping in aortic surgery.

POSITIONING

Positioning of the patient undergoing vascular surgery is of particular importance because of restricted circulation distal to the area of arterial obstruction and the fact that many vascular patients have systemic vascular disease. Particular care must be exercised in positioning elderly patients. Awareness of joint range of motion limitations caused by immobility or joint surgery is critical even for a procedure as routine as Foley catheter insertion. Preoperative assessment can prevent injury and decrease OR time. Whenever possible, have the patient demonstrate the ability to assume the position for the proposed procedure while they are awake and can provide feedback. A foot board may be applied to the operating room bed to prevent the weight of drapes resting on the patient's lower extremities. For a carotid endarterectomy, the patient's head may be supported on a doughnut or a head support. A roll may be placed between the scapulae. For surgical procedures involving a lower extremity, the patient's thigh may be externally rotated and abducted with the knee flexed. A small bolster may be used under the knee to support the patient's leg. Proper skeletal alignment during surgery prevents injury to the neuromuscular system. Attention to the skin overlying bony prominences, especially the heels, sacrum, and elbows, and the use of proper supports and pads prevent injury to the patient. Because of the lengthy nature of these procedures, an egg crate mattress or gel-filled pad can be placed on the operating room bed to help prevent patient injury. For the same reasons, members of the scrubbed team should also be cognizant of heavy instruments and drapes resting on the patient's body and take measures to avoid pressure injuries (MacVittie, 1995). A radiopaque OR bed should be used for all vascular procedures in the event that an angiogram must be done. The patient should be positioned carefully to allow x-ray access to the appropriate part of the body.

SKIN PREPARATION

Skin preparation for vascular surgery may be extensive. For abdominal aortic surgery, the patient's skin is prepared from the nipple line to the knees. For peripheral vascular surgery on the extremities, the patient is prepped from the umbilicus to the feet. The patient's legs are prepared circumferentially. For carotid surgery, the patient is prepped from the ear and chin on the affected side to below the clavicle. Draping should permit the surgeon free access to involved areas. For example, abdominal surgery may also require exposure of the groin region for possible exploration of the femoral arteries. A femoral-popliteal bypass on one leg may require access to the other leg

for harvesting of the saphenous vein. AORN Recommended Practices for Skin Preparation of Patients (1995) describes sound practice to include assessment of the skin, cleanliness, careful hair removal only where needed, and the use of an antimicrobial agent. The antimicrobial agent must be allowed to air dry before draping for maximal duration of effect. Measures should be taken to prevent or correct any pooling of prep solutions under the patient. Pooled fluid can cause a skin reaction from lengthy contact with the agent, possibly from a reaction to the bleach or detergent residue in the linen, and can promote skin breakdown from the presence of moisture. Impervious drapes should be used to prevent contamination of the surgical field from blood and irrigation fluids.

A urinary catheter should be inserted, especially if the proposed procedure involves the renal arteries or clamping the aorta above the renal arteries, if considerable blood loss is anticipated, if the planned procedure time is lengthy, or whenever spinal or epidural anesthesia is used because they delay the patient's ability to void voluntarily. Urinary catheterization facilitates accurate hourly measurements of urine during and after the surgical procedure and assists in the assessment of renal perfusion and fluid status.

A thorough discussion of all that is involved with aseptic technique is beyond the scope of this book. Asepsis is a team effort but the circulating nurse is usually the most knowledgeable and in the best position to monitor the aseptic practices intraoperatively. Limiting the number of personnel and visitors, limiting traffic through the OR, and good organizational skills to limit the transport of supplies and equipment are a few of the things that can minimize breaks in aseptic technique. Unnecessary movement and talking should be discouraged. Universal precautions must be practiced by all personnel to protect the patients and personnel. Nurses are usually responsible for monitoring the environment for cleanliness, safety, and comfort.

COUNTS

Another area of safety involves the counting of items used intraoperatively to ensure that nothing is left in a patient unintentionally. All operating rooms must have policies in place to cover counting of instruments, sponges, sharps, and other small items used on the sterile field (AORN Recommended Practices for Sponge, Sharps, and Instrument Counts, 1996). Counts are performed to prevent leaving an item in a patient that could cause infection or other injury. Patient safety is an important role of the professional nurse. The counts are an example of accountabilty for optimal patient outcomes. Counts may also be justifiable to ensure inventory control and prevent loss through careless handling. Some institutions elect not to count instruments in procedures where no body cavity is entered and therefore there is no possibility of loss of an object in the patient. The time savings may be justified in these instances. However, if instrument sets are streamlined and the instrument lists efficiently organized, counting instruments should take only minutes. Sponges and other items must be counted initially on all procedures and the nurse may decide to discontinue unnecessary counts before closure if the procedure does not warrant one. Policies should state specifically when and how counts are performed. Safe practice includes the following: the scrub nurse and circulating nurse count together, aloud, as the scrub nurse points to each item. Interruptions of the counting process can lead to errors or omissions. Counts are done to protect the patient as well as the staff and hospital. Incorrect counts require immediate action. The nurse must inform the surgeon, who should search the field and wound as soon as possible. The nurse must search the room, trash, and linen hampers. Assistance should be obtained to prevent prolonging the patient's time under anesthesia or time in the OR. Items that are already counted and off the sterile field, such as sponges, should be carefully recounted. An x-ray should be taken for any item that is radiopaque. The results are documented according to policy (Pierson, 1995).

BLOOD LOSS

All surgical patients should have accurate intraoperative intake and output assessment and documentation. Fluid administration may be controlled and documented by anesthesia personnel but the circulator must maintain an awareness of intake. The circulator will also ensure that urinary output is monitored and will monitor and communicate fluid loss. This requires the scrub nurse to communicate accurate use of irrigation fluids. An experienced nurse may be able to estimate blood loss visually when it pools on the drapes and floor. Using a scale to weigh sponges is advisable to prevent miscalculation. One g is estimated as 1 ml of blood. The weight of a dry sponge and a saline-moistened sponge should be posted so that the sponge weight can be subtracted from the total weight (Atkinson & Fortunato, 1996: Pierson, 1995). Writing the blood loss on a board visible to the surgical and anesthesia teams can be helpful during cases with massive blood loss. This allows all members to have the information without interrupting anyone's work at a crucial time. Heavy blood loss can be anticipated in some vascular surgeries. Heavy blood loss can be anticipated for procedures that are near or involve the aorta, thrombectomies, trauma to an artery, or anytime the surgeon communicates the anticipation of a potentially difficult case.

HOMOLOGOUS BLOOD

Homologous blood donation (drawn from one person and transfused into another) has become a major public concern since the advent of the HIV epidemic. Patients do not always trust banked blood and verbalize requests that they not receive blood transfusions. Public concern has driven improvements in screening, collection practices, and research for alternatives. Investigation of methods to stimulate a patient's own bone marrow to avoid transfusion have received more attention (Nielsen, 1995). The actual risk of AIDS is low statistically but any risk is unacceptable to the public. Hepatitis transmission, at a rate of about one case per 6000 units transfused, is more common than AIDS. Cytomegalovirus is increasing as a risk factor as a result of the increase in immunosuppresssed transplant and cancer patients (Perkins, 1995). Institutions have developed stricter guidelines and policies for the criteria for transfusion during surgery. Quality improvement strategies are often very strict and specific about these parameters. Fourteen million units of blood are transfused into 13.2 million patients in the United States annually. Of these, there are approximately 120,000 adverse reactions. Acute hemolytic reactions have been reported as occurring 1 in every 25,000 units of red blood cells as a result of clerical errors of incorrectly identified blood samples or incorrectly identified patients. The risk of renal failure or death is fairly high for the transfusion of incompatible blood. True anaphylactic reactions have an occurrence rate of 1 in every 150,000 units transfused. Bacterial contamination is rare in units of red blood cells (RBCs) (1 in 2.5 million) but increases to 1 in 350 units for platelets. This has been attributed to the fact that platelets are stored at 22° C (71.6° F) (Sloop & Friedberg, 1995). Research indicates that blood transfusions, both homologous and autologous, carry an increased risk of infectious complications related to a triggered immunosuppression. Surgery seems to trigger immune responses; minor surgeries may stimulate the immune system and major surgeries and recent traumas may suppress the immune system for periods that range from days to weeks. In comparison, transfusions to nonsurgical patients have been found to cause an immune response for unknown reasons. The timing of a blood transfusion may be very critical to this process; this has been most impressive in the intraoperative phase to about 48 hours postoperative. This immunosuppression phenomenon has been linked to surgical wound infections but more research needs to be done in this area (Nielsen, 1995). Immediate reactions that should cause concern include hemolytic, febrile, allergic, and fluid overload. Symptoms vary and can be masked by anesthesia and the inability of the anesthetized patient to communicate subjective responses (Tranter, 1995).

AUTOLOGOUS BLOOD

For the reasons just described, alternatives to homologous blood replacement have been investigated (Box 7-3). For volume expansion, crystalloids and colloids are infused (Williamson, 1994). Autologous blood is blood recovered and returned to the same patient. The process is referred to as autotransfusion. In some instances, Jehovah's Witness patients may accept this form of blood replacement (Atkinson and Fortunato, 1996). Preoperative blood donation has become increasingly popular. Patients who can tolerate this may donate as often as every 4 days up to 72 hours before elective surgery. Whole blood may be stored for 35 days and RBCs for 42 days. The same safety precautions and procedures must be followed as for other donated blood products (Atkinson and Fortunato, 1996). Since clerical error could result in this blood reaching the wrong patient, this is still not risk free and is not given to the patient unless needed.

Hemodilution is another means to avoid blood transfusion. The anesthesiologist removes and stores 500 to 1000 ml of blood from the patient at the time of the induction of anesthesia. Colloids are infused to place the patient's HCT at 25% to 30%. This reduces the number of RBCs lost during surgery. The patient's blood is then reinfused at the conclusion of the surgical procedure or sooner if needed (Williamson, 1994; Atkinson and Fortunato, 1996).

Medications may help reduce the need for blood transfusions. Vasodilators to lower blood pressure may be used to decrease blood loss but is not the first choice in most vascular patients. Aprotinin, a serine protease inhibitor, has been used primarily in cardiac patients to reduce blood loss during surgery (Levy et al, 1995).

Box 7-3 Alternatives to Banked Blood

Volume expansion
   cystalloids (e.g., Lactated Ringers)
   colloids (e.g., albumin)
Autologous RBCs
   preoperative donation
   perioperative hemodilution
   intraoperative or postoperative cell salvage
Medications to decrease blood loss
   aprotinin
   desmopressin acetate (DDAVP)
   vasodilators or hypotensive anesthesia
Meticulous surgical technique
Blood substitutes or "artificial blood"
   hemoglobin solutions* (derived from outdated blood
   products)
   per fluorocarbons* (low oxygen-carrying ability)

Adapted from Williamson, 1994; and Atkinson & Fortunato, 1996.
*Still in trial phase.

Intraoperative blood salvage is another means to recover blood from surgical procedures. There are systems that use a dual lumen suction tubing to collect the blood from the surgical field. The dual lumen allows an anticoagulant (heparinized saline or a citrate phosphate dextrose solution) to run continuously, mix with the blood at the suction wand, and collect in a sterile cannister. This filtered (140 µm filter) blood may be given directly to the patient or processed. It could be processed by the blood bank or on site in a centrifuge processor. This separates out most drugs, debris, white cells, and plasma. WARNING: Do not salvage blood when microfibrillar collagen has been used because it does not wash out and has been implicated in disseminated intravascular coagulation (DIC) and adult respiratory distress syndrome (ARDS) (Atkinson and Fortunato, 1996). The red cells are then drawn off into a sterile IV bag and returned to the patient intravenously (see Figure 8-10). Massive blood transfusion increases the risk of the patient developing a coagulopathy. Some studies have defined massive as 10 units of blood or more but no clear correlation exists between the number of transfusions and the development of a severe coagulopathy. The causes appear to be multifactorial (Harvey, Greenfield, Sugrue, & Rosenfeld, 1995).

DEATH IN THE OPERATING ROOM
Staff Considerations

Death in the operating room is infrequent. In emergency situations it may be sudden and totally unanticipated by family and, at times, by staff. Nurses may experience grief when a patient dies whether or not they had extensive contact or knowledge of the patient. The nurse's own unresolved grief may prevent or at least inhibit the ability to support the grieving family members. Nurses must develop awareness of their beliefs and abilities in order to be able to utilize therapeutic listening skills. Awareness of one's limitations will allow mature responses that assist the

family in coping with their immediate grief. Lack of self-awareness may result in the staff member personalizing the experience rather than detaching from it. Many health care providers have not had extensive experience in dealing with death and may experience feelings of helplessness, anger, fear, denial, or detachment. The nurse needs to recognize when it is necessary to seek time away and provide self-care (Potter & Perry, 1993). Self-care strategies include acknowledging the positive efforts made by oneself and other team members, sharing feelings, crying, and bringing the event to closure (Atkinson & Fortunato, 1996). Knowing what is helpful and what is not helpful can make a difference in the successful resolution of grief by the family (Box 7-4). The nurse is legally accountable for treating a body with dignity and respect (Potter & Perry, 1993). Postmortem care of the body is particularly distressing to OR nursing personnel because of the quiet that descends (monitors and ventilators stop) and the fact that the majority of team members leave. Surgeons must inform families and anesthesiologists no longer need to provide care. The nurses are left to wash the patient and place identification markers on the body for transfer to the morgue.

Family Considerations

It is important to understand the grieving process, especially in acute loss situations, and recognize the many forms of grief reactions. Patient and family behavior must be accepted as long as a safe situation exists and no harm will come to self or others. If the family wishes to see the patient, the nurses are present to provide support (Atkinson & Fortunato, 1996). It is best to move the patient to a room less intimidating than the OR. The nurse should provide a quiet, private environment with chairs, tissues, and spirits of ammonia available.

END OF PROCEDURE: ASSESSMENT, REPORT, DOCUMENTATION

Documentation of patient problems and nursing actions addressing these identified problems is important. Nursing assessments and interventions are recorded. Every patient is identified and assessed for allergies. The surgical procedure is verified and any other interventions performed by the nurse for patient safety and mandated by institution policy are documented. A brief mental status examination and neurologic check is especially important for vascular patients who are at risk for stroke. For a patient undergoing vascular surgery, possible areas to document include the preoperative and postoperative assessment of the integrity of the patient's skin, the presence or absence of peripheral pulses, the surgical position and positioning devices used, fluid intake and output, and the progress made toward the achievement of patient goals. During surgery various local anesthetic drugs and irrigating solutions, such as thrombin, antibiotic, and heparin solutions, may be used. The scrub nurse should label each container with the solution type and strength. The circulating nurse maintains an accurate record of the solutions used and the amounts administered. The type, size, and serial and lot numbers of vascular implants should be documented according to institutional policy and procedure (MacVittie, 1995). (Refer to the chapters on specific surgeries for additional documentation needs.)

Box 7-4 Suggestions for Verbal Support

WHAT TO SAY

1. I wish there was something I could say or do to ease your pain.
2. I am so sorry. I am so sad for you.
3. Tell me about your son/daughter/husband/wife.
4. I know you hurt terribly right now. This situation must seem unbearable.
5. Do you have any questions about the death?
6. Discuss the death with the family: e.g., While she was in the operating room she was asleep under anesthesia so she had no pain at the end.
7. Talk about the patient's last words if appropriate.
8. If guilt feelings are expressed: This is not your fault.

WHAT TO AVOID SAYING

1. Be strong. Pull yourself together.
2. It is God's will.
3. I know how you are feeling.
4. Go ahead and cry, it's okay to cry (if they are not crying).
5. To parents: You're lucky you have other children.
6. Do not talk about *your* experiences.

Adapted from Watson, 1994; Mian, 1990; Gifford & Cleary, 1990; Antonacci, 1990; Bolton, 1996.

The circulating nurse must plan ahead for transferring the patient to the appropriate unit. If the patient's acuity changes and he or she requires intensive care nursing that was not anticipated, the nurse should coordinate communication with the appropriate personnel to provide a smooth transition. Documentation is important but verbal communication is essential to ensure that priorities are maintained. Adequate time must be given for the receiving nurses and other personnel to be ready. It may be necessary to obtain a respirator or alter personnel assignments to provide adequate coverage for patient care. The patient should have a general assessment by the nurse just before transfer. Skin integrity must be assessed and noted, the patient should be clean, and dressings should be intact . A comfortable position should be attempted if possible. If the patient has been supine for a long period it would be helpful to position them on their side to relieve the pressure that has been on their back, heels, and other pressure areas. Care is taken to prevent respiratory compromise or limit immediate access to the surgical incision. Send the patient to the receiving nurse in the condition you would like to receive them. Unless patient transfer would be hampered or delayed, OR staff should strive to:

- Wash prep solutions, blood, and any other drainage from the skin
- Check that dressings are clean and intact
- Secure catheters and drains as appropriate
- Untangle and secure IVs, arterial lines, etc.
- Maintain patient dignity and privacy by using adequate covers
- Check that the medical record is intact and with the patient

- Check that transport equipment is functioning (O_2 tank, monitors, etc)
- Ensure that a cooler of blood for transfusion accompanies the patient if needed.

References

Atonacci M. (1990). Sudden death: Helping bereaved parents in the PICU. *Critical Care Nurse*, 10(4): 65-70.

Association of Operating Room Nurses (1996). Recommended practices for monitoring the patient receiving local anesthesia. In *AORN standards and recommended practices for perioperative nursing.* Denver: The Association.

Association of Operating Room Nurses (1996). Recommended practices for skin preparation of patients. In *AORN standards and recommended practices for perioperative nursing.* Denver: The Association.

Association of Operating Room Nurses (1996). Recommended practices for sponge, sharp, and instrument counts. In *AORN standards and recommended practices for perioperative nursing.* Denver: The Association.

Atkinson, L. J., & Fortunato, N. H. (1996). *Operating room technique* (8th ed.). St. Louis: Mosby.

Bolton, V. (January 1996). Personal communication.

Brumfield, V. C., Kee, C. C., & Johnson, J. Y. (1996). Preoperative patient teaching in ambulatory surgery setting. *AORN Journal*, 64(4): 941, 943-946, 948.

Canobbio, M. M. (Ed.) (1990). Diagnostic procedures. In *Cardiovascular disorders* (pp 41-60). St. Louis: Mosby.

Carton, R. W., & Brown, M. D. (1993). Ethical considerations and CPR in the elderly patient. *Clinics in Chest Medicine*, 14(3):591-599.

Cheblowski, S. (January, 1996). Personal communication.

Clark, G. D., Lucas, K., & Stephens, L. (1994). Ethical dilemmas and decisions concerning the do-not-resuscitate patient undergoing anesthesia. *American Association of Nurse Anesthetists Journal*, 62(3):253-256.

Cohen, C. B., & Cohen, P. J. (1991). Do-not-rescuscitate orders in the operating room. *New England Journal of Medicine*, 332:1879-1882.

Docker, C. S., Muthusamy, R., Balasundaramy, S., & Duran, C. (1992). Intra-operative echocardiography: An essential tool in cardiac surgery...epicardial...echocardiography...transesophageal echocardiography. *AORN Journal*, 55(1), 167, 169-170, 172-173.

Eldor, J., & Frankel, D. Z. N. (1991). Intra-anesthetic awareness. *Resuscitation*, 21(2-3): 113-119.

Golanowski, M. (1995). Do not resuscitate: Informed consent in the operating room and postanesthesia care unit. *Journal of Post Anesthesia Nursing*, 10(1): 9-11.

Gifford, B. J., & Cleary, B. B. (1990). Supporting the bereaved. *American Journal of Nursing*, 90(2): 48-55.

Guzzetta, C. E., & Dossey, B. M. (1992). *Cardiovascular nursing: Holistic practice.* St. Louis: Mosby.

Harvey, M. P., Greenfield, T. P., Sugrue, M. E., & Rosenfeld, D. (1995). Massive blood transfusions in a tertiary referral hospital: Clinical outcomes and haemastatic complications. *Medical Journal of Australia*, 163(7): 356-359.

Heneghan, C. (1993). Clinical and medicolegal aspects of conscious awareness during anesthesia. *International Anesthesiology Clinics*, 31(4):1-11.

Hoffer, J. L. (1995). Anesthesia. In M. H. Meeker, & J. C. Rothrock (Eds.), *Alexander's care of the patient in surgery* (10th ed., pp. 143-181). St. Louis: Mosby.

Levy, J. H., et al (1995). A multicenter, double-blind, placebo-controlled trial of aprotinin for reducing blood loss and the requirement for donor-blood transfusion in patients undergoing repeat coronary artery bypass grafting. *Circulation*, 92(8): 2236-2244.

Mian, P. (1990). Sudden bereavement: Nursing interventions in the ED. *Critical Care Nurse*, 10(1):30-41.

MacVittie, B. A. (1995). Vascular surgery. In M. H. Meeker, & J. C. Rothrock (Eds.), *Alexander's care of the patient in surgery* (10th ed., pp. 1033-1057). St. Louis: Mosby.

Nielsen, H. J. (1995). Detrimental effects of perioperative blood transfusion. *British Journal of Surgery 82*(5): 582-587.

Perkins, H. (1995). Transfusion reactions: The changing priorities. *Immunological Investigations, 24*(1-2): 289-302.

Pierson, M. A. (1995). Patient and environmental safety. In M. H. Meeker, & J. C. Rothrock (Eds.), *Alexander's care of the patient in surgery* (10th ed., pp. 19-34). St. Louis: Mosby.

Pokalo, C. (1992). Understanding the Patient Self-Determination Act. *Journal of Gerontological Nursing, 18*(3): 47.

Potter, P. A., & Perry, A. G. (1993). Loss, death and greiving. In P. A. Potter, & A. G. Perry (Eds.), *Fundamentals of nursing: Concepts, process, and practice* (3rd ed.). St. Louis: Mosby.

Sloop, G. D., & Friedberg, R. C. (1995). Complications of blood transfusions: How to recognize and respond to noninfectious reactions. *Postgraduate medicine, 98*(1): 159-162, 166, 169-172.

Staff (1995a, October). Declining hospital inpatient days are creating bed oversupply. *OR Manager, 11*(10), p 25.

Staff (1995b, October). Interactive informed consent. *OR Manager 11*(10), p 34.

Tranter, J. (1995). Making sense of blood transfusions. *Nursing Times, 91*(36): 34-36.

Watson, M. A. (1994). Elder care: Bereavement in the elderly. *AORN Journal, 59*(5): 1079-1084.

Williamson, L. (1994). Homologous blood transfusions: The risks and alternatives. *British Journal of Haematology, 88*(3): 451-458.

8 Equipment, Supplies, and Instrumentation

THE OPERATING ROOM

The OR needs to be designed to consider traffic flow and efficient access for the equipment and personnel that enter for temporary tasks without requiring the sterile field to be rearranged for each situation. Depending on the hospital construction, a writing surface for the nurse may take the form of a computer, a built-in recessed desk, or use of a prep table or case cart top (Figure 8-1)

Communication systems are a critical component of every OR. Telephones in the OR may be positive or negative depending on their use. They are a negative if abused, such as requiring the performance of routine secretarial duties for the surgical team that draw the circulating nurses' attention from the patient. Nonessential incoming calls from patient units, offices, or personal calls may be difficult to restrict. The OR telephone may be very helpful if it is used to give direct patient reports to the PACU or ICU or communicate directly with the blood bank or other patient services. This direct communication allows accurate and timely information to be relayed avoiding the inaccuracies that can occur from speaking with a third party. This also permits the in room staff to remain in the OR and continue to supervise patient care. Any laboratory data that must be relayed over the phone must be done with the inclusion of the patient's name for accuracy. Unless the OR is equipped with computers, the phone may be the fastest way to receive laboratory results such as blood gas analysis. Intercoms may compromise patient care when calls are either inappropriate or poorly timed. Inappropriate calls include roll call of surgical team members, pathology results that could be inadvertently directed to the wrong room, or ill-timed broadcasts, e.g., at the time of anesthesia induction when sounds are increased, disturbing, and often misinterpreted by the patient. Atkinson (1992) suggests that intercoms may best be situated in areas adjacent to the OR such as the substerile area where the surgeon and patient will not be disturbed. Policies need to be established to define the appropriate utilization of communication tools and personnel need to be oriented to safe practices.

Operating Room Furniture

The vascular OR needs to be equipped with the basic furniture (Box 8-1). This includes a patient OR bed that is **radiopaque** and adaptable for full body fluoroscopy capabilities (Figure 8-2). Many vascular interventions may require the planned or unplanned need for an intraoperative angiogram. The optimal size of the room has been described as between 400 and 600 square feet (Atkinson, 1992). The increased technology demanded in today's ORs may require more space until more compact units, e.g., portable fluoroscopy and transesophageal echocardiogram (TEE) machines, are developed (Figures 8-3 and 8-4). The electrical outlets need to be plentiful. Anesthesia equipment that requires electrical outlets include the anesthesia machine, ECG monitor, pulse oximeter, activated clotting time (ACT) machine, TEE unit, automatic medication delivery units, and rapid infusion systems (Figures 8-5, 8-6, and 8-7). Aside from the anesthesia equipment, the following items are

Text continued on p. 89

Box 8-1 **Basic Operating Room Furniture**

OR bed
Arm boards
Safety belt
Instrument table (one or more)
Mayo stand
Ring stand
Prep table
Arm table for arm procedures (Figure 8-12)
Bovie or electrosurgical unit
IV poles or ether screen to hold drapes off patient
Trash hamper
Kickbucket (optional)
Linen hampers
Sitting stools
Standing platforms
In addition, the following are basic requirements and often built in:
Suction; this must include at least four suction lines (anesthesia needs one, two may be needed for the surgical field, and one for a cellsaver)
X-ray view box
Clock with a second hand and a stop clock with warning signals
Air line for tourniquet (some are powered electrically)
Nitrogen line or tank for power saw
Oxygen lines
Communication for emergency needs (may be an emergency alarm panel, intercom system, or call light that may be foot or hand activated to alert a control desk to summon assistance)

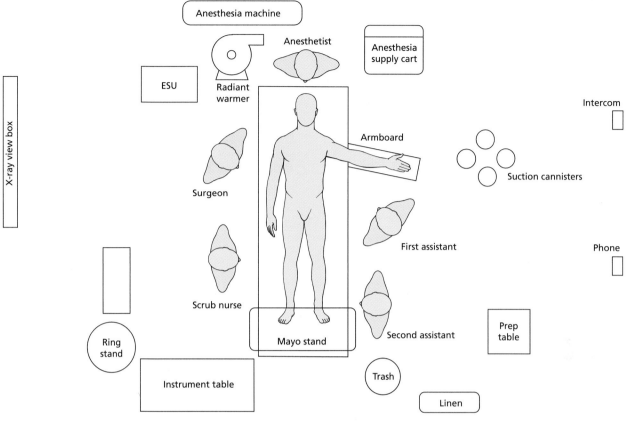

Fig. 8-1 Operating room set-up.

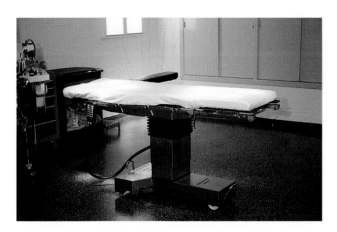

Fig. 8-2 Radiopaque bed.

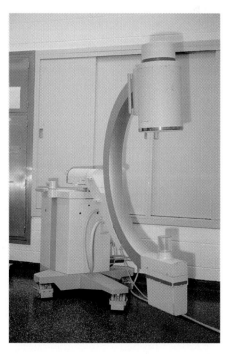

Fig. 8-3 C-arm or x-ray fluoroscopy machine.

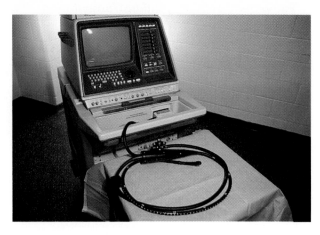

Fig. 8-4 Transesophageal echocardiography (TEE) machine and esophageal transducer probe.

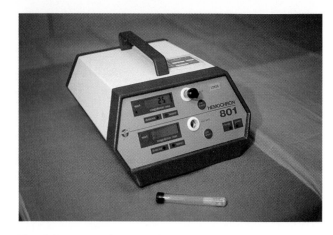

Fig. 8-5 ACT machine: used to measure bedside activated clotting time for titrating systemic anticoagulation and reversal intraoperatively.

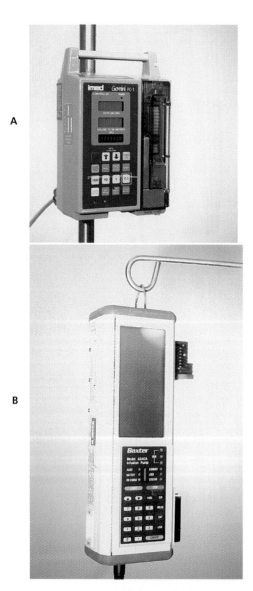

A

B

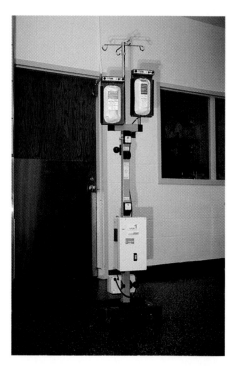

Fig. 8-7 Rapid infuser: provides a means for infusing and warming massive quantities of fluid or blood products.

Fig. 8-6 I-Med: useful for continuous infusion of medications such as heparin, Dextran, or antithrombolytic therapy. **A,** The pump can be programmed to control rate and volume and trigger alarms when air enters the line or infusion is complete or interrupted. **B,** A smaller infusion pump can be used with a syringe to infuse small amounts of medications.

frequently used simultaneously: electrosurgical unit (ESU), headlights, blood warmers, blood salvage machine, hypothermia machines or radiant heater, video camera, light source and viewer, and a fluoroscopy unit and monitor screen (Figures 8-8 to 8-11).

Equipment for Direct Patient Care

Because of the typical patient profile (see Chapter 5), the vascular patient is at risk for inadequate tissue perfusion, hypothermia, excessive blood loss, and pressure injury. Altered tissue perfusion results from both venous and arterial disease as well as from the decreased blood flow that results from the application of surgical clamps. Many of the patients are diabetic or have a history of smoking. Meticulous attention must be paid to positioning. Skin assessment is critical preoperatively to plan for individual patient needs. The presence of skin ulcers is a frequent finding in patients with lower extremity vascular disease. A full length gel mattress or similar OR bed mattress may aid in the prevention of intraoperative tissue damage. Positioning devices should be clean, appropriate and readily available (AORN Standards and Recommended Practices on Positioning, 1995) (Box 8-2). Although the chronic application of heating devices that patients with impaired circulation sometimes use for extremity warmth may be detrimental, the application of a warm blanket in the OR is a benign but essential comfort measure. A warmer for blankets and solutions should be available. A refrigerator is also needed in the OR suite for storing medications that must remain refrigerated, e.g., topical thrombin and cold physiologic solutions. Cold Normosol or Ringer's lactate may be the surgeon's choice for vein graft preservation. Certain technologies require the use of cold sterile saline such as the insertion of the Simon-Nitinol vena cava filter (see Chapter 18).

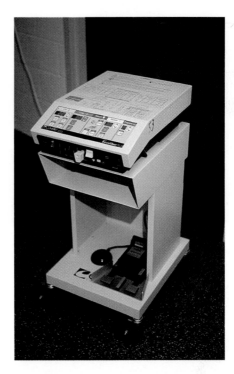

Fig. 8-8 Electrosurgical unit (ESU), also known as cautery or "Bovie."

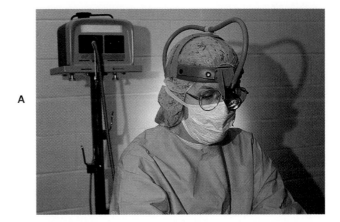

A

Fig. 8-9 Improved visibility can be augmented by the, **A,** headlights worn on the head by the surgeon with a fiberoptic cord going to a mobile light source and

---

Box 8-2 **Positioning Devices**

Arm boards
Gel pads
Axillary roll and gel ring for lateral positioning (Figure 8-13)
Sheep skin booties
Pillows
Warm blankets
Extremity holder for leg preps (Figure 8-14)
Bean bag positioner (conform to desired shape for support
   and apply suction; the bean bag becomes rigid (Figure 8-15)

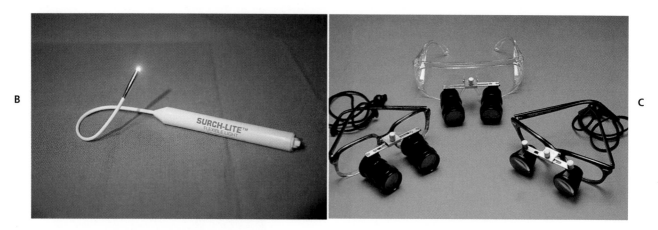

B

C

Fig. 8-9 cont'd B, A sterile, single-use, battery-powered, flexible light. **C,** Magnifying loupes. *(C courtesy Scanlan International, St. Paul, Minn.)*

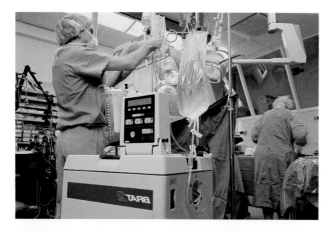

Fig. 8-10 BRAT blood salvage machine. *(Courtesy COBE Cardiovascular, Arvada, Colo.)*

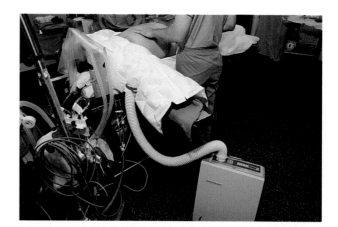

Fig. 8-11 Gaymar blanket and radiant warmer unit: useful in preventing hypothermia.

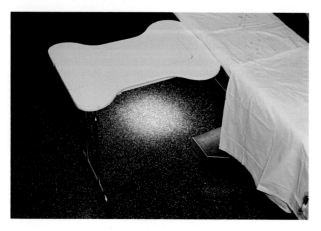

Fig. 8-12 Arm table.

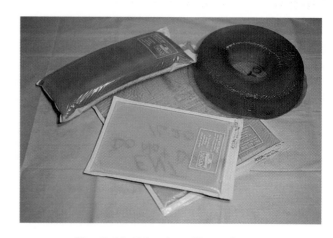

Fig. 8-13 Gel pads, axillary roll, ring.

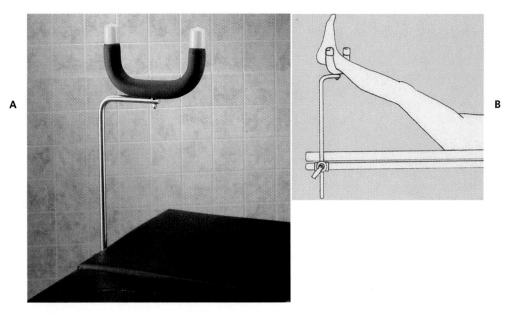

Fig. 8-14 **A,** Leg prep holder. **B,** Proper positioning. *(Courtesy OR Direct, Acton, Mass.)*

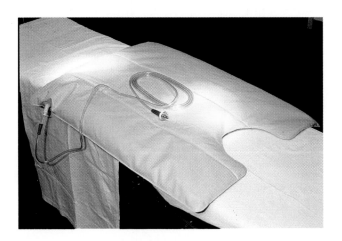

Fig. 8-15 Bean bag positioner.

STERILE SUPPLIES

The OR is a specialty area that is known for the utilization of supplies. Sterile supplies that are needed for or are unique to vascular surgery are described and depicted to familiarize nursing staff with basic requirements (Box 8-3).

Suture and Pledget Material

The choices of suture material are based upon the surgeon's preference, the nature of the tissue, the characteristics of the suture material, and the purpose of the suture. Custom suture packs may be helpful in some specialty procedures but the basic suture needs of most peripheral vascular procedures are best kept simple and to a minimum. **Polypropylene** suture (Prolene, Surgilene, Deklene) is the most commonly used suture for the suturing of blood vessels. It is one of the least reactive of materials, maintains its tensile strength, and may be used even in the infected wound. Its property of being inert is surpassed only by stainless steel. Polypropylene has excellent handling properties and as a monofilament strand glides through tissue (Atkinson, 1992). Typically, a 3-0 suture will be used on the aorta, 5-0 and 6-0 on the carotid, femoral, and popliteal arteries, and down to a 7-0 or 8-0 on the smaller vessels of the lower extremity. Other vascular suture materials include Dacron (polyester) and PTFE (GoreTex). The sizes manufactured range from 10-0 to #2 (Olsen, 1995).

Handling of vascular sutures is an important aspect of the scrub nurse's role. The suture is usually swaged on (needle preattached to the thread) to make it as atraumatic as possible and double-armed (a needle on both ends of the thread) to permit back to front suturing of an anastomosis. The polypropylene suture maintains some memory of its curled packaging, but it should be handled as little as possible to prevent weakening it. Most important, the suture must never be passed to the surgeon with a knot in it. Some surgeons or situations require the suture be double-loaded, or prepared with a needle holder on each needle. This makes it faster for the surgeon to switch needles. Others may prefer the application of a rubbershod clamp to keep the second end of the

Box 8-3 Routine Sterile Items for Vascular Surgery

Knife blades #11, #15, #10, #20
Microsurgical blade, e.g., ophthalmic knife or fine Beaver
    blade
Rubbershods or suture boots (Figure 8-16)
Kittner dissectors (for blunt tissue dissection) (Figure 8-17)
Vessel loops (for identification, retraction or occlusion of a
    vessel) (Figure 8-18)
Umbilical tapes (for vessel retraction or as a permanent tie)
Fogarty inserts of varying sizes (Figure 8-19)
Vessel clips or hemoclips in three sizes (Figure 8-20)
Syringe for irrigation with heparin solution
Asepto for wound irrigation and wetting surgeon's hand
    for tying a vascular suture
Marking pen (for labeling solutions)

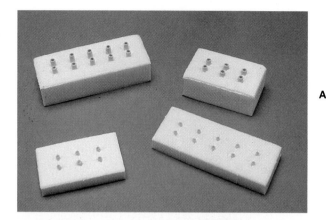

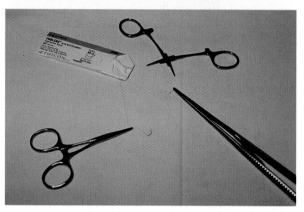

Fig. 8-16 **A,** Suture boots, also called rubbershods, are placed on the tips of clamps to protect the suture material from being damaged by the metal of the clamp. **B,** An alternative to rubbershods are small, smooth-jawed clamps. (*A courtesy Scanlan International, St. Paul, Minn.)*

suture from drifting or tangling or to weight it for counter-traction while sewing. **Rubbershods** or **suture boots** may be purchased in varying sizes to fit standard crile or mosquito clamps. Suture boots pad the clamp to prevent damage or breakage to the suture. These are best if they are radiopaque so they may be counted and retrieved if they inadvertently come off a clamp. Tiny metal clamps that do not injure the suture may also serve the same function (see Figure 8-16). Tying a polyprolylene suture is facilitated if the suture or the surgeon's hand is wet. The scrub nurse usually moistens the tying hand or suture with saline to allow a smoother tying action (Figure 8-21). Surgeons will often wear magnifying glasses called loupes which allows greater visualization of vessels when operating (see Figure 8-9, *C*). The scrub nurse should be aware that this limits the surgeon's peripheral vision. Items passed to the surgeon need to be placed in his or her line of vision and increased vigilance for breaks in aseptic technique may be needed.

Vascular sutures may need to be "pledgeted." Pledgets serve to prevent the suture from tearing through friable tissue or may be used when an anastomosis leaks and needs a better seal. Teflon felt pieces may be cut to size or purchased commercially precut in a variety of shapes and sizes (Figure 8-22). Alternately a leftover segment of vein graft or a piece of graft material may be used. The pledget may be loaded onto the suture before passing it to the surgeon or added by the surgeon to a stitch in progress (MacVittie, 1995). An additional pledget should always be ready on a clamp (straight crile or mosquito, depending on the size of the pledget). This may be referred to as a "free" or "blank" pledget. Preparing a suture with a pledget is a skill that takes practice and patience to master since it is usually needed when the patient is bleeding or the anastomosis is difficult.

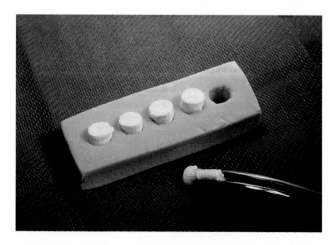

Fig. 8-17 Kittners are tightly rolled gauze "peanuts" used on the end of a clamp for blunt tissue dissection.

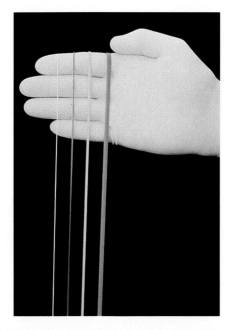

Fig. 8-18 Vessel loops or Silastic loops used to gently retract or identify a structure. *(Courtesy Scanlan International, St. Paul, Minn.)*

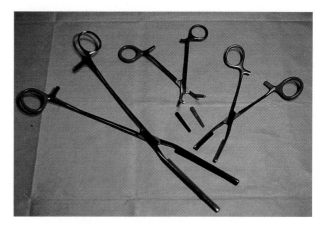

Fig. 8-19 Fogarty inserts are fitted into slots on Fogarty clamps, atraumatic vascular clamps. Inserts are disposable.

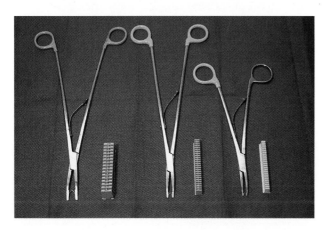

Fig. 8-20 Hemoclip racks and appliers.

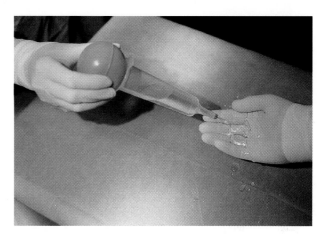

Fig. 8-21 The scrub nurse uses an asepto of saline to wet the surgeon's hand to facilitate the tying of Prolene suture.

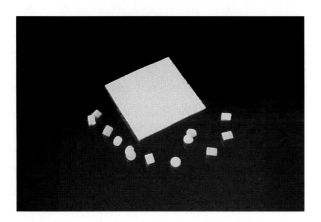

Fig. 8-22 Teflon pledgets in a variety of commercially prepared sizes. *(Courtesy Meadox Medical, Oakland, NJ.)*

There are different ways to load a pledget (Figures 8-23 and 8-24). The experienced scrub nurse will often unconsciously develop strategies to cope with the stress and resultant tremors by bracing the hand or instrument in order to work with safety and speed (Figure 8-25). The commercially prepared pledgets, which come in a variety of sizes, can be of great value in eliminating the time-consuming step of cutting a pledget to size from a large piece. Because the preparation of a pledgeted suture may be time consuming when speed is imperative, a general rule in vascular surgery is to prepare a minimum of one suture ahead. This allows the scrub nurse to have a suture immediately available.

Basic ties include nonabsorbable silk suture, sizes 2-0 and 3-0. Sizes 3-0 or 4-0 silk controlled-release suture ligatures may be used as a suture ligature or with blunt tip needles to quickly pass the tie around a vessel branch. Blunt tip needles can lessen the

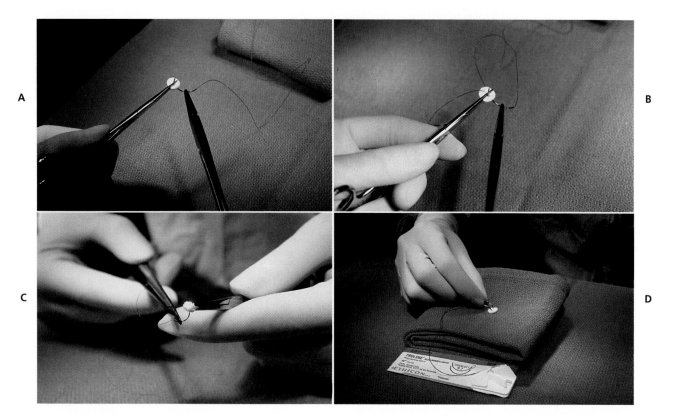

Fig. 8-23 A, A "blank" pledget, or pledget on a clamp, held for surgeon to pass needle into. **B,** Step two: second suture needle passed through pledget. This technique is used when the suture has already been passed through tissue and the pledget is added. Sutures are prepared with a pledget before passing it to the surgeon. Two preparation methods are shown: **C,** Folded pledget and suture being placed, and **D,** Pledget on towel and 2 needle insertion.

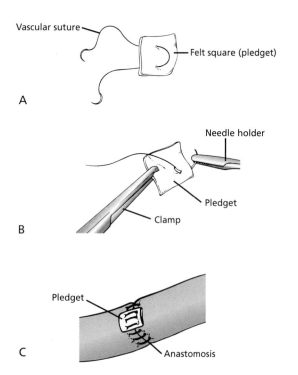

Fig. 8-24 Pledgeted suture. *(From Meeker, M. H., & Rothrock, J. D. [1995]. Alexander's care of the patient in surgery [10th ed.]. St. Louis: Mosby.)*

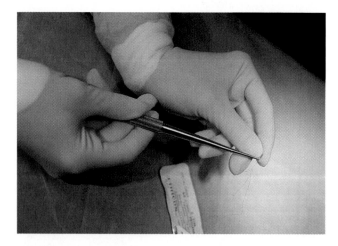

Fig. 8-25 Scrub nurse loading vascular suture and bracing hand to minimize movement and maximize accuracy of needle placement on needle holder.

incidence of staff injuries. Wound closure sutures will also vary with the surgeon, procedure, and anatomy. Absorbable subcuticular closure versus skin staple closure continues to be a subject of debate and research for closure of extremity wounds. Many surgeons use an absorbable suture (2-0 Vicryl) to close subcutaneous tissue in either a continuous (running) or interrupted method. Then 3-0 or 4-0 Vicryl may be used to close the subcuticular layer. Alternately, staples may be used to close the skin. Patients often complain about discomfort with staples while they are present and particularly when they are removed. The ultimate cosmetic result has been reported to be equal after about 6 months (East, 1995). Closure of abdominal wounds is done routinely according to surgeon protocol and patient needs.

Custom Packs

Custom packs are a unit of preselected sterile items that are used routinely for standard procedures (Box 8-4). A custom pack for vascular surgery may be worth considering when the volume of surgery can justify this (Figure 8-26). Custom packs have many advantages for the circulating nurse and the patient. Time savings or labor savings can be measured by considering the time it takes to order, inventory, shelve, and then select and open each item for a surgical procedure. Having custom packs may save on storage space because the entire kit may preclude the need for multiple drawers or shelves for all the individual items. They may streamline the ordering process and make inventory more efficient. Cost savings may be realized when OR staff is unfamiliar with all the needs of the surgical procedure. Staff may be confident that the basics are available while they learn and avoid the costly opening of unnecessary supplies. Custom packs may also free the circulating nurse and scrub nurse to devote their time to tasks and responsibilities other than package opening. This may also assist in reducing OR turnover time. The nurse may have more time for direct patient care activities and interactions. Custom packs are ideal for emergency situations. The packs can be designed to promote efficiency of motion and ensure a rapid set up for the emergency. It is possible that the minimal need to handle supplies contributes to improved asepsis. Each item opened could be a

potential opportunity for contamination (Atkinson, 1992). Multiple packages also contribute to lint and particulate matter becoming airborne, and multiple wrappers are undesirable from an environmental standpoint.

INSTRUMENTATION

Instrumentation covers a broad range of topics. Because of the long and hard work that instruments are required to perform, it is important that they be properly selected and handled. Many surgical instruments are handmade by master craftsmen. The material used must withstand years of daily use, washing, steam sterilization, and possible rough handling. Many factors must be considered when purchasing instrumentation. Surgeon preference must be considered. When multiple surgeons are working at an institution, they bring varied training backgrounds. Many will require the instrumentation that they used in their training programs. Budget constraints also influence instrument selection. Because the instruments are individually crafted, they may vary in certain details. The vascular nurse may have to blend the preferences of many surgeons and surgical procedures in order to put together a usable instrument set. It may or may not be possible to accommodate all the specific requests of every surgeon. Sets must be practical and readily available for emergencies. There are probably as many ideas for the ideal instrumentation as there are operating rooms. The number of surgical procedures, types of procedures, and number of surgeons will influence the design of instrument sets. One method of creating a vascular set is to have a basic vascular instrument set that requires a few additions for specific surgical procedures. Another method is to have a set for various body regions. This might include a set for abdominal procedures, one for extremities, and one for microvascular work (Box 8-5). Instruments may be wrapped individually to accommodate either specific surgeons or specific procedures. AORN and some regulatory agencies recommend that instruments be wrapped and sterile for each surgical procedure. The number of sets available may be dependent upon the capabilities of the sterile processing department and the number of procedures performed.

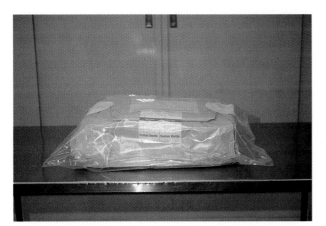

Fig. 8-26 Custom pack of sterile supplies.

Box 8-4 **Example of Contents of a Custom Pack for Vascular Surgery**

Laparotomy drape	Electrocautery pencil
8 cloth towels	Marking pen and labels
3 gowns	Sharps container
Prep kit, gloves, sponges	Asepto
Sponges	50 cc syringe
Blades, 1 each	Suture boots
of #10, #11, #15, #20	4 vessel loops
2-0 silk ties	
3-0 silk ties	
3-0 silk pop-offs	
(controlled-release needles)	
Surgical clips, small and medium	
Suction tubing	
Suction tips	

Box 8-5 **Equipment and Supplies for Specific Procedures**

ANGIOGRAPHY
Sterile C-arm drape for fluoroscopy machine (Figure 8-27)
Lead aprons as appropriate for protection of staff and
   patient

ANGIOSCOPY (SEE FIGURE 8-59)
Angioscope
Video camera
Camera cover
Light source and fiberoptic cord
Irrigation pump and tubing
Video monitor and cassette recorder

EMBOLECTOMY/THROMBECTOMY
C-arm cover
Arterial embolectomy catheters (Figure 8-28)

DOPPLER FLOW DETECTION
Doppler flow detector (amplifier)
Sterile Doppler probe (Figure 8-29)
Gel (for Doppler detection over intact skin), sterile and
   unsterile

DUPLEX ULTRASONOGRAPHY (FIGURE 8-30)
Duplex machine
Intraoperative probe
Sterile probe covers with gel inside cover

CAROTID ENDARTERECTOMY
Shunts (Figure 8-31)
Patch material (see Chapter 11)

AORTIC SURGERY
Vessel occlusion catheter for aortic tamponade (Figure 8-32)
Foley catheter with large balloon (30 or 75 cc) for aortic
   tamponade
Vascular grafts (see Chapter 9)
Dual lumen suction tubing for blood salvage (Figure 8-33)
Cell saver machine

VENOUS ULCER
Alternating compression stockings (Figure 8-34)
For split-thickness skin graft (STSG), dermatome, mineral
   oil, mesher, and skin carrier for mesher

VARICOSE VEIN SURGERY
Vein strippers, disposable or reusable (Figure 8-35)

INFRAINGUINAL ARTERIAL RECONSTRUCTION
Clear, sterile plastic bag to drape foot (isolates aseptically
   and permits view of tissue perfusion)
Sterile tourniquet cuffs (Figure 8-36)
Extension tubing for tourniquet (optional)
Sterile cotton padding
Esmarch bandage for limb exsanguination
Tourniquet box and tester (tester not required for all models)
   (see Figure 8-36)
Radiopaque ruler (Figure 8-37)

IN SITU VEIN GRAFT (SEE FIGURE 8-58)
Fluid infusion machine
Valvulotomes (disposable)

PERCUTANEOUS BALLOON ANGIOPLASTY (FIGURE 8-38)
Seldinger needle
Guidewires
Introducer sheath
Angioplasty balloons
Balloon inflators
Radiopaque ruler (either plastic rigid or disposable adhe-
   sive tape) (see Figure 8-37)

LASER-ASSISTED BALLOON ANGIOPLASTY
(SEE FIGURE 8-61)
(All items listed for percutaneous balloon angioplasty)
Laser machine
Laser probes
Protective eyewear specific to type of laser in use
Moist saline eye pads for sleeping patient (goggles for
   awake patient)

ENDOSCOPIC PROCEDURES (SYMPATHECTOMY)
(SEE FIGURE 8-60)
Lens
Fiberoptic carrier cord
Light source
TV monitors (2)
Sterile camera sheath
Trocars
Electrocautery tip
Endoscopic clip applier
Blunt dissector
Nerve hook
Endoscopic graspers
Coagulating scissors
Laparoscopic fan retractors

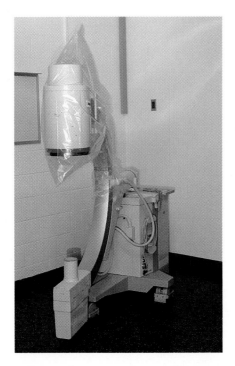

Fig. 8-27 C-arm to show sterile cover.

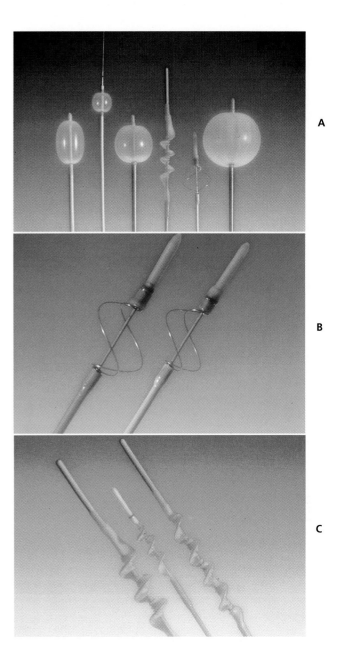

Fig. 8-28 **A,** Balloon embolectomy catheters. **B,** Graft thrombectomy catheter. **C,** Adherent clot catheter. *(Courtesy Baxter Vascular Systems Division, Irvine, Calif.)*

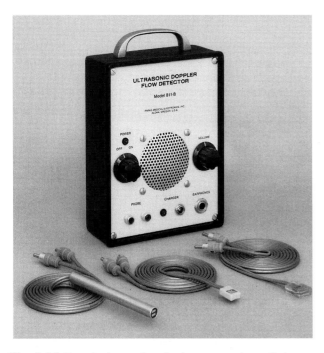

Fig. 8-29 Doppler box and probe *(Courtesy Parks Medical Electronics, Aloha, Oreg.)*

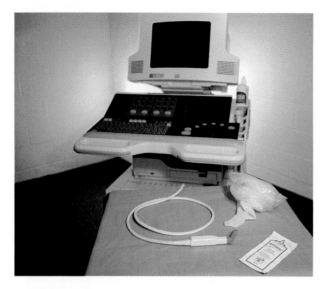

Fig. 8-30 Duplex ultrasound machine with probe, sterile sheath, and sterile coupling gel.

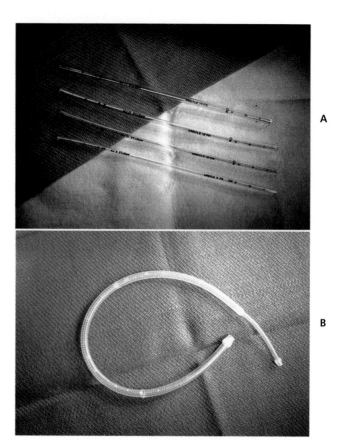

Fig. 8-31 Carotid artery shunts come in a variety of sizes and styles. **A,** Argyle shunts, packaged with radiopaque line on each shunt in sizes 8, 10, 12, and 14 FR. **B,** Sundt shunts.

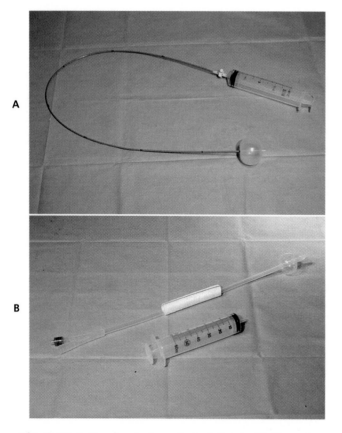

Fig. 8-32 A, Vessel occlusion catheter inflated with 45 cc of fluid. This catheter comes with a built-in locking mechanism to maintain balloon inflation. **B,** Large Foley catheter with large balloon for aortic tamponade.

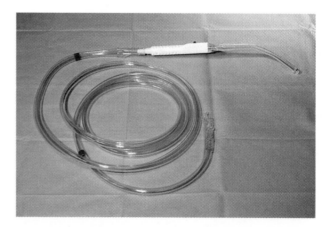

Fig. 8-33 Dual lumen suction tubing: heparinized saline is dripped into the small tubing lumen to mix at the junction where the blood is collected by the suction wand. The blood and heparinized saline mix and are collected into the blood salvage canister.

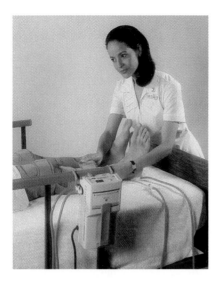

Fig. 8-34 Venous compression stockings, used in venous disease to assist in prevention and healing of venous stasis ulcers. *(Courtesy Huntleigh Healthcare, Manalapan, NJ.)*

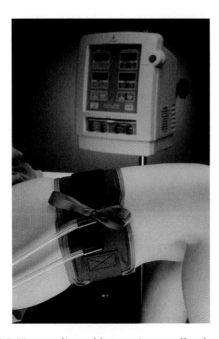

Fig. 8-36 Zimmer disposable tourniquet cuff and pneumatic inflation unit. Tourniquets may be used for varicose vein surgery or arterial reconstructive surgery on the leg to provide a bloodless operative field. *(Courtesy Zimmer, Dover, Ohio.)*

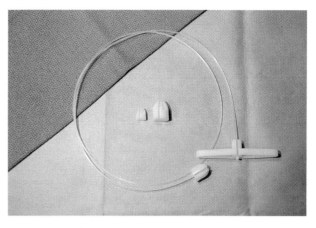

Fig. 8-35 Codman varicose vein strippers, with two plastic passers, three sizes of tips and handle (disposable).

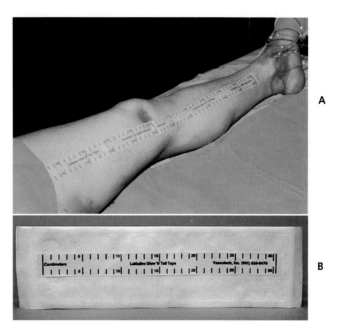

Fig. 8-37 **A,** Radiopaque ruler. **B,** Glow-N-Tell tape. Disposable adhesive strip with radiopaque ruler markings are used with fluoroscopy to identify the location of vessel branches (when harvesting vein grafts for bypass) or in identifying atherosclerotic lesions during balloon angioplasty. *(Courtesy Vascutech, North Andover, Mass.)*

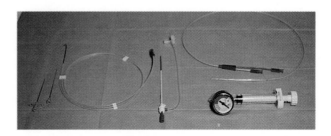

Fig. 8-38 Supplies for balloon angioplasty: left to right, seldinger needle (2 part, 18 gauge), guide wire, introducer sheath, angioplasty balloon; front, balloon inflator with pressure gauge.

Basic Vascular Set

A basic vascular set could be the simplest way to accommodate most peripheral vascular procedures (Box 8-6). This could be combined with a basic laparotomy or major or minor instrument set to accommodate abdominal surgery versus another set for extremity work (Boxes 8-7 and 8-8; see chapters on specific surgical interventions for unique instrumentation). Decisions to assemble instrument sets are based on the resultant weight of the pan. Very heavy sets can cause staff injury. It may make sense to separate delicate instruments from very heavy items that could damage them during processing. This can be accomplished by using small protective trays inside larger sets or by creating totally separate pans (Figure 8-43). Too many sets could lead to loss and fragmentation. Each work setting must be assessed for the correct balance of numbers and types of instrument sets.

Vascular Clamps

Vascular clamps are atraumatic or noncrushing to minimize injury to vessels. The Debakey teeth, common to forceps, occluding, and partial occluding clamps, are atraumatic (Figure 8-44). Clamps used on the aorta must be of a size and strength to withstand the pressure of the aortic blood flow. It is useful to have a variety of sterile, individually wrapped aortic clamps available to accommodate variations in anatomy (Figure 8-45). Total occluding clamps or "cross clamps" will completely stop blood flow through a vessel while partial-occluding clamps or "side-biting" clamps allow the blood to continue to flow but prevent blood flow to the clamped section where the surgeon is operating (Figure 8-46). Clamps are designed to not only occlude blood flow but configured so that the handle does not interfere with the surgery. The length, size, or angle may be important to permit easy access to the vessel. In addition to the Debakey configuration, soft, disposable inserts may be the most atraumatic means of vessel occlusion (see Figure 8-19). There are a variety of products available; some are reusable gel-filled inserts, some are disposable, and others are fibrous. These are

---

Box 8-6 **Basic Vascular Instrument Set (Figure 8-39)**

Clamps (24)
  2 aortic (giant Fogarty, giant DeBakey)
  2 iliac DeBakey
  1 large right-angled (long tip to go around large vessels)
  2 fine right-angled
  3 derra
  4 peripheral Debakeys (2 curved and 2 angled)
  4 peripheral Fogartys (2 straight and 2 angled)
  6 mosquito
Needle Holders (16)
  4 Castroviejo (Figure 8-40)
  4 long (10 ½ inch)
  4 medium length (2 medium tips, 2 finer tips)
  4 short (7 ¼ inch), 2 medium tips and 2 finer tips
Scissors (10)
  4 Potts (25-, 45-, 120-degree angle and 1 coronary
    Potts with a 45-degree angle)
  4 dissecting
  1 fine dissecting
  2 long Metzenbaum
Forceps (11)
  2 Potts
  2 Geralds
  2 fine-tipped Debakeys (7 ¾ inch)
  2 medium-tipped Debakeys (7 ¾ inch)
  2 long Debakeys
  1 micro
Hemoclip appliers (small and medium)
Miscellaneous
  4 deep self-retaining retractors
  1 Freer elevator (for endarterectomies)
  1 nerve hook (for snagging suture to untangle it)
Bulldog clamps (variety of sizes and strengths)
Disposable bulldog clamps may be helpful (Figures 8-41
  and 8-42)
Cannula (placed on syringe for irrigation of vessels)

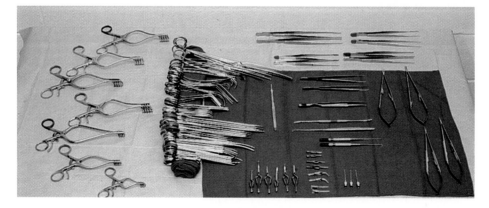

Fig. 8-39 Basic vascular instrument set.

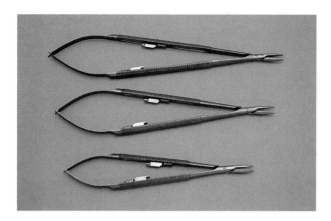

Fig. 8-40 Castroviejo needle holders. *(Courtesy Scanlan International, St. Paul, Minn.)*

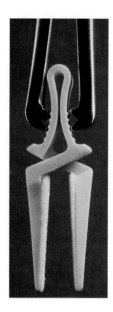

Fig. 8-41 Disposable bulldog clamps. *(Courtesy Scanlan International, St. Paul, Minn.)*

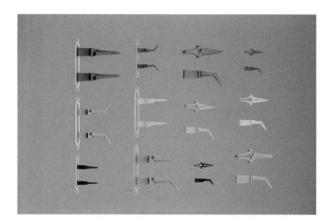

Fig. 8-42 Disposable bulldog clamps. *(Courtesy Scanlan International, St. Paul, Minn.)*

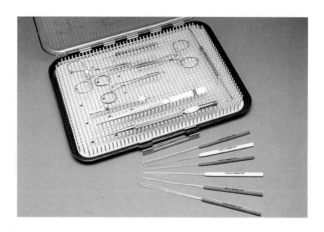

Fig. 8-43 Small protective set with microvascular instruments. *(Courtesy Scanlan International, St. Paul, Minn.)*

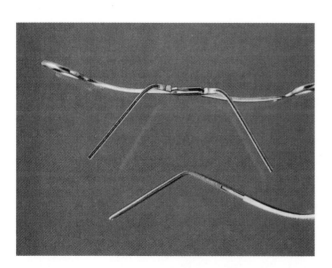

Fig. 8-44 DeBakey teeth on peripheral vascular clamp. *(From Brooks Tighe, S. M. [1994]. Instrumentation for the operating room: A photographic manual [4th ed.]. St. Louis: Mosby.)*

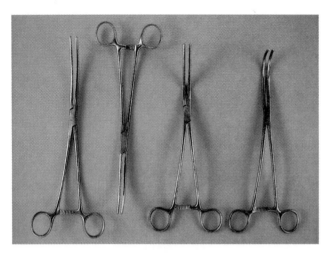

Fig. 8-45 Variety of aortic clamps to accommodate different needs. *(From Brooks Tighe, S. M. [1994]. Instrumentation for the operating room: A photographic manual [4th ed.]. St. Louis: Mosby.)*

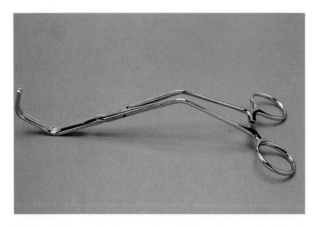

Fig. 8-46 Example of a partial occluding clamp or "side-biting clamp." *(Courtesy Scanlan International, St. Paul, Minn.)*

Box 8-7 **Basic Laparotomy Instrument Set (Figure 8-47)**

CLAMPS
12 curved Criles
4 straight Criles
4 Kelly
2 Babcocks
4 Allis
4 right-angled
8 cystics or tonsils
4 long Kellys
4 long Kochers
2 sponge sticks
4 towel

NEEDLE HOLDERS
2 long Mayo
2 short Mayo
2 French eye

FORCEPS
2 toothed Adsons
2 heavy-toothed
2 long-dressing
2 long Debakeys (10 inch)
2 medium Debakeys (7 inch)

KNIFE HANDLES
1 #7
1 #3
1 #4

SCISSORS
1 suture
1 straight Mayo
1 curved Mayo
1 7 inch Metzenbaum
1 10 inch Metzenbaum

RETRACTORS
Balfour and bladder blade
1 wide malleable
1 Harrington
3 Deavers
6 Richardsons
1 thyroid
2 right-angled
2 vein

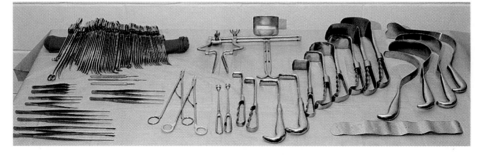

Fig. 8-47 Basic laparotomy set.

CLAMPS
Curved mosquitoes
Straight mosquitoes
Curved Criles
Straight Criles
Kellys
Kochers
Allia
Lahey
Right-angled
Cystic duct or tonsils
Sponge sticks

NEEDLE HOLDERS
Variety of delicate to heavy

FORCEPS
Brown Adsons
Toothed Adsons
Smooth Adsons
Debakeys
Bonnies

RETRACTORS
Thyroid
Right-angled
Vein
Army-Navy
Self-retainers (small and large)
Richardsons (variety)
Ribbon
Face lift
Senns
Skin hooks, double, single, Guthrie

SCISSORS
Straight Mayo
Curved Mayo
7 inch Metzenbaum
5 inch Metzenbaum
Sharp and blunt plastic

KNIFE HANDLES
2 #7
2 #3

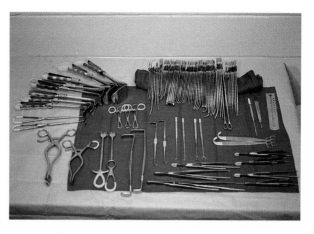

Fig. 8-48 Plastic or minor instrument set.

Microsurgical Instruments

Microsurgical work will require special, delicate instrumentation that is usually expensive and requires extra care. Needle holders may become magnetized, which results in the fine vascular needles adhering unpredictably. This can make it very difficult to properly position the needle for sewing. An instrument demagnetizer can quickly and easily correct this problem (Figure 8-50). Sterile water should be available for washing blood and body fluids from *all* instruments but especially for delicate items (Atkinson, 1992). A basin in a ring stand that is separate from irrigation basins may be one way to provide water for this purpose. Basins and bowls on the sterile field are used to hold drugs and solutions. Care should be taken to use clean irrigating solutions for wound irrigation. Solutions used for cleaning instruments should *not* be used for wound or vessel irrigation. Particles or clots rinsed from clamps may not be visible but could act as an embolism if introduced into a vessel during irrigation. Normal saline is physiologically similar to body fluids and will maintain the integrity of some blood components while sterile distilled water will not. The osmotic difference between the water and the blood cells causes the cell to be lysed. This lysing action speeds up the removal of blood from instruments. Instruments may be soaked temporarily in the water to clean them during surgery. Instruments of any kind, delicate or heavy, should never be soaked in saline. Instruments that are kept clean work better, last longer, require fewer repairs, and take less time to clean adequately after a case. Instruments must be inspected by the instrument processing personnel for adequate cleaning and proper functioning. A gauze sponge can be brushed over the tips of scissors, Debakey teeth, and other surfaces to detect any burrs that might interfere with proper function (Seifert, 1994). The scrub nurse can also perform this function routinely so that instruments do not get used that could cause damage to delicate tissue.

ususally radiopaque and counted as items that could be inadvertently left in a patient if not accounted for. These padded clamps are often the clamps of choice for clamping synthetic graft material, especially Gore-Tex (PTFE) that could be damaged even by the teeth of the Debakey clamps. Another way to control or temporarily occlude a vessel is by using a **Rummel** or **vascular tourniquet** with a suture or umbilical tape (Figure 8-49).

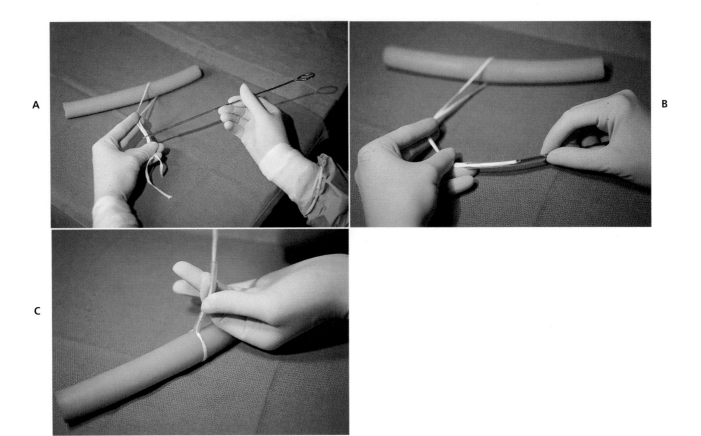

Fig. 8-49 Vascular tourniquet or Rummel tourniquet using a Rummel stylet or "slider." **A,** A temporary occlusive device may be used to control a vessel by placing a loop of suture, umbilical tape, or vessel loop around it(rubber tubing acting as vessel). **B,** It is then threaded through a segment of plastic tubing. **C,** The device is then cinched down on the vessel and secured with a clamp.

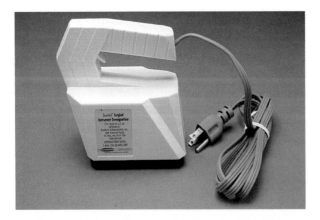

Fig. 8-50 Instrument demagnetizer is plugged into electrical outlet and moved in a circular motion over instruments for a few seconds to demagnetize the instrument tips. *(Courtesy Scanlan International, St. Paul, Minn.)*

Bone Instrumentation

Patients with arterial disease are at risk for amputation of toes or lower extremities. Therefore, instrumentation for bone surgery is also needed (Box 8-9). An appropriately sized soft tissue set is used with these. Few tissue clamps are needed for a toe amputation, while a leg amputation requires many.

First rib resections are performed to relieve compression on neurovascular structures of the arm (see Chapter 13). For a transaxillary approach, the wound is deep and narrow. Long instruments are often needed, e.g., long scissors, forceps, clamps, cautery tip, sponges on ring clamps. A variety of bone rongeurs, cutters, and elevators are needed for variations in anatomy (see Figure 8-53). This is a procedure that may be expedited by the use of auxiliary light sources. The surgeon may elect to use a headlight, a fiberoptic light to illuminate the wound, or a disposable battery powered light to illuminate the surgical site (see Figure 8-9, *A* and *B*).

Box 8-9 **Bone Instruments**

BONE INSTRUMENTS FOR SMALL BONES (FINGER OR TOE AMPUTATIONS) (FIGURE 8-51)
Periosteal elevator
Bone cutter
Bone rongeur
Currettes
Small rasp
Towel clip (to grasp toe)

BONE INSTRUMENTS FOR LARGE BONES (LEG AMPUTATIONS) (FIGURE 8-52)
Periosteal elevator
Bone hook
Bone cutters
Bone rongeurs
Large rasp
Saws:
   Gigli saw with handles
   Hand-held saw (e.g., Satterlee)
   Power saw (optional)
   Amputation knife (for soft tissue)

BONE INSTRUMENTS FOR FIRST RIB RESECTION (FIGURE 8-53)
Periosteal elevators: Cushing, Cobb
Bone cutters: straight, double-action angled, Bethune, guillotine, first-rib cutters (right, left, and angled)
Bone rongeurs: variety, include Kerrison

ADDITIONAL INSTRUMENTS
Narrow Deaver retractors
Narrow ribbon retractors
Long nerve root retractor (Roos)

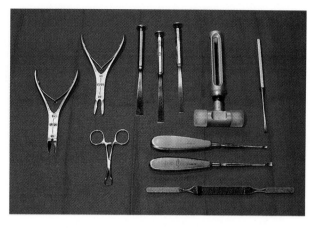

Fig. 8-51 Instrumentation for small bones (finger or toe amputations): periosteal elevator, bone cutter, small rasp, towel clip. *(Courtesy Scanlan International, St. Paul, Minn.)*

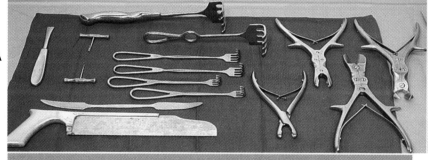
A

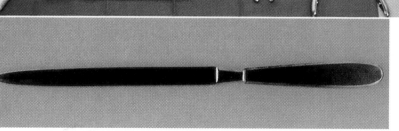
C

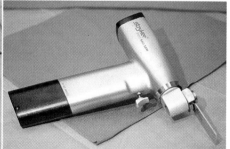
B

Fig. 8-52 Instrumentation for large bones: **A,** periosteal elevator (Cushing), bone cutters, bone rongeurs, bone hook, rasps; saws: gigli saw handles, Satterlee hand saw; **B,** power saw; **C,** Amputation knife. *(C from Brooks Tighe, S. M. [1994]. Instrumentation for the operating room: A photographic manual [4th ed.]. St. Louis: Mosby.)*

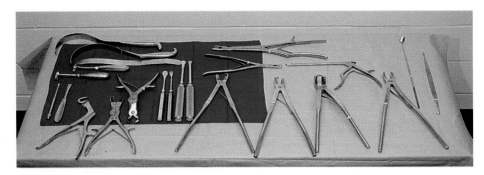

Fig. 8-53 Instrument set for first rib resection.

Miscellaneous Instrumentation

Abdominal surgery will require the addition of long soft-tissue instruments and an abdominal self-retaining retractor. A traditional Balfour retractor (Figure 8-54) may be used for exposure for an abdominal aortic aneurysm resection but it may be helpful to use a retractor that can be set up with a variety of blade sizes and retraction angles. An example is the Omni-Tract retractor (Figure 8-55).

The arterial reconstructive procedures for the lower extremity have several special instruments depending on the choice of graft. A prosthetic graft may need to be protected and carried by a "tunneler" (Figure 8-56). A variety of self-retaining retractors are needed for the multiple incisions made on the leg (Figure 8-57). When vein graft is used, the vein may be **reversed** or left in its bed, **in situ** (see Chapter 12). In situ vein grafts require instruments to disrupt the vein's valves that would interfere with arterial flow since the blood flow will be reversed. Many techniques and instrumentation have evolved because this surgery requires meticulous care to protect the intimal surface of the vein graft. Instruments that disrupt the valves are called **valvulotomes** (Figure 8-58).

Disruption of the valves with the previously described instruments is not performed under direct visualization. Using an angioscope allows direct visualization of the valves. Angioscopes, disposable and reusable, have been developed to permit their introduction into small caliber vessels. The scope provides access, illumination, and visualization of the vessel lumen (Figure 8-59). For in situ vein use, this means the valve is disrupted under direct visualization. A fluid irrigation system allows a controlled irrigation of the vessel. This may prevent fluid overload, which was a concern in earlier systems used with angioscopes. These scopes can also be used to verify the integrity of a vascular anastomoses and check for residual clot after thrombectomy.

Endoscopic surgery is increasing. The basic requirements include a lens or "scope," fiberoptic light carrier or cord, light source, and video monitor. Additional equipment will vary with the procedure and anatomy (Figure 8-60). Laser surgery may be a component of endoscopic surgery. This may be an adjunct to balloon angioplasty. The laser probe vaporizes atherosclerotic plaque and may increase the long-term patency of a vessel (Figure 8-61).

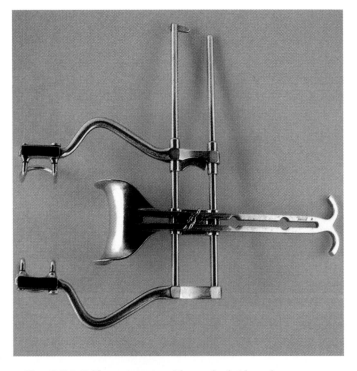

Fig. 8-54 Balfour retractor with standard side and center blades. *(From Brooks Tighe, S. M. [1994].* Instrumentation for the operating room: A photographic manual *[4th ed.]. St. Louis: Mosby.)*

Garrett dilators are usually composed of a set of nine dilators ranging from 1 mm to 5 mm in increments of 0.5 mm. They may be useful to measure the lumen diameter of vessels (for selection of correct size of valvulotome or angioscope), check a vessel for patency before and during an anastomosis, or occlude a vessel lumen to prevent back bleeding (Figure 8-62).

Occasionally, a vascular patient may need a skin graft to cover either a venous stasis ulcer or a defect from ischemic tissue loss. The donor skin site should be protected from contamination by the ulcerated area.

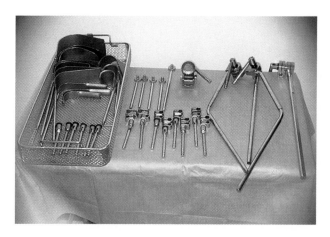

Fig. 8-55 Omni-Tract abdominal self-retaining retractor.

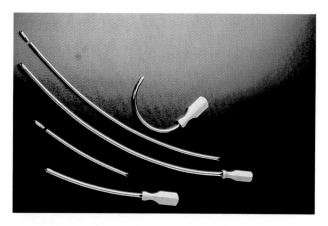

Fig. 8-56 Vascular tunnelers used as devices to create a path for a bypass graft and as a protective carrier for the graft. *(Courtesy W. L. Gore & Associates, Flagstaff, Ariz.)*

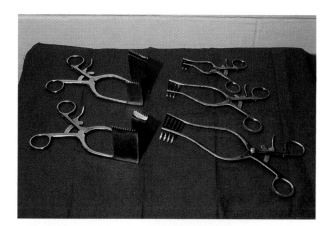

Fig. 8-57 Examples of self-retaining retractors: Darling popliteal retractor (*left*). Deep self-retainers, small self-retainers (*right*).

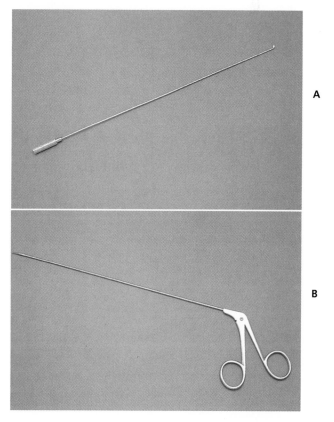

Fig. 8-58 In situ vein harvest instruments. **A,** Rigid valvulotome with retrograde micro-cutting blade. **B,** In situ valvulotome micro scissors.

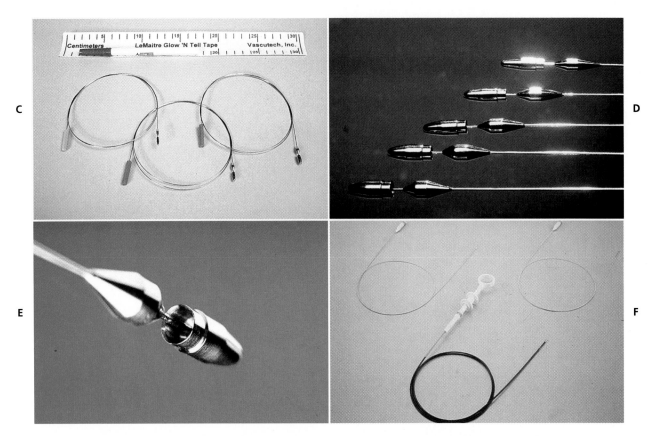

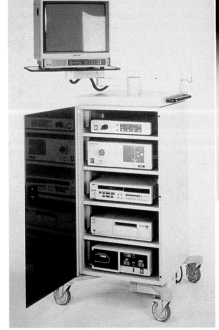

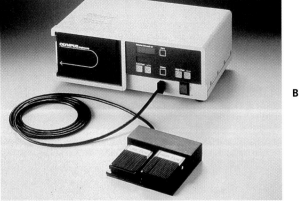

Fig. 8-58, cont'd. **C,** LeMaitre valvulotomes have a long, flexible wire configuration. **D,** These disposable valvulotomes are available in a variety of sizes to match the diameter of the vein graft. **E,** Magnified view to show blunt end that is advanced into the in situ vein graft and circular cutting blade that disrupts the valve leaflets. **F,** A valvulotome may also be used through an angioscope. This is an example of an endotherapeutic valvulotome. *(A and B courtesy Scanlan International, St. Paul, Minn. C to E courtesy Vascutech, North Andover, Mass. F courtesy Olympus America, Melville, New York.)*

Fig. 8-59 Angioscopy video cart can conveniently house and protect the units needed. **A,** These are units needed for angioscopy: light source, camera unit, angiofiberscope, and video monitor. **B,** A controlled fluid pump provides variable flow rate irrigation. This permits clear visibility for endoscopic surgery. *(Courtesy Olympus America, Melville, New York.)*

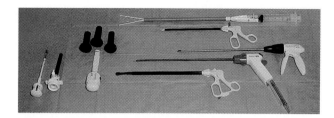

Fig. 8-60 Disposable endoscopic equipment: 10 mm trocar and sheath, trocar with three flexible sheaths (for thoracic or deeper abdominal), top to bottom: laparoscopic fan retractor, scissors, endoscopic clip applier, nerve hook with cautery, and endoscopic graspers. *(Courtesy Ethicon Endo-Surgery, Somerville, NJ.)*

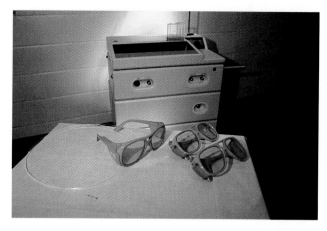

Fig. 8-61 Laser machine, laser probe, and laser goggles.

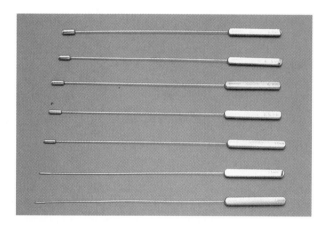

Fig. 8-62 Garrett dilators. *(Courtesy Scanlan International, St. Paul, Minn.)*

References

Atkinson, L. J. (1992). *Berry & Kohn's operating room technique* (7th ed.). St. Louis: Mosby.

Association of Operating Room Nurses (1995). Standards and recommended practices on positioning the surgical patient. In *AORN standards and recommended practices for perioperative nursing*. Denver: The Association.

East, S. A. (1995). The registered nurse first assistant role in surgical wound closure: An integrated review. *Journal of Vascular Nursing, 8*(3): 83-91.

Olsen, C. C. (1995). Sutures, needles, and instruments. In M. H. Meeker, & J. C. Rothrock (Eds.), *Alexander's care of the patient in surgery* (10th ed., pp. 113-142). St. Louis: Mosby.

MacVittie, B. A. (1995). Vascular surgery. In M.H. Meeker, & J. C. Rothrock (Eds.), *Alexander's care of the patient in surgery* (10th ed., pp. 1025-1057). St. Louis: Mosby.

Seifert, P. C. (1994). Environment, instrumentation, and equipment. *Mosby's perioperative nursing series: Cardiac surgery* (pp. 65-101). St. Louis: Mosby.

9 Vascular Grafts

HISTORY

Vascular grafting has only been a practical reality for about 30 years. Surgical techniques and prosthetic technology have developed rapidly and allowed life- and limb-saving surgical interventions that many people take for granted. Consider that there was no successful surgical intervention for replacement of the abdominal aortic aneurysm until synthetic grafts became available. Rigid plastic and fiberglass fabric tubes were tried in animals and found to be highly thrombogenic. Researchers tried preservation of cadaver homografts with gluteraldeyde and freeze-drying in the 1940s. Contamination and problems with processing led to infection and graft deterioration (Dennis, 1987). Although no perfect graft for replacement of diseased and occluded arteries of the leg exists, many patients have been spared amputations and retained their ability to walk pain free by the current routine bypass procedures.

The early innovations inevitably led to some failures but each step helped in the evolution toward the best graft possible. The mode of creation was one of trial and error initially. Grafts that were carefully tested in animal models sometimes behaved very differently in humans. No research animal has displayed the exact outcomes subsequently seen in people. Grafts that pass initial tests and seem successful in the early period of implantation may fail dismally in a couple years. Examples are the aneurysm formation in the original unreinforced umbilical cord vein grafts and the early trials that resulted in short-term patency of PTFE in distal bypass procedures (PTFE is currently having increased success in distal bypass procedures because of improved techniques and patient selection). Patient selection, meticulous and consistent surgical technique, and patient lifestyle compliance (smoking cessation) is critical to the success or failure of a graft trial (Wright et al, 1987) (Table 9-1).

THE IDEAL GRAFT

The search for the ideal vascular graft continues (Box 9-1). Some desired characteristics are that they are reasonably priced, readily available in a variety of sizes, and suitable for use anywhere in the body. They need to be biocompatible, hypoallergenic, and able to survive repeated sterilizations. The surgeon's preference also includes ease of handling, i.e., elastic, easy to sew, nonfraying. An implanted graft should last a lifetime and permit blood passage without clotting or infection (Kempczinski, 1995). The patency rate should be as close to 100% as possible and it should have a compliance as close to that of the vessel it is replacing (Wright & Hiratzka, 1983). Brewster (1995) believes grafts should be easy to manufacture and store. The graft should be impervious to blood leakage to prevent excessive blood loss and the development of a perigraft hematoma, which can interfere with healing and promote infection. He further describes ease of handling to include fabric that is strong enough to prevent suture tears but not so tough that the surgeon has difficulty passing a needle through it. A long held ideal was that grafts had to have porosity that promoted healing. This has been questioned because of the more recent experience with ePTFE (expanded polytetrafluoroethylene) grafts that have a small pore size that correlates with improved graft patency (White, RA, 1983). Porosity may only be essential for fabric and not for autogenous and other biologic grafts.

Table 9-1 **Grafts That Have Failed to Stand the Test of Time**

Large Vessel	Small Vessel
Vinyon-N	Dacron (below-knee)
Polyethylene	Bovine heterograft
Aortic homograft	Unsupported PTFE
Ivalon	Umbilical vein graft
Ultra-lightweight Dacron	Supported PTFE
Unsupported PTFE	
Bovine heterograft	

From Wright, C. W., et al (1987). The regulatory environment for vascular grafts. In P. N. Sawyer (Ed.), *Modern vascular grafts* (pp. 105-114). New York: McGraw-Hill.

Box 9-1 **Characteristics of the Ideal Graft**

- Reasonably priced
- Readily available
- Variety of sizes
- Easy to store
- Easy to manufacture
- Durable (survives repeated sterilization, long life in body)
- Suitable for use throughout body
- Biocompatible
- Nontoxic
- Nonallergenic
- Nonthrombogenic
- Infection resistant
- Easy to handle:
  - Easy to pass suture needle
  - Pliable
  - Elastic
  - Does not fray
  - Does not kink

BIOLOGIC GRAFTS

Vascular grafts may be biologic or synthetic. Biologic grafts may be **autologous** (tissue taken from one part of the body and moved to another part) or **homologous** (transplanted from another individual). There are three categories of biologic grafts: autologous arterial and vein grafts, allografts, and heterografts. Autologous grafts (tissues taken from one part of the body and moved to another part) are the most desirable. They are not rejected as a foreign substance, they heal well, and are less prone to infection than synthetic replacements. Artery to replace artery is also a goal but most arteries are not expendable. No vessels, arteries, or veins are large enough to replace the aorta and iliac arteries. Synthetic grafts for these vessels have been very successful. **Allografts or homografts** are tissue from one person transplanted into another. One currently useful allograft for peripheral vascular disease (PVD) is the human umbilical cord vein graft. These are costly and not as conveniently available as other options. Because they are preserved with glutaraldehyde, the manufacturer's instructions for rinsing must be followed. The graft must be rinsed for 3 minutes in three separate basins of sterile normal saline. These grafts were disappointing when they were initially used in humans because they became aneurysmal in the early postoperative period. They have since been improved with a Dacron outer mesh layer. A second type of allograft that is being used in infrainguinal arterial bypass procedures is the cryopreserved human saphenous vein graft (Shah, 1993). **Heterografts** are tissue from another species that are transplanted into a human. Porcine cardiac valves are an example of a widely used and successful heterograft.

Vein Grafts

Vein graft has been a successful substitute for arteries in many areas of the body as both a conduit and a patch. In infrainguinal bypass procedures, the method of using the saphenous vein graft has generated controversy. The vein can be removed from its bed and reversed to allow arterial flow. Removing the vein from its bed disrupts the vasovasorum and sometimes results in a size discrepancy since the vein typically tapers distally in the leg. Another method for using saphenous vein graft is to perform an in situ bypass. The vein remains in place, the branches ligated, and the valves disrupted by special instrumentation. This is a time-consuming surgery and some centers have better success than others (see Chapter 12). Dr. Charles Rob first performed in situ bypasses in London but soon abandoned the practice. This was started again with better techniques and delicate instrumentation for valve disruption. Because the vasa vasorum remains intact, the vein graft has reduced ischemia time. This has been implicated in the success of the graft patency and claims of the in situ procedure being superior to the reversed saphenous vein graft (Benson & Karmody, 1987). A reversed saphenous vein graft is a vein graft harvested from its bed, reversed (the distal end becomes the proximal end), no valve disruption is needed, and the graft is anastomosed to the artery for bypass. Arm veins (basilic and cephalic) may be used when the saphenous vein is either unsuitable or unavailable. 20% to 30% of cephalic veins are unusable either because of inadequate size or damage. Damage may be attributed to venipuncture and fluid or drug infusion, diffuse vasculitis, and endothelial disruption (Apyan, Schneider, & Andros, 1992).

SYNTHETIC GRAFTS

In the 1950s and 1960s many different grafting materials were tried and all except Dacron (polyester) and Teflon (polytetrafluoroethylene) were rejected (Figures 9-1 and 9-2; Table 9-2). Grafts of 10 mm in diameter and larger are usually Dacron and those smaller are Teflon (PTFE or polytetrafluoroethylene) (Turner, 1987). Although PTFE grafts are used for aortic surgery with less frequency, they appear to have equal patency rates to those of Dacron (Green & Ouriel, 1994) (Figure 9-3).

Table 9-2 **Early Graft Materials**

MATERIAL	YEAR STUDIED	COMMENT
Vinyon-N	1952	Unstable above 60° C
Orlon	1955	Fatal hemorrhage
Ivalon	1955	Inflammatory reaction
Marlex	1961	Kinked easily
Teflon	1960	Satisfactory
Dacron	Late 1950-1961	Satisfactory

From Turner, R. I. (1987). Vascular graft development: An industrial perspective. In P. N. Sawyer (Ed.), *Modern vascular grafts* (pp. 75-103). New York: McGraw-Hill.

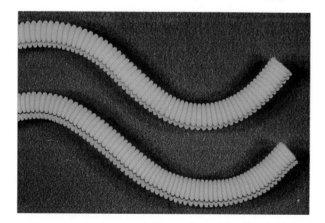

Fig. 9-1 Example of Dacron vascular graft. *Top,* Hemashield Microvel double velour vascular graft. *Bottom,* Microvel double velour vascular graft. *(Courtesy Meadox Medicals.)*

The method of construction of the grafts has been evolving and is critical to its function. Braiding was tried for a period and discarded because the fabric frayed enough to make it unworkable. Researchers tried woven cylindrical or tube grafts (Figure 9-4). Woven fabric is strong but also stiff. This stiffness makes it harder to handle because it does not conform to the tissue and is harder for the surgeon to suture. Woven grafts have a lower porosity, which is a desirable characteristic, especially in thoracoabdominal aortic replacements (Figure 9-5). High porosity permits greater fluid leakage through the graft interstices (Table 9-3). Grafts placed above the diaphragm are subject to higher pressures and therefore have a greater potential for blood loss.

Thoracoabdominal grafting may also be performed during cardiopulmonary bypass using high-dose heparin, which may also increase the bleeding through high-porosity graft material.

Some knowledge of the weaving process is helpful in understanding the choice of graft. Weaving is done on a loom and the first threads strung on it are called the **warp**. Standing in front of the loom, these would be the threads going away from you. The threads that are placed on next at a 90-degree angle, that go over and under the warp, are the **weft**. Compare the fabric in a woven article of clothing with a knitted one such as a sweater. The knitted fabric is more pliable. This characteristic makes it more user friendly but also increases the porosity (Figure 9-6). An early

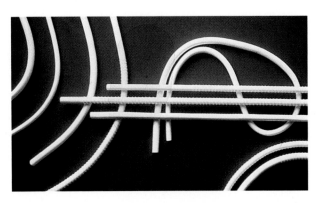

Fig. 9-2 Examples of Teflon grafts. *(Courtesy W. L. Gore & Associates.)*

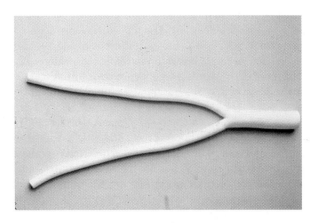

Fig. 9-3 Bifurcated Gore-Tex graft. *(Courtesy W. L. Gore & Associates.)*

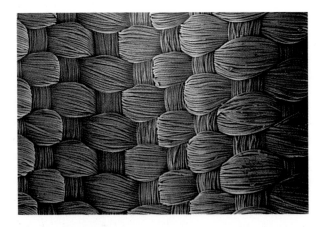

Fig. 9-4 Magnification of woven graft. Internal surface of a woven vascular graft at 50 × magnification. *(Courtesy Meadox Medicals.)*

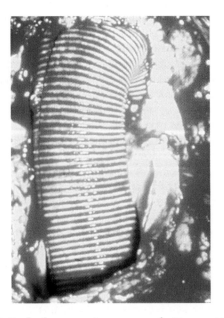

Fig. 9-5 Cooley low-porosity woven graft. *(Courtesy Meadox Medicals.)*

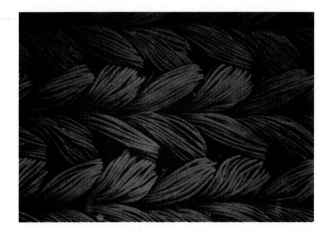

Fig. 9-6 Example of knitted graft wall. *(Courtesy Meadox Medicals.)*

Table 9-3 **Porosity of Prosthetic Grafts*****

FABRIC	MEAN POROSITY
WOVEN FABRIC (DACRON)	
Low-porosity woven (Cooley) Fabric patch Tube graft Intraaortic (ringed) graft	(Less than) 50 ml/min/cm^2
Woven (Cooley) Tube graft	(Less than) 100 ml/min/cm^2
KNITTED FABRIC (DACRON)	
Meadox knitted (Cooley) Fabric patch Tube graft	2000 ml/min/cm^2
VELOUR FABRIC (DACRON)	
Single-velour	3000 ml/min/cm^2
Double-velour	4750 ml/min/cm^2
FELT (DACRON)	
Patch graft	Not measured
Pledgets	Not measured

From Seifert P. C. (1994). *Cardiac surgery.* St. Louis: Mosby.
*Porosity is measured as the flow of distilled water through the fabric, at a pressure of 120 mmHg, expressed in milliliters per minute per square centimeter.

pioneer in graft development, Wesolowski, discovered that the greater porosity encouraged better healing and less porosity increased the chance for calcification on the inner surface of the graft. Tightly woven grafts also limited healing and there was concern that the poorly attached surface elements secondary to smaller interstices could slough and lead to graft failure. They developed weft knitting to improve compliance. This process uses only the fiber that goes in the direction of the weft on a loom, hence its name. Bifurcated grafts were developed that started as tubes with seams at the "legs," and then were seamless as the knitting technology gleaned from the pantyhose industry was utilized. Warp knitting was used also but despite the intricate possibilities of structure that this allowed, it was problematic for the construction of bifurcated grafts. Today, all knitted grafts are warp knitted. Liotta (1966, cited in Snyder, 1987) began the use of the **velour** or loop construction that lined the inner lumen of grafts to promote better adherence of a healing surface. Internal velours preceded external velours followed by internal *and* external or **double velour** grafts (Snyder, 1987). The internal loops of the velour are slightly smaller than the loops on the external surface. The external velour promotes good perigraft attachment and the inner loops act as a pseudo-intimal layer (Figure 9-7).

Dacron grafts are subjected to various procedures before they are packaged and ready for use. They are "compacted," which serves to improve durability and reduce the porosity. "Crimping" is done to improve handling (Figure 9-8). Both procedures may involve chemical additives, therefore the final step is to thoroughly clean the graft (Snyder, 1987). Sealing a graft with albumin to decrease the porosity was sometimes done in the operating room at the time the graft was needed. The scrub nurse would soak the selected Dacron graft in a basin of 10% human albumin and the graft was steam sterilized by the circulating nurse. The result was a foul smelling graft with an excess of a beige coagulum that had to be scraped from the graft. This was not only messy but time consuming. In 1983 Meadox introduced the first factory-sealed *knitted* graft as the "Hemashield Microvel Double Velour Vascular Graft." This graft was impregnated with bovine collagen, which decreased the permeability enough to eliminate the need for preclotting. In 1988 Meadox marketed the first sealed *woven* graft. Both types of graft (knitted and woven) heal well, maintain their patency, and have proven that the human body will completely replace the bovine collagen. Four hundred thousand Hemashield grafts have been sold since their introduction. It is helpful to visualize the complexity of structure to appreciate the efforts that continue to be applied to graft development (Figures 9-9 and 9-10). Because it is critical that a graft not be twisted during implantation, a line has been added to the construction of the graft to allow easy visual detection (see Figure 9-1). Twisting could cause graft occlusion and place tension on the anastomoses. Before this improvement was made some surgeons used a skin marker to mark the graft intraoperatively.

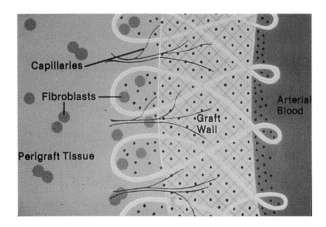

Fig. 9-7 Double velour construction; diagram of internal and external loops of graft wall. *(Courtesy Meadox Medicals.)*

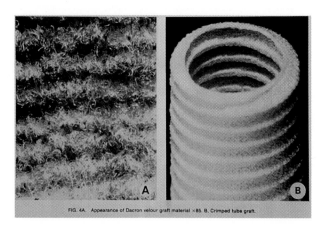

Fig. 9-8 Examples of a knitted and crimped velour graft. *(Courtesy Meadox Medicals.)*

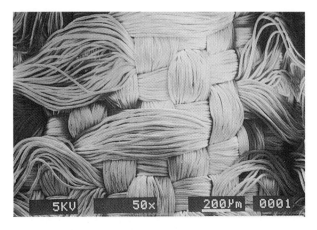

Fig. 9-9 Internal surface of a woven double velour graft magnified × 50. *(Courtesy Meadox Medicals.)*

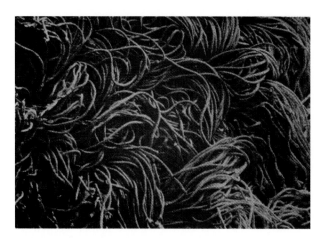

Fig. 9-10 Internal surface of a woven double velour graft magnified × 100. *(Courtesy Meadox Medicals.)*

PTFE Grafts

The Dacron grafts have worked very well in the high-flow states of the aorta. However, in low-flow states, such as axillofemoral bypasses or bypasses in the lower extremity (infrainguinal), they have functioned less well in some instances. PTFE is not considered a fabric but is an extruded *plastic*. Because of the small pore size compared with woven or knitted Dacron, PTFE may be less likely to develop long-term stiffening and contracture (Figure 9-11). This has been attributed to the pore size resisting the development of highly organized tissue healing (White, 1983).

W. L. Gore & Associates invented the process for making PTFE porous by "expanding" it. The wall of the graft is now 85% air. The addition of an outer layer that is perpendicular to the fibrils of the rest of the graft corrected early problems with aneurysm formation. Blood pressure will not expand the graft more than 14% over the life of the patient. The graft is soft and

pliable and until the recent introduction of the "stretch" grafts did not stretch. Care must be exercised in handling to cut it the exact length and avoid a suture larger than size 4-0 (Cannon, 1983). Needle holes can bleed and prolong operating time. Some surgeons use PTFE sutures to eliminate this nuisance bleeding (Figure 9-12). These grafts were used successfully in dogs in 1973 for the first time (Matsumoto, Hasegawa, & Fuse, 1973) and have had promising to dismal results depending on the data reported, patient selection, and many other variables that make judgment difficult. The reports of patency rates vary with the location of placement and technique. It was believed that PTFE and vein graft were about equal in the above-the-knee femoropopliteal procedures. Some authors have opted for sparing the saphenous vein graft by using synthetic grafts in above-the-knee surgery to have vein to use below the knee for subsequent procedures. Controversy exists about the patency rates of vein grafts versus synthetic grafts (NYC Conference).

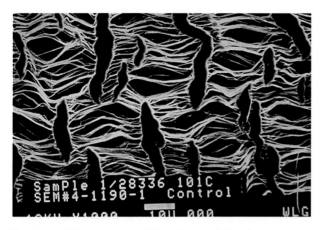

Fig. 9-11 Microstructure of Gore-Tex graft, luminal surface of stretch graft magnified × 1000. *(Courtesy W. L. Gore & Associates.)*

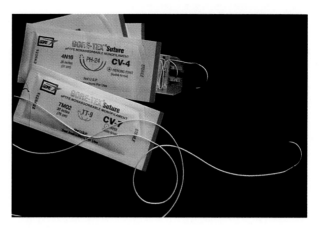

Fig. 9-12 Gore-Tex suture. *(Courtesy W. L. Gore & Associates.)*

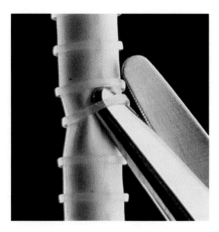

Fig. 9-13 Externally supported or ringed Gore-Tex graft. Rings may be removed by cutting or grasping with a clamp. *(Courtesy W. L. Gore & Associates.)*

Patients who need hemodialysis access fistulae are preferentially started with one of native vessels. For those patients whose vessels are too small or that later fail, PTFE has worked well and seems to resist infection because of its structure (Turner, 1987). The original Gore-Tex graft wall or *standard* wall is 0.65 mm thick. The *thin-walled* graft walls are 0.39 mm thick. The thin walled grafts are the graft of choice for vascular reconstruction or bypass procedures, while the standard wall grafts are better suited for dialysis access.

REGULATIONS

The Association for the Advancement of Medical Instrumentation (AAMI) has a Vascular Prostheses Committee composed of physicians and manufacturers with representation from the Food and Drug Administration (FDA). The committee drafted standards to serve as a guide for industry and health care providers in the early 1980s. The standards are not intended to discourage innovation but to encourage and facilitate dialogue and comparisons. The standards define terminology and describe uniform testing procedures employed in prostheses research and development. The committee also addressed concerns and needs regarding packaging, labeling, and package insert information. Emphasis was placed on the inclusion of a means to specifically identify each prosthesis by a lot or batch number for tracking purposes (Brewster, 1995).

In 1983 a pacemaker battery series was discovered to be defective after implantation. No practical means to track these devices existed. The estimated 1% to 2% morbidity and mortality rate of the device failing was lower than that for reoperation and replacement. The public was understadably disturbed by this situation and demanded a better way to address this problem. The manufacturer of the Bjork-Shiley artificial heart valve discovered the device was prone to a life-threatening fracture. The device was implanted in 23,000 patients but only 50% of the tracking forms that are included with the device were returned to the manufacturer. As a result, only 61% of the patients were located (ECRI, 1992). The 1990 passage of the Safe Medical Devices Act resulted. This legislation has been amended to allow a recall in 10 business days. Currently there are 26 items on a list that must be tracked and reported to the FDA. Vascular grafts are on the list (Weed, 1995).

The concept of tracking is simple: document the item and its specific identifier and communicate the information to a central data system. *It is important to document the catalog number of the implant and the serial or batch number that identifies it.* This allows identification of the specific item or a batch or group of items that are made from the same material and have undergone identical processing. Graft manufacturers have developed tracking forms to facilitate the process (Figure 9-14). The information requested included the patient's Social Security number, which may require patient permission. Some institutions have developed their own forms for generic tracking of all implants. It is possible to have secretarial and administrative staff transmit the required data electronically from the documentation already generated by the circulating nurse.

This device must be tracked by FDA Regulation. Compliance is mandatory. Please carefully read instructions contained in the package. Failure to comply will result in being in violation of the Food and Drug and Cosmetic Act.

MEDICAL DEVICE REGISTRATION FORM

COMPLETE AT TIME OF SURGERY

CATALOG/MODEL SIZE

PRODUCT NAME

BATCH/LOT NUMBER

**AFFIX LABEL
PROVIDED WITH DEVICE
HERE**

(If label in not available, complete information at right)

**AFFIX BAR CODE LABELS
PROVIDED WITH DEVICE HERE**

IMPLANT SITE (TYPE OF SURGICAL PROCEDURE) | DATE IMPLANTED

PATIENT INFORMATION

LAST NAME (INCLUDE SUFFIX: SR., JR., ETC.) | FIRST NAME | M.I.

ADDRESS | TELEPHONE NUMBER ( )

CITY | STATE | ZIP CODE | COUNTRY ☐U.S.A.

DATE OF BIRTH (MM-DD-YY) | GENDER ☐ MALE ☐ FEMALE | SOCIAL SECURITY NUMBER | PATIENT I.D. NUMBER | DATE DEVICE PROVIDED

HEALTHCARE FACILITY INFORMATION

NAME OF FACILITY | TELEPHONE NUMBER ( )

ADDRESS | FAX NUMBER ( )

CITY | STATE | ZIP CODE | COUNTRY ☐U.S.A.

COMPLETED BY | DEPARTMENT

IMPLANTING/PRESCRIBING PHYSICIAN INFORMATION

LAST NAME (INCLUDE SUFFIX: SR., JR., ETC.) | FIRST NAME | M.I. | TELEPHONE NUMBER ( )

ADDRESS | FAX NUMBER ( )

CITY | STATE | ZIP CODE | COUNTRY ☐U.S.A.

ATTENDING/FOLLOW-UP PHYSICIAN INFORMATION

LAST NAME (INCLUDE SUFFIX: SR., JR., ETC.) | FIRST NAME | M.I. | TELEPHONE NUMBER ( )

ADDRESS | FAX NUMBER ( )

CITY | STATE | ZIP CODE | COUNTRY ☐U.S.A.

EXPLANT IMFORMATION

WAS EXPLANT PERFORMED? ☐NO ☐YES *COMPLETE EXPLANT INFORMATION FORM. IF SAME MANUFACTURER AS IMPLANTED DEVICE, ATTACH FORM TO THIS FORM. IF DIFFERENT MANUFACTURER FROM IMPLANTED DEVICE, MAIL TO MANUFACTURER.*

FCE 96010272

Fig. 9-14 Example of device tracking form. *(Courtesy Meadox Medicals.)*

Multiple self-adhesive implantation labels may assist in maintaining accurate, legible documentation and save time for the circulating nurse, and eliminate costly work duplication. The employing institution bears the responsibility to adequately inform the staff of policies and procedures to assure compliance. A policy to address the method of compliance with the regulation is necessary. The professional RN also has the responsibility for keeping current about legislation and policies and for accurate and complete record keeping. This is ultimately for consumer protection.

When a hospital purchases a graft, it is a requirement that they track the graft from receipt to implantation, explantation, and destruction. If a hospital borrows a graft or returns a graft to another institution, it is necessary to notify the manufacturer. Some institutions find it simpler to obtain the graft directly from their sales representative rather than borrowing. The manufacturer must be notified even when a graft is opened and not implanted (discarded because it was mistakenly requested or inadvertently contaminated). Grafts that are removed or explanted for any reason (amputation or infection) require manufacturer notification.

The regulations for prosthetic devices are increasing as the public demands greater assurance of quality and safety. The adverse reactions to silicone breast implants led to unprecedented legislation and increased public awareness. This inevitably increases the costs of research and development. Stricter requirements will necessarily demand more extensive testing via larger or longer clinical trials. The liability that manufacturers face also drives the cost of business upward but hopefully will improve safety. Innovations need appropriate testing even if the time required precludes many patients from benefitting in the interim. Quality assurance has become increasingly important as an industry standard.

NURSING RESPONSIBILITIES

The circulating nurse has responsibility for overseeing the safe-handling of the vascular prostheses. The surgeon communicates the type and size of the graft. The nurse obtains the appropriate graft and verifies the correct selection visually and verbally with both the surgeon and the scrub nurse. The act of verification as well as the identification numbers, size and type of graft must be documented (AORN, 1996). Institutional policies must be followed for handling and tracking mechanisms. Although vascular fabric patches are not on the FDA mandatory tracking list, it may be prudent to follow similar procedures for documentation and maintenance of a log book.

Safe-handling also entails familiarity with specific manufacturers' recommendations. PTFE grafts must be protected as much as possible from contact with iodophor prep solutions (breakdown) and skin (bacterial contamination). "Preclotting" of knitted grafts is sometimes necessary. Knitted grafts have greater porosity than woven. Their interstices must be soaked or coated by blood to limit the porosity and subsequent bleeding. The degree of healing and calcification have been related to the pore size of the graft and yarn flexibility. Velour grafts are easier to preclot than nonvelour (Snyder, 1983). There are different "preclotting" procedures. Low-porosity grafts can be simply coated with blood or allowed to sit in a basin of nonheparinized blood until sewn in place. A more porous graft may have the blood forcefully and repeatedly flushed until visible leaking decreases as fibrin fills the spaces. Obvious adherent clot should be removed with gentle suction. Preclotting can be done with heparinized blood but it takes more time. Topical thrombin added to a basin of blood may also assist in the procedure (Brewster, 1995). The scrub nurse must handle the graft with care, protecting it from contamination or loss.

Institutional variations will determine the responsibilities for purchasing, stocking, and inventory levels. Stock may be purchased or maintained on a consignment basis. A manufacturer's representative can be very valuable in assisting with these needs.

FUTURE

Researchers (industry and physicians) are conducting graft research on existing materials to decide their best use and to determine innovative ways to combat various problems. Graft infections do not occur frequently, but they can be threatening to life or limb. Grafts bonded with antibacterial agents have been tried unsuccessfully but new work is being done using metals to assist in the adherence of the drug to the graft. Bandyk (1994) suggests that antibiotic impregnated grafts will probably have little impact on the *rate* of graft infections but may be useful in immunodepressed patients. No antibiotic impregnated grafts are available for human implantation at this time (Kempczinski, 1995). Studies have been performed using carbon-lined grafts to address the need for a nonthrombogenic luminal (inner) graft surface. Two forms of carbon have been used, vitreous and turbostratic. Thermal degradation is used to create vitreous carbon. Turbostratic carbons are formed into a lattice arrangement by heat under pressure. Both have shown some feasibility in animal and human subjects (Sharp, 1987). The most valuable aspect of the carbon grafts may be more related to the ability to be treated in such a way as to bind heparin (Kempczinski, 1995).

Healthy endothelial cells that line a native vessel have the ability to prevent thrombosis and infection. Humans do not line artificial grafts with endothelium as some animal models have. Another growing area of graft research is in "seeding" graft fabric with endothelial cells to promote the growth of an endothelial lining throughout the intraluminal graft surface. Both PTFE and Dacron grafts have seeded successfully in experiments (Kempczinski, 1995).

In 1976 Herring reported the first work in seeding. He scraped endothelial cells off a vein surface into a solution that was then mixed with blood to preclot a graft (Glover, 1987). Herring, Gardner, and Glover (1978) published their results of seeding knitted Dacron aortic grafts in dogs. They found that the grafts developed a psuedointimal lining throughout, which was their goal. The lack of endothelium has been considered one of the reasons that small diameter grafts thrombose. Unfortunately, this endothelialization has not occurred as readily in the human population. Heralded as the most important advances since the start of prosthetic graft usage, the results are complex. Studies are showing that transplanted endothelial cells may have altered function that exhibits unfavorable reactions (Libby, Birinyi, & Callow, 1987). If this process does become more feasible, it could mean that prostheses for venous construction could be more viable also (Tabbara & White, 1994). The smaller diameter grafts, 6 mm or less, are at high risk for failure. An important area of research will include work to discover the best conduit for these small vessel replacements. Information about materials, thrombosis, and endothelial cell biology are a few of the areas in which research is needed to solve the problems encountered with small grafts (Tabbara & White, 1994).

Another area that may bear investigating is the possibility of synthetic grafts that are radiopaque (the currently available synthetic grafts are not radiopaque). This could prove useful in endovascular procedures that include stent placement. Endovascular procedures are receiving renewed interest and grafts are an integral component of this. Work is currently underway on the placement of aortic grafts through a simple groin incision (Mathias, 1994). This work includes modifications of the graft to conform to small carriers and the addition of attachment mechanisms similar to those found on the Greenfield vena cava filters (see Chapter 18). The grafts used for endovascular implantation may need special modifications.

It was originally believed that an inert material that was passively resistant to any immune or foreign body reaction by the body was the desired trait for grafts. Research has not borne this out and now there is the potential for an "active" graft. Trials are underway in New England to use an endothelial growth factor. An angioplasty balloon is dipped into a growth factor and an angioplasty performed. The intent is to stimulate the growth of collateral vessels in the surrounding tissue (Dr. Jean Goggins, personal communication).

References

AORN Recommended Practices for Documentation of Perioperative Nursing Care (1996). *AORN standards and recommended practices* (pp. 151-153). Denver: AORN.

Apyan, R. L., Schneider, P. A., & Andros, G. (1992). Preservation of arm veins for arterial reconstruction. *Journal of Vascular Nursing, 10*(2);pp. 2-5.

Bandyk, D. F. (1994). In-situ prosthetic graft replacement for coagulase-negative Staphylococci infection. In K. D. Calligaro, & F.J. Veith (Eds.), *Management of infected arterial grafts* (pp. 185-201). St. Louis: Quality Medical Publishing.

Bensen, J. L., & Karmody, A.M. (1987). In situ artery bypass: Surgery for leg salvage. *AORN Journal, 45*(1); 40-55.

Brewster, D. C. (1995). Prosthetic grafts. In R. B. Rutherford (Ed.), *Vascular surgery* (4th ed) (pp. 492-521). Philadelphia: W. B. Saunders.

Cannon, J.A. (1983). The expanded reinforced polytetrafluoroethylene prosthetic vascular graft (ERPTFEVG). In C. B. Wright, R. W. Hobson III, L.F. Hiratzka, & T.G. Lynch (Eds.), *Vascular grafting: Clinical applications and techniques* (pp. 31-42). Boston: John Wright, PSG.

Curl, R. J., & Ricotta, J. J. (1994). Total prosthetic graft excision and extra-anatomic bypass. In K. D. Calligaro, & F. J. Veith (Eds.), *Management of infected arterial grafts* (pp. 82-94). St. Louis: Quality Medical Publishing.

Dennis, C. (1987). Brief history of development of vascular grafts. In C. B. Wright, R. W. Hobson III, L.F. Hiratka, & T. G. Lynch (Eds.), *Vascular grafting: Clinical applications and techniques* (pp. 1-26). Boston: John Wright, PSG.

ECRI (Emergency Care Research Institute) (1992). ECRI advisory: Safe medical devices act of 1990. Pennsylvania: ECRI.

Glover, J. L. (1987). Historical perspectives on endothelial seeding. In M. Herring, & J. L. Glover (Eds.). *Endothelial seeding in vascular surgery* (pp. 1-6). Orlando: Grune & Stratton.

Goggins, J., Meadox Medical (August 1995). Personal communication.

Green, R. M., & Ouriel, K. (1994). Peripheral arterial disease. In S. I. Schwarz, G. T. Shires, & F. C. Spencer (Eds.), *Principles of surgery* (pp. 925-987). New York: McGraw-Hill.

Herring, M., Gardner, A., & Glover, J. (1978). A single-staged technique for seeding vascular grafts with autogenous endothelium. *Surgery, 84*(5):498-504.

Kempczinski, R. F. (1995). Vascular grafts. In R. B. Rutherford (Ed.), *Vascular surgery* (4th ed., pp. 470-474). Philadelphia: W. B. Saunders.

Libby, P., Birinyi, L.K., & Callow, A. D. (1987). Functions of endothelial cells related to seeding of vascular prostheses: the unanswered questions. In M. Herring & J.L. Glover (Eds.), *Endothelial seeding in vascular surgery* (pp. 17-35). Orlando: Grune & Stratton.

Liotta, D., et al (1966). A pseudoendocardium for implantable blood pumps. *Transcripts of the American Society of Artificial Internal Organs, 12*: 129-137.

Matsumoto, H., et al (1973). A new vascular prosthesis for a small caliber artery. *Surgery, 74*(4): 518-523.

Mathias, J. M. (1994). Aortic aneurysm repair made less invasive. *OR Manager, 10*(9): 22-23.

Ouriel, K., & Geary, K. (1994). When can a vein graft be preserved and when should it be excised? In K. D. Calligaro, & F. J. Veith (Eds.), *Management of infected arterial grafts* (pp. 212-218). St. Louis: Quality Medical Publishing.

Sharp, W.V. (1987). Update on carbon-coated grafts. In P.N. Sawyer (Ed.), *Modern vascular grafts* (pp. 215-224). New York: McGraw-Hill.

Snyder, R.W. (1983). Fabrication and testing of textile vascular prostheses. In C. B. Wright, R. W. Hobson III, L.F. Hiratzka, & T. G. Lynch (Eds.), *Vascular grafting: Clinical applications and techniques* (pp. 13-22). Boston: John Wright, PSG.

Tabbara, M., & White, R. A. (1994). Biologic and prosthetic materials for vascular conduits. In F.R. Veith, R. W. Hobson, R. A. Williams, & S.E. Wilson (Eds.), *Vascular surgery: Principles and practices* (2nd ed., pp. 523-535). New York: McGraw-Hill.

Turner, R.I. (1987). Vascular graft development: An industrial perspective. In P.N. Sawyer (Ed.), *Modern vascular grafts* (pp. 75-103). New York: McGraw-Hill.

Weed, P. (1995). A successful device tracking program. *AORN Journal, 62*(2): 260-265.

White, R.A. (1983). Evaluation of small diameter graft parameters using replamineform vascular prostheses. In C.B. Wright, R.W. Hobson III, L.F. Hiratzka, & T.G. Lynch (Eds.), *Vascular grafting: Clinical applications and techniques* (pp. 315-325). Boston: John Wright, PSG.

Wright, C.W., et al (1987). The regulatory environment for vascular grafts. In P.N. Sawyer (Ed.), *Modern vascular grafts* (pp. 105-114). New York: McGraw-Hill.

Fundamentals of Vascular Surgery

INTRODUCTION

Fundamental techniques of vascular surgery include the intraoperative techniques that are basic to surgery involving blood vessels. These include principles of selecting incision site, techniques of dissection, and vessel control. Understanding of these basic techniques will enhance the role of the perioperative nurse, RNFA, and operating room technician. Many vascular procedures can be categorized as reconstructive interventions. **Reconstruction** encompasses the **bypass** of blocked vessels (anatomic and extraanatomic) and the **restoration of blood flow** as in endarterectomy, patch angioplasty, balloon angioplasty, and embolectomy. These are divided into open versus endovascular procedures (Box 10-1). Some of these techniques are the primary surgical intervention or may be utilized as an adjunct to the scheduled intervention. An example of this is endarterectomy. A carotid endarterectomy may be the primary intervention or may be required in a lower extremity bypass as an ancillary procedure (see Chapter 11).

MISCELLANEOUS PRINCIPLES

Incisions

The skin incision for a vascular surgery is based on providing the best visualization of the relevant anatomy. Preoperative angiograms may assist in selecting the best site. When possible, the incision is placed directly over the vessel. When a bypass graft is being placed, the best path for the graft or the site of harvest

of a vein graft also determines the incision to follow. Smaller incisions that still permit adequate surgical access and avoid creating a skin flap are important for wound healing. When abnormal anatomy or pathology is encountered, a basic principle is to work from known structures to unknown. This allows control of vessels and avoidance of damage to nerves by using the familiar or normal anatomy as landmarks. Other factors that may modify the incision are obesity, scarring from previous surgeries, infection, or prior radiation treatment.

Dissection

Sharp dissection is generally employed (a scalpel for the skin and scissors for the perivascular tissue). Numerous #15 blades may be used for careful dissection in a "redo" procedure to dissect the scarred, adhered tissue. When working with atherosclerotic arteries, the lack of a clearly defined sheath may complicate dissection. The perivascular area may be fibrotic and vascular. Injecting 1 or 2 ml of saline around the vessel to lift the sheath may be helpful to define the tissue planes (Haimovici, 1996b). Meticulous attention is paid to achieving hemostasis (clamps, ties, suture ligatures, manual compression, packs, clips, cautery) since anticoagulation of the patient is often employed during vascular surgery. Anticoagulation can cause bleeding that would not be problematic in the nonheparinized patient. Ligation of lymphatics is required, especially in groin dissection, to prevent lymph leakage that may complicate wound healing.

Vessel Control

There are a variety of techniques for controlling or occluding vessels. Once the vessel is identified, it must then be "mobilized." A normal (disease free) vessel usually has a "sheath" around it that can be lifted and incised. After freeing the vessel from surrounding tissue, a right-angled clamp may be passed under the vessel and a tie, umbilical tape, or elastic vessel loop is passed around it. This loop can be used to lift the vessel for better visualization of any posterior branches of the vessel (Haimovici, 1996b). A loop or tie may be left as a single pass (for vessel identification or manual retraction) or passed around the vessel a second time to permit occlusion of the vessel. This double loop is called a **Potts** tie (Figure 10-1). A small clamp or tag may be placed on the ends of the single loop or Potts tie to provide retraction or counter traction during further dissection. The Potts loop may be cinched to occlude the vessel and the clamp fastened to the drapes to maintain occlusion. Another means of controlling a vessel is by placing a vascular or Rummel tourniquet around it (see Figure 8-49). Adequate proximal control is required before any intervention. In instances of traumatic injury (including iatrogenic vascular

Box 10-1 **Revascularization and Reconstructive Techniques**

OPEN PROCEDURES
Bypass grafts (synthetic and autogenous materials)
Interposition grafts
Endarterectomy
Patch angioplasty
Ancillary techniques
    Embolectomy
    Angioscopy

ENDOVASCULAR PROCEDURES
Seldinger technique
Balloon angioplasty
Stents
Stent-grafts
Laser
Atherectomy

puncture) the existence of a hematoma or inflammatory reaction may make vessel dissection and control more difficult. A remote incision may be needed for adequate control.

Clamping is another means of vessel control. Vascular clamps are available in a variety of sizes and styles. The small bulldog clamps are even available by the amount of pressure they exert (see Chapter 8). The size of the clamp must be appropriate for the size of the vessel, have a shape that is suitable for the depth of the wound, and permit adequate access. Clamps are also selected on the basis of configuration for the purpose of total occlusion ("cross-clamp") or partial occlusion ("side-biting") (Figure 10-2). This configuration is also important when the surgeon elects to place the clamp to occlude the vessel from side to side or from anterior to posterior. The anterior-posterior placement is often preferred in diseased vessels because the plaque usually lies on the posterior vessel wall. The surgeon tries to avoid placing a clamp on an area of plaque. Clamping directly on plaque could fracture the plaque and send debris distally, occluding a vessel or branch. Clamping on plaque may not effectively prevent bleeding. A basic technique for placement of a vascular clamp is to seek a soft or plaque-free point of the artery. Manual compression of traumatized, diffusely diseased, or tiny vessels may be less damaging than clamping. Use of an extremity tourniquet has been advocated as another alternative to clamping that may prevent endothelial damage to distal extremity vessels (Green, 1993) (see Figure 8-36 and see Chapter 12).

Vessel control can be accomplished by temporarily "plugging" the vessel. A Garrett dilator, a commercially created soft vessel occluder, or a "balloon" may be used. A venous occlusion catheter or a balloon embolectomy catheter makes use of a flexible balloon (see Figure 8-28, *A*). The embolectomy catheter can be adapted to maintain the balloon inflation by simply placing a stopcock on the balloon port, inflating it, and closing the stopcock (Figure 10-3). This technique is used in working with tiny vessels to avoid the trauma of clamping and prevent back bleeding during an anastomosis. Balloon occlusion is also useful in the event of inadvertent entry into an undissected artery, to control a ruptured artery (such as during a percutaneous intervention or a ruptured aortic aneurysm), or to avoid clamping a calcified vessel (see Figure 8-32). This technique may be helpful when using an extremity tourniquet, which does not always provide complete control of bleeding.

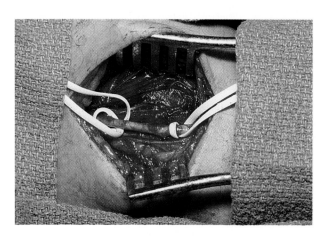

Fig. 10-1 Vessel loops around a vessel.

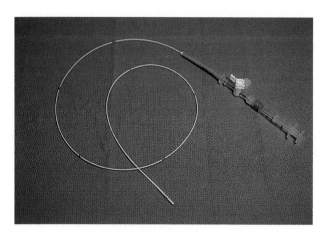

Fig. 10-3 Embolectomy catheter.

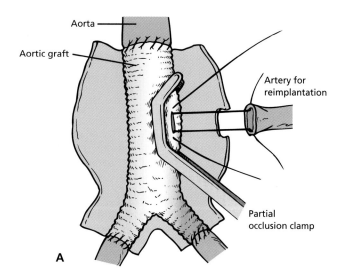

A

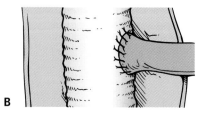

B

Fig. 10-2 **A,** This shows the technique of using a side-biting or partial occlusion clamp on the aortic graft for reimplantation patch angioplasty. This technique permits blood flow to continue through the aorta while the small area needed for the anastomosis is occluded. This may be used for reimplanting the renal or mesenteric artery. **B,** The completed reimplantation anastomosis.

REVASCULARIZATION AND RECONSTRUCTIVE TECHNIQUES

Open Procedures

Bypass

Bypass procedures are performed to provide blood flow around an obstructed or diseased vessel. "Inflow" and "outflow" are selected by angiography. The graft material options include autologous, homologous, and synthetic conduits (see Chapter 9).

Vascular Anastomoses. The incision into a vessel may be transverse or horizontal. Horizontal incisions are made to transect a vessel in preparation for an end-to-end anastomosis, for placement of an interposition graft, reimplantation of a vessel, or access to the lumen for embolectomy (Figure 10-4). A longitudinal incision is better for visualizing the lumen. The longitudinal incision can be enlarged as needed. It is used for end-to-side anastomoses. Closure of a longitudinal incision may narrow the lumen and increase the possibility of thrombosis. To prevent these problems, especially in vessels <5 mm, a **patch closure** may be used (Dzsinich & Gloviczki, 1993).

Three basic anastomoses are used routinely in vascular surgery: **end to end, end to side,** and **side to side.** A transected vessel may be repaired with an end-to-end anastomosis. An end-to-end anastomosis is performed when placing an interposition graft such as an aortic graft (Figure 10-5). An end-to-side graft may be used in procedures such as reimplantation of the renal artery in a suprarenal aortic aneurysm resection (Figure 10-6) or a renal artery bypass (see Chapter 15). Arterial reconstructions or arterial bypass procedures may use an end-to-side anastomosis (e.g., femorofemoral bypass, axillofemoral bypass, femoral-popliteal bypass). Side-to-side anastomoses (Figure 10-7) are used for creating arteriovenous (AV) fistulae (Dzsinich & Gloviczki, 1993) (see Chapter 16).

Ancillary techniques to improve the patency of prosthetic grafts also use concept of AV fistulae. This technique incorporates an adjacent vein into the anastomosis. This may be a temporary measure to increase graft patency. It is a minor procedure to ligate the fistula at a later time. Incorporation of a vein segment is also used to improve graft patency. Two examples of this are the **Taylor patch** and the **Miller cuff.** The

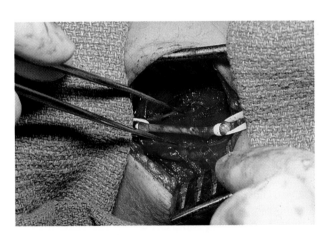

Fig. 10-4 Arteriotomy.

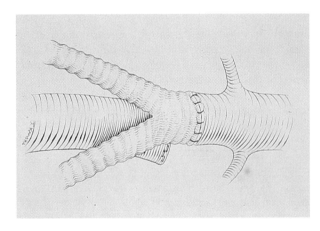

Fig. 10-5 End-to-end anastomosis. *(Courtesy Meadox Medicals.)*

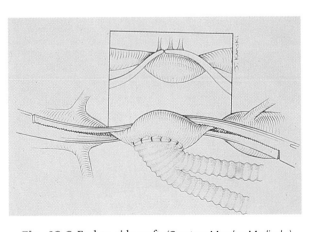

Fig. 10-6 End-to-side graft. *(Courtesy Meadox Medicals.)*

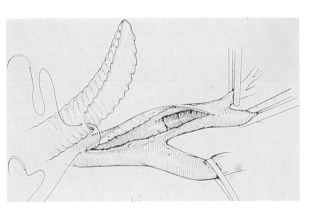

Fig. 10-7 Side-to-side anastomosis. *(Courtesy Meadox Medicals.)*

Taylor patch is used in distal lower extremity bypass with PTFE (Taylor, et al, 1992). The heel of the PTFE graft is sewn to the native (outflow) vessel and vein patch incorporated into the anastomosis (Figure 10-8). A Miller cuff is created with a tubular segment of vein interposed between vessel and PTFE graft. This may be useful when a vein graft to a distal bypass fails. A segment of the initially placed vein graft is left and the PTFE graft sewn to it.

Suturing techniques. End-to-end anastomoses may be performed with a continuous over-and-over style of suturing. The two ends to be approximated are tacked with a stay stitch at two equidistant points. A running suture is then used to sew the visible half of the anastomosis, the vessel is rotated 180 degrees, and the remaining half is sewn in the same manner. Another technique for an end-to-end anastomosis is to sew the posterior walls together through the lumen; the anterior walls are then sewn. End-to-side anastomoses can be accomplished by sewing the posterior wall by the intraluminal method and the anterior wall on the outside. Another method is to use four "guy" sutures to approximate the vessels or graft and a continuous over and over extraluminal technique. A side-to-side anastomosis can be accomplished by placement of two stay sutures at the tips of the openings and two stay sutures to retract the centers of the openings. The intraluminal technique is used on the back wall, the two sutures tied together, and the closure completed with an extraluminal technique (Haimovici, 1996b). When creating an anastomosis, the two edges are everted in order to bring intima in contact with the graft lining (Greenhalgh, 1989). Interrupted suturing may also be used to approximate an anastomosis. This technique is indicated to permit growth, such as in repair of coarctation of the aorta in children (Eastcott & Thompson, 1985).

Suturing with monofilament polypropylene suture is facilitated by wetting the hand of the person tying (surgeon or RNFA). The scrub nurse uses an asepto syringe with saline to "splash" the tying hand. This permits the gloved hand to slide easily on the suture (see Figure 8-21).

Interposition graft

An interposition graft is the replacement of a segment of a vessel. The procedure is similar to a bypass except that the diseased or injured portion of the native vessel is removed. Autologous or synthetic graft may be used as replacement and an end-to-end anastomosis is employed at both ends. A modification of this is used in repair of abdominal aortic aneurysm repair. The outer wall of the aorta remains and is used to cover the interposition graft.

Endarterectomy

The terms *endarterectomy* and *thromboendarterectomy* are used synonymously to refer to a technique of removing an obstructing atherosclerotic plaque (Figure 10-9) and thrombus from an artery. The term *endarterectomy,* strictly refers to the concomitant removal of the endothelial layer but in fact also removes the inner media as well. A plane is seen between the artery wall involved and the disease-free area. The nature of atherosclerotic pathophysiology is such that it usually does not involve the adventitia or outer portion of the media (Stoney & Thompson, 1995). This cleavage plane exhibits variations depending on the structure of the vessel involved. Haimovici (1996a) describes three planes: subintimal, transmedial, and subadventitial. The subintimal is just under the intima and subintimal endarterectomy is usually avoided because it may lead to postoperative thrombosis. The transmedial plane is found at three quarters of the depth of the media. The subadventitial is between the media and adventitia. Plaque often tapers to an endpoint that lends itself to a cleaner removal. In instances where the endpoint does not taper ideally or is inaccessible the plaque can be sutured in place. This suturing is called a **tacking** stitch and prevents the remaining plaque from lifting and obstructing blood flow (Stoney & Thompson, 1995).

Aneurysmal disease is a contraindication to endarterectomy. The residual media and adventitia in the nonaneurysmal artery maintain enough strength that the technique does not threaten their structural integrity. However, in aneurysmal disease, degeneration of the adventitia increases the risk of dilation and subsequent rupture (Stoney & Thompson, 1995).

Open endarterectomy is the most common method. An arteriotomy is performed with a # 11 blade and the opening enlarged longitudinally with Potts scissors (see Figure 10-9, *B*). An elevator or a clamp may be used to remove the plaque from the artery (see Figure 11-4). A semi-closed or "blind" endarterectomy is used on an arterial branch. Arterial loop strippers are selected by the size of the diseased artery and the plaque is removed by feel (Figure 10-10). Another example of this is an

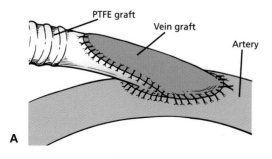

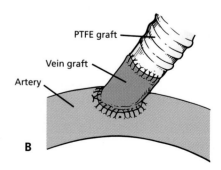

Fig. 10-8 **A,** Taylor patch. **B,** Miller cuff.

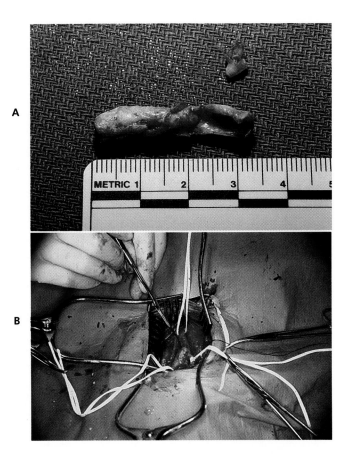

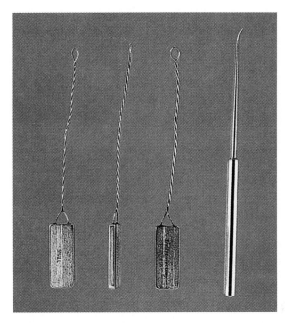

Fig. 10-10 Endarterectomy loops. *(From Brooks-Tighe, S. [1994]. Instrumentation for the operating room [4th ed.]. St. Louis: Mosby.)*

Fig. 10-9 A, Atheromatous plaque: Whitish with yellow streaks, it is often tubular and may contain thrombus or ulceration. It may have a fibrous feel to it or contain segments of calcification that feel hard and inflexible. The vessel layers are usually not identifiable. **B,** A fine-tipped knife, such as a # 11 blade, is used to make the initial arteriotomy, which is enlarged with a Potts scissors.

eversion technique commonly seen during carotid endarterectomy. The external carotid is partially visualized and the plaque grasped and everted.

Patch angioplasty

Closure of a longitudinal incision that was made into a vessel may compromise the lumen diameter and result in stenosis, which is undesirable. A **patch graft angioplasty** may prevent stenosis. Patch material may be either autogenous or synthetic. Autogenous grafts have been formed from arterial, venous, and peritoneal tissue. Many surgeons prefer *veins* for autogenous patches because they are more readily available and expandable. Autogenous *arterial* patches have shown fewer degenerative changes but are not always readily available, nor do they expand like a vein patch (Haimovici, 1996c). Obtaining autogenous material may require a separate incision for graft harvest, which may be undesirable in terms of wound healing in a compromised patient, incisional discomfort, or additional surgical time.

Synthetic patch material may be made of PTFE (polytetrafluoroethylene) or Dacron (polyester) (see Figure 11-3). Patches may be purchased in flat pieces of fabric or cut from a tube graft. The patch is cut to fit the arteriotomy and may be oval, rectangular, or Y-shaped (such as at a bifurcation). In transplantation or reimplantation, a portion of native vessel from the original implant site may be left on the end of the vessel to be reimplanted to create its own patch (see Figure 10-2, *B*).

Ancillary techniques (embolectomy, angioscopy)

Fogarty catheter embolectomy. Fogarty catheter (balloon) embolectomy is the removal of a clot from a vessel. A transverse arteriotomy is made (see Figure 10-4), a balloon catheter is inserted directly into the vessel past the obstructing clot (Figure 10-11), the balloon is inflated, and the catheter is withdrawn with the balloon inflated to remove the clot (Figure 10-12). The more common sites for arterial embolectomy include the femoral artery (50%), popliteal artery (15%), iliac artery (15%), and aorta (10%). Embolectomies can be performed under local anesthesia.

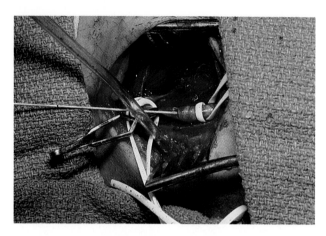

Fig. 10-11 Shows balloon catheter inserted into arterial opening.

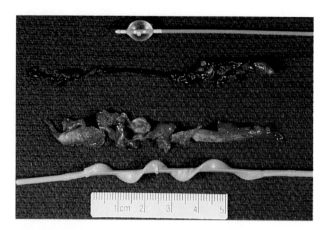

Fig. 10-12 Two catheters with resultant thrombus and plaque. *(Courtesy Baxter Vascular Systems Division.)*

For a femoral or arctic embolectomy, an arteriotomy is made into the femoral artery for removal of an embolus from the aorta and the arteries of the lower extremity (Myhre & Saether, 1989). Embolectomy may be performed as a separate surgical procedure or in conjunction with reconstructive interventions. The standard Fogarty embolectomy balloon catheter designed in the early 1960s has remained a significant and widely used technology. The balloons are made of latex, which continues to provide the best balloon strength and feel for the procedure (Fogarty, et al, 1991). These embolectomy catheters are available in sizes from 2 Fr to 7 Fr. Variations have been developed. Balloon embolectomy catheters were originally developed for arteries and modified to have a very soft, flexible leading tip for venous embolectomies (see Figure 8-28, *A*). The modified tip prevents the catheter from becoming caught on the valves (Fogarty, et al, 1991). More recently, two special catheters were designed for thrombectomies. These are more aggressive in extracting material lodged in either a native vessel or a graft. The adherent clot catheter has a corkscrew-like balloon with a wire framework inside a latex covering that retracts to provide a scraping maneuver (see Figure 8-28, *C*). A graft thrombectomy catheter is similar to the adherent clot catheter but has the spiral wire configuration without the latex covering (see Figure 8-28, *B*). This is the more aggressive of the two items and is used only in synthetic grafts (Fogarty & Hermann, 1991).

Angioscopy. Angioscopy, sometimes called microendoscopy, allows the surgeon to visualize the intraluminal surfaces of a vessel at a point remote to the surgery and as a means to perform procedures under indirect visualization. The angioscopes available in the 1980s have been replaced by the improved angioscopes of the 1990s. Improvements were made in the quality of the fiberoptic fibers. The newer scopes provide better image resolution, particularly when combined with special lenses that are available as small as 0.3 mm in diameter. The fiberoptic cords are also very flexible and soft, making them easier to work with and possibly less likely to cause endothelial damage. Some scopes can be "steered" but this steering mecha-

nism takes up space and may not allow room for operating channels. Steering may allow better control and access to small vessels and branches. The complete system for an angioscope requires a large capital investment. The scopes are fragile and require patient, skillful use and handling. They are available as both single use and multiple use. Staff need adequate training for using the scope, light source, video system, and fluid pump. Crystalloid solutions under pressure may be used in the pump to maintain a clear view of the vessel lumen (Grundfest, 1996) (see Figure 8-59)

Endovascular Procedures

Percutaneous transluminal angioplasty (PTA)

Percutaneous transluminal angioplasty includes a variety of methods for restoring patency to an obstructed or stenosed vessel. The procedure may be performed using local anesthesia under fluoroscopic guidance. It may be performed in the radiology suite by a radiologist, in the cardiac catheterization suite by a cardiologist, or in the OR by a surgeon. Sometimes PTA is done in conjunction with other surgical interventions. PTA includes atherectomy, placement of an intraluminal stent, balloon angioplasty, and laser-assisted balloon angioplasty (Box 10-2). It may be prudent to have equipment and supplies readily available for an open surgical intervention in the case of vessel perforation and hemorrhage (Atkinson & Fortunato, 1996).

Seldinger technique

The Seldinger technique is the percutaneous placement of a large bore needle into a vessel (vein or artery) followed by a guidewire. The needle is removed and a vessel sheath dilator may be introduced over the guidewire. This sheath is usually a flexible plastic tube that both guides the introduction of subsequent catheters or instruments and protects the vessel wall at the entry site region. This technique is used in a number of percutaneous interventions, including the placement of vena cava filters (see Chapter 18), balloon angioplasties, and insertion of central monitoring lines (Figure 10-13).

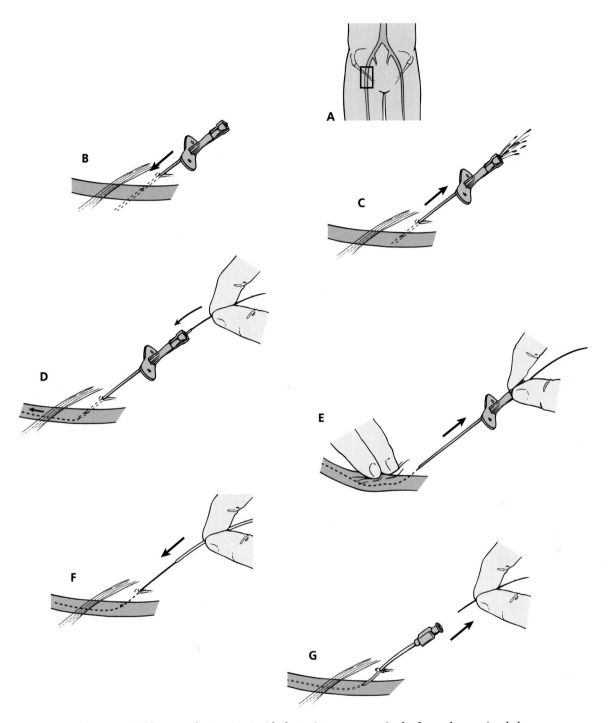

Fig. 10-13 Seldinger technique. **A,** An ideal arteriotomy occurs in the femoral artery just below the inguinal ligament. **B,** A beveled compound needle containing an inner cannula pierces through the artery. **C,** The needle is withdrawn until good blood return occurs. **D,** The needle's inner cannula is removed, and a flexible guide wire is inserted. **E,** The needle is removed; pressure fixes the wire and reduces hemorrhage. **F,** The catheter is slipped over the wire and into the artery. **G,** The wire guide is removed, leaving the catheter in the artery. *(From Ballinger, P. W. [1995].* Merrill's Atlas of radiographic positions and radiologic procedures *[8th ed.]. St. Louis: Mosby.)*

Balloon angioplasty

Balloon angioplasty is a percutaneous transluminal technique to open the lumen of an atherosclerotic vessel stenosis. The balloon is at the end of a catheter that usually has two lumens. One lumen is open at the distal end of the catheter to permit irrigation and injection of x-ray contrast. The second lumen is to the balloon to permit balloon inflation with saline or x-ray contrast (or a mixture of both). These specially designed balloon catheters are made of polyvinyl that allows expansion of the balloon against a plaque without the balloon rupturing or conforming to the plaque. The balloon is usually marked by radiopaque dots that allow the physician to visualize the balloon placement within the stenotic area of the vessel. The catheter lengths vary and the balloon varies in length (2 to 10 cm) and width at inflation (3 to 12 mm). Selection of the balloon catheter is based on the size of the vessel and the lesion. Angioplasty is accomplished by rupturing the atheromatous plaque and endothelium and rupturing and stretching the media (McIvor, 1989) (see Figure 8-38 and Box 8-5).

Laser-assisted balloon angioplasty (LABA)

In laser-assisted balloon angioplasty the same technique for balloon angioplasty is used with the addition of a laser probe to open a path for the balloon by vaporizing a segment of the lesion. The use of laser-assisted balloon angioplasty (LABA) to recanalize stenotic arterial lesions has remained controversial. The FDA approved the use of the laser in iliac and femoropopliteal lesions in 1987 (White, 1996). However, the constantly evolving technologies to address problems with early restenosis, vessel perforation, and heat injury have made evaluation of the technology difficult. Until randomized, multicenter trials are conducted to determine the optimal patient selection and indications for intervention, the use of LABA is considered an evolving technology (Green & Ouriel, 1994).

Intraluminal stents

Intraluminal stent placement is the catheter-guided implantation of a remote device to maintain vessel patency. It can be permanent or temporary (resorbable) and is usually a mesh configuration made of metal or other materials. The device is designed to prevent collapse of the vessel and provide a nonthrombogenic surface. The devices being used most often are balloon expandable or self-expanding. The balloon-expandable stent (e.g., Palmaz stent) is deployed on an angioplasty balloon and opened up and fixed in place by the inflation of the balloon (Figure 10-14). Advantages of balloon-expandable stents include accurate placement and exact diameter expansion. The self-expandable stent (e.g., Gianturco stent) expands without balloon inflation and has the reported advantage of placement via a smaller profile introducer (Casteneda, 1996).

Indications for stent placement are generally for vessel restenosis, failure, or intimal flap creation after PTA. This is an evolving technology and placement of stents in the iliac, renal, and lower extremity arteries are being performed in Europe and the United States (Casteneda, 1996). Intraluminal stent placement is evolving in response to the problems of reclosure of a vessel after balloon angioplasty. The vessel reclosure may be attributed to vessel spasm, dissection, recoil, or thrombosis.

Atherectomy

Atherectomy is performed using a catheter-mounted device that has a side-biting cutter or a rotational burr or cam that cuts or shaves the atheromatous plaque from the vessel wall. A variety of manufacturers and subsequent styles have been marketed. Atherectomy devices come in different sizes and may be designed with a balloon at the tip to prevent particles of plaque from migrating distally and causing further occlusion. Initial results have been favorable with few complications from the procedure. Long-term patency rates have yet to be conclusive and define optimal patient selection (Fogarty, Biswa, Hermann, & Newman, 1996).

INFECTION
Incidence

The incidence of *vascular graft infections* is reported as between 1% and 6%. It is difficult to obtain a clear picture of this because of the variation in follow-up data and the variation in the time of onset. The onset may vary from the immediate postoperative period to as late as 10 years after implantation (Goldstone & Bowersox, 1996). Although the incidence is relatively low, the impact can be devastating and result in loss of life

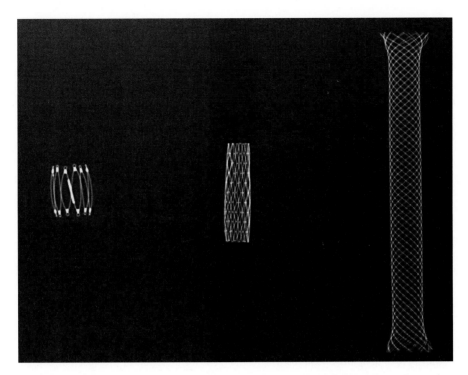

Fig. 10-14 Vascular stents. **A,** Gianturco-Rosch Biliary Z-stent. **B,** Palmaz. **C,** Wallstent. *(From Ballinger, P. W. [1995]. Merrill's atlas of radiographic positions and radiologic procedures [8th ed.]. St. Louis: Mosby.)*

or limb. The incidence of infection is higher in synthetic vascular grafts. Even atherosclerotic arterial vessels maintain an ability to protect against infection. The intraluminal blood flow and flow from the vasa vasorum provide ready access to white blood cells. The endothelial lining prevents bacteria from adhering to the vessel wall. The endothelium also defends against invasion to the subendothelial space. The periarterial lymphatic network provides an additional means to transport and filter bacteria from the vessel. The vessel media provides a mechanical barrier to bacterial migration (White, Nessel, & Whang, 1994). Vascular grafts lack these defenses until healing occurs. As a result, grafts increase the likelihood of infection.

Richet, et al (1991) studied vascular surgical patients for factors associated with *surgical wound infection.* They identified risk factors for infection as surgery on the lower extremity, insulin dependent diabetes, past history of vascular surgery, and a delay in surgery. Most of these factors cannot be altered but they can be used to identify those patients at risk. They concluded that lower extremity surgery combined with only one other risk factor or patients with four of the risk factors benefited from a course of antibiotics of 48 hours. A surgical wound infection places a vascular graft at risk and prevention or prompt recognition and treatment of wound infections may reduce the incidence of more serious infections.

Diagnosis

Ultrasonography is the first test utilized to diagnose a vascular graft infection. It has the advantages of being simple, noninvasive, and readily available. A CT or MRI may be ordered in more difficult cases. Angiography is *not* ordered to diagnose an infected graft, but may be helpful in planning a subsequent surgery by showing the run-off vessels, especially when graft excision is needed (Murray & Goldstone, 1994; Hollier, 1989).

It can be difficult to diagnose a vascular graft infection and delay of diagnosis can increase patient morbidity. The timing of the infection assists in the assessment of the probable extent. Infection in the early postoperative period usually involves the entire graft because the normal healing process of tissue incorporation and resolution of the perigraft space and fluid has not occurred. Infection that occurs months or years after implantation is usually localized to a graft segment. (Hollier, 1989).

Diagnostic tests should be performed with the understanding that negative findings do not rule out graft infection. Physical examination, especially in patients with groin incisions, is often the best means of diagnosis of a perigraft infection (Goldstone & Bowersox, 1996). Diagnosis of graft infection can be made on the basis of a draining sinus in the groin in patients with an aortofemoral graft (Hollier, 1989). These patients rarely are toxic and have the expected signs and symptoms of sepsis less than half the time. Patients with aortoenteric fistulas are difficult to diagnose on physical examination but usually present with signs of systemic infection. CT scan and MRI are used to diagnose graft infection in these patients. CT scan augmented with contrast may be used to detect false aneurysms or graft occlusion. CT scan is less reliable for detection of an aortoenteric fistula. Aortic grafts normally have fluid accumulations up to 4 weeks postoperatively, and an MRI is superior to a CT scan for differentiating between graft hemorrhage and other fluids around the graft. Ultrasonography is not as useful for diagnosing infection because it does not provide adequate visualization of nonvascular structures. It may be used initially to detect a mass or fluid accumulation because it is readily available, noninvasive, and relatively inexpensive. Needle aspiration may be helpful in diagnosing early perigraft infections. Needle aspiration may be performed under the guidance of ultrasound, CT scan, or MRI (Goldstone & Bowersox, 1996).

Cultures

Preoperative and intraoperative cultures correlate about 72% of the time. One study showed that cultures of the surrounding tissue were positive for *S. epidermidis* in 11% of patients and 83% when broth cultures of the actual prosthetic fabric were taken (Bandyk, et al, 1984). *S. aureus, S. epidermidis, Streptococcus viridans,* and *S. faecalis* are gram-positive bacteria most frequently responsible for graft infections. *Pseudomonas aeruginosa, Proteus mirabilis,* and *E. coli* are the gram-negative organisms most often associated with infected grafts (Calligaro, DeLaurentis, & Veith, 1995). Coagulase-negative *S. epidermidis* is a slime-producing bacteria that is relatively benign but may be difficult to culture using routine methods. The slime produced causes the organism to be more adherent to the graft material (Groschel & Strain, 1994). Swabs of the infected area may be inadequate to collect bacteria that create a biofilm. Anaerobic cultures should be obtained. Aspiration of pus and tissue or graft biopsy increase the chances of successful organism identification. Grinding or sonication of tissue or graft may be required for adequate culture results when a biofilm is present. It may also be helpful to maintain cultures for up to 4 weeks to identify slow growing organisms. Prophylactic antibiotics do not appear to interfere with intraoperative culturing (Groshel & Strain, 1994).

General Principles of Surgical Management of Infected Grafts

Prevention of infection is the underlying goal of any procedure. Using a site two or more times for surgical access is associated with increased risk of infection. Prophylactic IV antibiotics administered within 1 hour of the incision have been shown to be effective (Calligaro, DeLaurentis, & Veith, 1995). Prosthetic grafts must be protected from contamination that may occur by contact with the skin during implantation (Jicha & Stoney, 1995). Draping the skin with an adherent plastic drape, with or without iodophor incorporated in it, may decrease graft contact with skin.

Basic treatment of synthetic graft infections includes removal of the infected material and tissue. This is considered the gold standard for treatment of an aortic graft infection. These patients are at risk for increased mortality from sepsis but

also from graft rupture and hemorrhage. There are four basic options: (1) An extraanatomic bypass, e.g., an axillofemoral bypass, may be scheduled at the time of graft excision (Curl & Ricotta, 1994). (2) Infected grafts are sometimes replaced with PTFE grafts at the same time as graft excision. (3) Staged surgical intervention may be excision of the infected graft followed by replacement at a later date or (4) extraanatomic bypass at a later date. Peripheral graft infections that are localized to any area, excluding the anastomosis, may be treated with local wound care or replacement of a segment with an interposition graft. Local wound care may include catheter and drainage placement for continuous wound irrigation using Gentamicin or antibiotic treatment based on cultures and sensitivities. Infection surrounding an anastomosis increases the risk of anastomotic rupture and bleeding (Bunt, 1994).

When an autogenous graft becomes infected the course of treatment is aimed at saving the graft and clearing the infection. Wound cultures that are either negative or grow *S. epidermidis* require local wound care, which may include a rotational muscle flap for coverage of the graft area or a split-thickness skin graft. If a more aggressive approach is needed, free-flap tissue coverage may be an option. Wounds tend to recover faster with the introduction of this vascular tissue (Ouriel & Geary, 1994). The sooner this approach is instituted, the better the outcome (Bunt, 1994). Free tissue transfers are generally performed by plastic surgeons.

OR Supplies

Separate vascular set-ups may be needed if both infected graft removal and placement of new grafts are scheduled for the same time in order to contain the infection and protect the new graft. Infected tissue is more friable than healthy tissue and dissection must be meticulous. These surgeries may be time consuming and the patient must be positioned carefully to prevent tissue damage and measures to prevent hypothermia instituted. The team must plan for possible heavy blood loss. Blood replacement should be available in the form of banked blood or the availability of blood salvage equipment. Extra suction set-ups should be readily available. When two surgical set-ups are needed the nursing team must plan carefully to coordinate the timing of the transition to the second surgery. Double set-ups demand vigilance in maintaining accountability for counted items, strict adherence to sterile technique, and efficient reprepping, gowning, and draping.

Supplies for culturing (swabs, culture media, sterile containers, patient labels, requisitions) must be available for rapid collection and accurate documentation. Special requests for sonication of cultures or longer culture times should be communicated to the appropriate laboratory personnel. When continuous antibiotic irrigation is desired, a variety of catheters and drains adaptable to a collection system may be used.

When a prosthetic graft is removed from a patient, documentation of the explant must be sent to the graft manufacturer, who reports this information to the FDA. This information is also documented in the patient's medical record.

Box 10-3 **RNFA Considerations Basic to Peripheral Vascular Surgery**

Knowledge of pertinent anatomy for proposed surgical procedure.

Anticipation of every step of the procedure (Camishion, Brown, & Spence, 1993)

Capability of performing and assisting in all perioperative nursing care functions (specific role will vary with particular work setting).

Role complements role of the circulating nurse (RNFA capable of performing as circulator; role depends on setting).

Role is differentiated from that of scrub nurse and is *not* that of scrub nurse *and* first assistant.

Able to perform well under stress and in emergencies.

Retractor selection is based on knowledge of the procedure, anatomy, characteristics of the wound (depth), length of time, and effort required. Selection of a hand-held retractor versus a self-retaining retractor depends on knowledge of the surgical procedure. Safe retractor placement requires care to avoid injury to tissues or organs (Davis, 1993).

Controlling blood loss.

Tissue dissection and suturing.

SPECIFIC VASCULAR DUTIES

Use right-angled clamp to pass ties or loops around vessel.

Pass tie or vessel loop with clamp or forcep to surgeon.

Vascular suture: prevent tangling or knotting of suture in use.

"Follow suture" by holding suture loop out of surgeon's way when suturing.

Prevent suture from catching on instruments by "following" and/or placing a towel over the instruments as possible.

Following is done with just enough *tension* to prevent distortion of the tissue, leaving adequate length of suture for the surgeon to work easily and timing the release for optimal results (Rothrock, 1987). Provide counter-traction on suture outward from vessel in radial direction.

Place tag on vessel loops or umbilical tapes and rubber-shod clamp on vascular suture as needed.

Provide visibility of tissue being sutured by gently and steadily irrigating with heparinized saline syringe when bleeding interferes with visibility.

Assist in hemostasis by applying pressure, clamping, applying Hemoclips or sutures or using the electrocautery.

Assist with or close wound.

References

Atkinson, L.J., & Fortunato, N.H. (1996). Peripheral vascular surgery. In L.J. Atkinson, & N.H. Fortunato (Eds.), *Operating room technique* (pp. 817-829). St. Louis: Mosby.

Brandyk, D. F., Berni, G. A., Thiele, B. Z., & Towne, J. B. (1984). Aortofemoral graft infection due to staphylococcus epidermidis. *Archives of Surgery, 119*(1):102-108.

Bunt, T.J. (1994). Current review. In K.D. Calligaro, & F.J Veith (Eds.), *Management of infected arterial grafts* (pp. 163-184). St. Louis: Quality Medical Publishing.

Calligaro, K. D., DeLaurentis, D.A., & Veith, F. J. (1995). Infected infrainguinal grafts. In K. Ouriel (Ed.), *Lower extremity vascular disease* (pp. 267-274). Philadelphia: W.B. Saunders.

Camishion, R. C., Brown, A. S., & Spence, R. K. (1993). Principles of tissue handling. In J.C. Rothrock (Ed.), *The RN first assistant: An expanded perioperative nursing role* (pp. 147-165). Philadelphia: J. B. Lippincott.

Castendea, F. (1996). In H. Haimovici, et al, *Vascular surgery* (4th ed., pp. 311-333). Cambridge, MA: Blackwell Science.

Curl, R. J., & Ricotta, J. J. (1994). Total prosthetic graft excision and extra-anatomic bypass. In K. D. Calligaro, & F. J. Veith (Eds.), *Management of infected arterial grafts* (pp. 82-94). St. Louis: Quality Medical Publishing.

Davis, N.B. (1993). Providing exposure: Retractors and retraction. In J. C. Rothrock (Ed.), *The RN first assistant: An expanded perioperative nursing role* (pp. 167-185). Philadelphia: J.B. Lippincott.

Dzsinich, C., & Gloviczki, P. (1993). Principles of vascular surgery. In D. L. Clement, & J. T. Sheperd (Eds.), *Vascular diseases in the limbs: Mechanisms and principles of treatment* (pp. 259-278). St. Louis: Mosby.

Eastcott, H. H. G., & Thompson, A. E. (1985). Arterial suture and anastomoses. In J. A. DeWeese (Ed.), *Rob & Smith's operative surgery: Vascular surgery* (4th ed., pp. 63-69). Boston: Butterworth.

Fogarty, T .J. (1995). In R .B. Rutherford (Ed.), *Vascular surgery* (4th ed., pp. 410-414). Philadelphia: W. B. Saunders.

Fogarty, T. J., Biswa, A., Hermann, & Newman, C. E. (1996). The role of atherectomy in the treatment of occlusive arterial disease. In H. Haimovici, E. E. Strandness, & J. B. Towne (Eds.), *Vascular surgery* (4th ed., pp. 304-310). Cambridge, MA: Blackwell Science.

Fogarty, T. J., & Hermann, G. D. (1991). New techniques for clot extraction and managing acute thromboembolic limb ischemia. In F. J. Veith (Ed.), *Current critical problems in vascular surgery* (Vol. 3, pp. 197-203). St. Louis: Quality Medical Publishing.

Fogarty, T. J., et al (1991). New techniques and instrumentation for the management of adherent clot in native and synthetic vessels. *Current surgery, 48*(2); 123-126.

Friedman, S. G. (1989). *A history of vascular surgery.* New York: Futura Publishing.

Goldstone, J., & Bowersox, J. C. (1996). Infected prosthetic arterial grafts. In H. Haimovici, et al (Eds.), *Vascular surgery* (4th ed.) (pp. 725-739). Cambridge, MA: Blackwell Science.

Green, R. M. (April 29, 1993). Personal communication.

Green, R. M., & Ouriel, K. (1994). Peripheral arterial disease. In S.I. Schwarz, G. T. Shires, & F. C. Spencer (Eds.), *Principles of surgery* (pp. 925-987). New York: McGraw-Hill.

Greenhalgh, R. M. (1989). Techniques of anastamosis. In R. M. Greenhalgh (Ed.), *Vascular surgical techniques: An atlas* (2nd ed.) (pp. 4-12). Philadelphia: W. B. Saunders.

Groschel, D. H. M., & Strain, B. (1994). Arterial graft infections from a microbiologist's view. In K. D. Calligaro, & F .J. Veith (Eds.), *Management of infected arterial grafts* (pp. 3-15). St. Louis: Quality Medical Publishing.

Grundfest, W. S. (1996). Angioscopy and laser angioplasty. In H. Haimovici, et al (Eds.), *Vascular surgery* (4th ed., pp. 334-347). Cambridge, MA: Blackwell Science.

Haimovici, H. (1996a). Endarterectomy. In H. Haimovici, et al (Eds.), *Vascular surgery* (4th ed., pp. 294-303). Cambridge, MA: Blackwell Science.

Haimovici, H. (1996c). Patch graft angioplasty. In H. Haimovici, et al (Eds.), *Vascular surgery* (4th ed., pp. 250-256). Cambridge, MA: Blackwell Science.

Haimovici, H. (1996b). Vascular sutures and anastomoses. In H. Haimovici, et al (Eds.), *Vascular surgery* (4th ed.) (pp. 239-249). Cambridge, MA: Blackwell Science.

Hollier, L.H. (1989). Management of aortic graft infection. In R.M. Greenhalgh (Ed.), *Vascular surgical techniques: An atlas* (pp. 18-27). Philadelphia: W.B. Saunders.

Jicha, D. L., & Stoney, R. J. (1995). Infected aortic grafts. In K. Ouriel (Ed.), *Lower extremity vascular disease* (pp. 253-265). Philadelphia: W.B. Saunders.

Ketch, L. K. (1995). Microvascular surgery. In R. B. Rutherford (Ed.), *Vascular surgery* (4th ed., pp. 405-410). Philadelphia: W. B. Saunders.

Ouriel, K., & Geary, K. (1994). When can a vein graft be preserved and when should it be excised? In K. D. Calligaro, & F. J. Veith (Eds.), *Management of infected arterial grafts* (pp. 212-218). St. Louis: Quality Medical Publishing.

McIvor, J. (1989). Percutaneous transluminal angioplasty. In R. M. Greenhalgh (Ed.), *Vascular surgical techniques: An atlas* (pp. 310-318). Philadelphia: W. B. Saunders.

Murray, S. P., & Goldstone, J. (1994). Diagnostic advances. In K. D. Calligaro, & F. J. Veith (Eds.), *Management of infected arterial grafts* (pp. 43-53). St. Louis: Quality Medical Publishing.

Myhre, H. O., & Saether, O. D. (1989). Embolectomy for acute lower-limb ischaemia. In R. M. Greenhalgh (Ed.), *Vascular surgical techniques: An atlas* (pp. 205-211). Philadelphia: W. B. Saunders.

Richet, H. M., et al (1991). Analysis of risk factors for surgical wound infections following vascular surgery. *The American Journal of Medicine, 91*(suppl 3B): 170S-172S.

Rothrock, J. D. (1987). *RN first assistant: An expanded perioperative nursing role*. Philadelphia: J. B. Lippincott.

Rutherford, R. B. (1995). Basic vascular surgical techniques. In R. B. Rutherford (Ed.), *Vascular surgery* (4th ed., pp. 395-405). Philadelphia: W. B. Saunders.

Shah, R. M., et al (1993). Early results with cryopreserved saphenous vein allografts for infrainguinal bypass. *Journal of Vascular Surgery, 18*(6): 965-971.

Stoney, R. J., & Thompson, R. W. (1995). Endarterectomy. In R. B. Rutherford (Ed.), *Vascular surgery* (4th ed., pp. 414-420). Philadelphia: W. B. Saunders.

Taylor, R. S., et al (1992). Improved technique for polytetrafluoroethylene bypass grafting: Long-term results using anastomotic vein patches. *British Journal of Surgery, 79*: 348-354.

Veith, F. J. (1994). Presidential address: Transluminally place endovascular stented grafts and their impact on vascular surgery. *Journal of Vascular Surgery, 20*(6): 855-860.

White, J. V., Nessel, C. C., & Whang, K. (1994). Differential effect of type of bacteria on peripheral graft infections. In K. D. Calligaro, & G. J. Veith (Eds.), *Management of infected arterial grafts* (pp. 25-42). St. Louis: Quality Medical Publishing.

White, R. A. (1996). Application of laser technology to vascular disease. In F. J. Veith, R. W. Hobson, R. A. Williams, & S. E. Wilson (Eds.) *Vascular surgery: Principles and practice* (2nd ed., pp. 318-330). New York: McGraw-Hill.

Additional Reading

Calligaro, K. D., & Veith, F. J. (Eds.) (1994). *Management of infected arterial grafts*. St. Louis: Quality Medical Publishing.

R. E. Vaiden, V. J. Fox, & J. C. Rothrock (Eds.) (1994). *Core curriculum for the RN first assistant*. Denver: Association of Operating Room Nurses.

RN first assistant: Practice resources (1995). Denver: Association of Operating Room Nurses.

J. C. Rothrock (Ed.) (1993). *The RN first assistant: An expanded perioperative nursing role*. Philadelphia: J.B. Lippincott.

11 Carotid Endarterectomy

CAROTID ENDARTERECTOMY

Description

The term *carotid* derives from the Greek word **karoo**, to stupefy (Donayre, Wilson, & Hobson, 1994). Carotid endarterectomy is the removal of an atheroma at the carotid artery bifurcation and internal carotid artery origin to increase cerebral perfusion and decrease the risk of embolization. It is performed to prevent stroke. However, transient or permanent neurologic deficit may complicate carotid endarterectomy in 2% to 5% of cases (Executive Committee for ACAS Study, 1995). To lessen the likelihood, it may be necessary to use a temporary carotid artery shunt in order to maintain cerebral blood flow during the surgery (see Figure 8-31). The patient will have either a transverse or vertical neck incision and a groin or ankle incision if the saphenous vein is harvested for patch closure.

Pathophysiology

Atherosclerotic lesions at the carotid bifurcation exhibit characteristic patterns. The intima typically thickens in this area at an early age. Complex lesions develop around the bifurcation and sinus but usually end proximal to the common carotid and just distal to the sinus in the internal carotid. The sinus is twice the cross sectional area of the artery immediately proximal to it and has characteristic turbulent flow. The shear forces generated by this turbulence damage the intima, predisposing it to atheromatous changes. High grade, or complex, stenotic lesions tend to have irregular surfaces, which may hemorrhage or ulcerate and embolize or thrombose (Glagov & Zarins, 1989) (Box 11-1).

Cerebrovascular disease is the third leading cause of death in the United States (Donayre, Wilson, & Hobson, 1994). Four hundred fifty thousand people suffer a stroke each year in the United States. Three quarters of these are attributed to thromboembolic events (Hobson, 1996). Terms that describe ischemic strokes include transient ischemic attack, reversible ischemic neurologic deficit, stroke in evolution, and completed stroke.

A stroke is an event that interrupts blood flow to an area of the brain (Box 11-2). It may be due to an embolus, thrombosis, or hemorrhage. Symptoms may include paralysis, parasthesias, speech disorders, loss of consciousness, visual disturbances, and confusion and/or changes in mentation. When these symptoms resolve in 24 hours or less, they are called **transient ischemic attacks (TIAs)**. When any of the symptoms last for more than 24 hours with minimal residual effect after 7 days it is referred to as a **reversible ischemic neurologic deficit (RIND)**. When symptoms do not resolve within 7 days, it is called a **stroke** or **cerebrovascular accident (CVA)** (Donayre, Wilson, & Hobson, 1994). It is estimated that one third of strokes are preceded by TIAs (Kyriazis, 1994).

On routine physical examination auscultation may reveal a bruit over the carotid artery. A bruit reflects turbulent flow, which can occur within a lumen stenosed as little as 20% to 30% (Hobson, 1996). A bruit, then, is not specific to hemodynamically significant lesions, but can be a sensitive indictor of vascular pathology. Hollenhorst plaques are retinal emboli that may be found on routine ophthalmoscopic examination. These appear as bright yellow-orange crystals that arise from an ulcerative carotid plaque (Hollenhorst, 1961). Patients with any of these findings need to be referred for further work-up (Box 11-3).

Box 11-1 **Risk Factors for Atherosclerosis**

Hypertension
High blood cholesterol
Diabetes
Heart disease
Obesity
Family history of arterial disease
Smoking
Age >70 years

Box 11-2 **Warning Signs of a Stroke**

VISUAL DISTURBANCES
Amaurosis fugax: momentary monocular blurring or vision loss.
Loss of vision in all or part of the visual field, classically described as a shade being pulled down over one eye.
Weakness or numbness in hand, leg, or both.
Speech alteration: inability to speak or garbled speech.
Brief episodes of memory loss.
Loss of consciousness.
Facial droop on one side or mouth turning downward on one side.

Indications

Indications for medical management versus surgical intervention have been controversial. A large randomized prospective study published in 1970 compared patient outcomes of surgery and medical management. The conclusion was that the 12% perioperative stroke rate did not justify the lowered risk of stroke and death after carotid endarterectomy. In 1982 Rand Corporation reviewed medical records and concluded that the procedure carried significant risk of major complications. Patient selection and case volume was questioned, and the procedure fell into disrepute. The Rand Corporation study also concluded that carotid endarterectomy should only be performed by surgeons with low complication rates.

In response to this the **North American Symptomatic Endarterectomy Trial** (NASCET) was started. This study showed that surgery reduced the risk of stroke by 17% after two years. It also concluded that patients with a 70% to 79% stenosis of the carotid artery had less to gain by surgery. Still it was not clear whether patients with symptomatic but moderate stenoses or asymptomatic patients benefit from surgery (Donayre, Wilson, & Hobson, 1994). In an attempt to further refine patient selection for carotid endarterectomy the **Asymptomatic Carotid Atherosclerosis Study** (ACAS) was initiated in 1987 to determine whether carotid endarterectomy is indicated for asymptomatic patients (Box 11-4). The trial clearly showed the advantages of surgical intervention in selected patients. This landmark research was halted because the results indicated that surgery significantly reduced the risk of stroke in patients with a stenotic carotid lesion of >60% (Executive Committee for ACAS Study, 1995)

Preoperative planning

Preoperative testing. **Noninvasive testing** Testing for carotid disease must include an ultrasound examination. With acoustic gel on the patient's neck, a Doppler probe is lightly placed on the skin to interrogate blood flow. A duplex scanner, which provides both Doppler signal and real time image information, is becoming the standard for diagnosis and management of carotid artery disease. In experienced hands, duplex scanning allows accurate localization of a lesion, permits determination of the degree of stenosis, and differentiates stenosis from total occlusion (Zierler & Sumner, 1995).

Invasive testing. An arteriogram may be required for more specific planning of the surgical procedure (Figure 11-1). Arteriography had been considered the study of choice for obtaining accurate anatomical information. Known adverse effects associated with arteriography (stroke, discomfort, technical problems, contrast reactions, complications at arterial puncture site) and cost have decreased its use in the wake of noninvasive studies. In some centers arteriography has been replaced almost exclusively by ultrasonography (Horn, Greisler, Littoy, & Baker, 1994). MRI may be superior to duplex scanning because it is not operator dependent and provides very accurate information about calcified vessels, the intracranial circulation, and aortic arch. However, limited access and high cost prohibit its use for routine screening (Donayre, Wilson, & Hobson, 1994).

Anesthetic considerations. The major goal of anesthetic management during carotid surgery is to protect the brain and heart from ischemia (Roizen & Ellis, 1992). The anesthesiologist strives to maintain blood glucose level and blood pressure at optimal levels. Control of blood sugar in diabetic patients is important because hyperglycemia is linked to cerebral ischemia. Hypertension increases the afterload of the heart and increases the risk of cerebral edema and bleeding (Chlebowski,

---

Box 11-3 **Indications for Carotid Endarterectomy**

URGENT NEED FOR CAROTID ENDARTERECTOMY
Critical stenosis (80% to 99% occlusion of internal carotid artery).
Crescendo TIAs
Stroke in evolution
(Surgery is contraindicated for neurologically unstable patients with evidence of intracranial bleeding or infarct on MRI or CT scan)

CRITICAL STENOSIS WITH STROKE
Surgery after 6 weeks
Asymptomatic with 60% stenosis or more (in an otherwise healthy patient) per ACAS trial.
Asymptomatic with hemodynamically significant lesion.
Symptomatic (TIAs, amaurosis fugax, stroke in preceding 3 months) with critical stenosis >80% per NASCET
Vertebral basilar insufficiency with critical stenosis (vertebral basilar ischemia symptoms: drop attacks, vertigo, dizziness, imbalance after postural changes, e.g., standing up or rotating neck).
Hollenhorst plaque

(Berman, et al, 1994; Imparato, 1996)

Box 11-4 **Asymptomatic Carotid Atherosclerosis Study (ACAS)**

The Asymptomatic Carotid Atherosclerosis Study was conducted between 1987 and 1993. Thirty-nine clinical sites in the United States and Canada were part of a prospective, randomized trial. The study randomly assigned 1662 patients with asymptomatic carotid artery stenoses of 60% or more to either medical or surgical treatment. The medical treatment was administration of daily aspirin and management of risk factors. The surgical group received the medical management interventions and underwent carotid endarterectomy. The surgical group had a 5% risk of stroke and the medical group had an 11% risk. Surgical intervention is clearly indicated for patients with a 60% or greater carotid artery stenosis if the patient's general health status is not a contraindication (Executive Committee for ACAS Study, 1995).

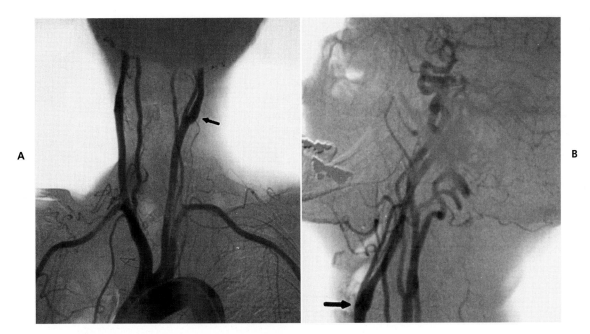

Fig. 11-1 Cerebral angiography, photographic subtraction technique. **A,** AP and **B,** AP oblique (RPO position) of aortic arch demonstrating excellent visualization of extracranial carotid and vertebral arteries. Normal left common carotid bifurcation (*arrows*). *(From Ballinger [1995]. Merrill's atlas of radiographic positions and radiologic procedures [8th ed.]. St. Louis: Mosby.)*

1996). Patients on antihypertensive medications should be instructed to take these the day of surgery. This assists with the intraoperative goal of maintaining the patient at his normal blood pressure in order to protect cerebral and myocardial perfusion.

Based on patient assessment and input from the surgeon the anesthesiologist will decide whether to use regional (cervical block) or general anesthesia. Advantages of cervical block include continuous CNS monitoring and lessened hemodynamic lability. In addition, awake patients can report anginal symptoms, and pulmonary complications from general anesthesia are avoided.

Using a cervical block requires a willing patient who can tolerate the awareness of surgery and maintenance of the surgical position. Sedation must be carefully titrated to balance comfort while preventing apnea, possible confusion, and movement. With CNS changes during the procedure there is a risk that the patient could move and disrupt the surgery. Any subsequent need to convert to general anesthesia with oral intubation may be more difficult because of patient panic or seizure once the surgery has started (Roizen & Ellis, 1992).

General anesthesia provides some cerebral protection by decreasing cerebral metabolic demands. It also may improve BP control intraoperatively. EEG may assist in determining the depth of anesthesia (Blume & Sharbrough, 1993). An arterial line is often inserted to monitor these patients, 50% to 75% of whom are hypertensive. This provides constant pressure and pulse surveillance, which is helpful in this population who tend to be hemodynamically labile. The arterial line also provides phlebotomy access for blood gas analysis and activated clotting time (see Chapter 5). Blood gas analysis is useful for maintaining optimal CO_2 levels. CO_2 alters the pH of arteriole smooth muscle, which can alter the cerebral blood flow. A decrease in CO_2 levels may lead to vasoconstriction and cerebral ischemia (Chlebowski, 1996).

The most critical time for the patient undergoing carotid endarterectomy is the time of the occlusion of the common carotid artery. Patients with adequate collateral blood flow to the brain by way of the Circle of Willis, contralateral carotid, and vertebral arteries will have no symptomatic response to clamping (Stoelting & Dierdorf, 1993). Two techniques that facilitate continual assessment of cerebral perfusion during surgery are the use of cervical block anesthesia and electroencephalographic monitoring. A conscious patient under cervical block anesthesia can be observed and assessed for neurologic deficits during the procedure. Assessment is made by noting changes in patient speech (no response or inappropriate response) and alterations in motor function on the contralateral side to the surgical site. Strength can be assessed by hand grip or patient's ability to continually squeeze a soft ball, observing for the lack of hand motion, or the ball dropping. A compressible squeaky toy may be taped to the patient's hand as another means of assessing movement (Imparato, 1996). This would require the cooperation of the entire team. The patient under general anesthesia can be monitored with an electroencephalogram (EEG) (Figure 11-2).

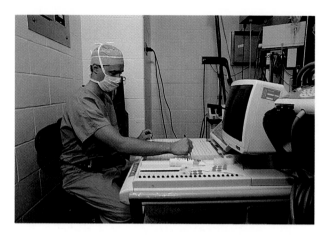

Fig. 11-2 EEG machine and technician.

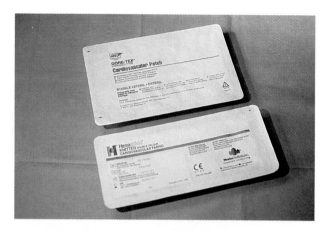

Fig. 11-3 Examples of synthetic patch material, commercially prepared to size (PTFE and polyester).

Equipment, instrumentation, medications, and solutions

Also refer to Chapter 8, Equipment, Supplies, and Instrumentation, and Chapter 4, Medications.

Contents of custom pack

Additional draping materials for leg incision site (optional saphenous vein harvest)

Routine sterile items for vascular surgery

Basic vascular instrument set

Major or minor instrument set

Sterile Doppler probe and Doppler amplifier

Duplex ultrasound machine

Duplex ultrasound probe sheath, sterile with gel

Vascular patch material, PTFE or Dacron (Figure 11-3)

Vascular suture: 6-0 polypropylene or PTFE for closure of arteriotomy and suturing patch in place; 7-0 polypropylene for "tacking" down intimal flap; 2-0 and 4-0 absorbable suture for wound closure

Adhesive strips for skin closure (optional)

Closed suction wound drain (optional)

Transparent dressing, gauze dressing (as needed or for drain site)

Critical items include:

Shunt clamps (Figure 11-4)

Carotid artery shunts

Endarterectomy dissector (Freer elevator, "spatula," "teaser")

Supplies for measuring "stump" pressures: butterfly needle (21 or 23 gauge), arterial pressure tubing, transducer, and monitor.

ACT machine

For the awake patient:

A soft rubber ball, compressible squeaky toy, or "clicking" device

Mayo stand to keep drapes off patient's face and permit eye contact with anesthesiologist

Intraoperative medications and solutions:

Saline for routine wound irrigation and for wetting surgeon's hand to facilitate tying polypropylene suture

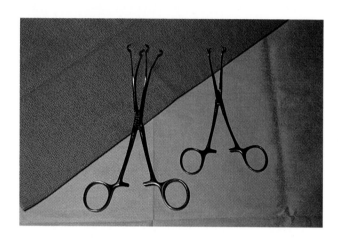

Fig. 11-4 Carotid shunt clamps.

Heparinized saline in syringe with 18 gauge cannula for irrigating intraluminal vessel and clearing surgical site of any bleeding during suturing

1% lidocaine:

As local anesthetic if needed to augment a cervical block

Used as needed to anesthetize carotid sinus if manipulation of carotid body causes bradycardia and hypotension or as prophylaxis for these symptoms

Procedural Steps

Two incision choices may be selected depending on surgeon preference, either transverse or longitudinal (vertical). The longitudinal approach is described and depicted in the following procedural steps. The transverse incision is made 2.5 fingerbreadths below the mandible. A subplatysmal skin flap is dissected to the mandibular angle (cephalad) and inferiorly to expose the sternocleidomastoid muscle. The remainder of the procedure is identical with either approach (Skillman, Kent, & Anninos, 1994).

RNFA CONSIDERATIONS

Maintain knowledge of pertinent anatomy: vascular structures, nerves, and carotid sinus reflex.

Protect patient from pressure on face and eyes during surgery by ensuring that protective eye coverings are in place before draping and by preventing any team members from leaning on patient's face.

Handle gently and carefully place retractors and forceps to prevent nerve injury and embolization of plaque.

Maintain awareness of patient's vital signs, and be prepared for injection of local anesthetic to carotid body as needed.

Assist in measurement of stump pressures as needed.

Assist in placement of carotid shunt as needed.

1. The patient is placed on the operating room bed in a supine position with the head supported on a head support as needed. The head is turned away from the operative side in a head-up tilt and the neck may be slightly hyperextended. A roll may be placed between the scapulae.

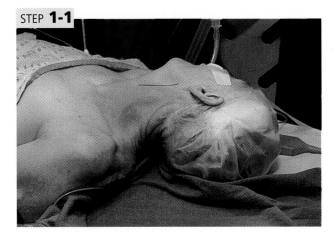

STEP **1-1**

Patient positioned for right carotid endarterectomy with incision marked. EEG leads are in place on head and covered with a protective plastic cap.

2. A longitudinal (vertical) incision is made over the area of the carotid bifurcation (along anterior border of sternocleidomastoid muscle). The Weitlaner or Travers self-retaining retractor is placed for exposure.

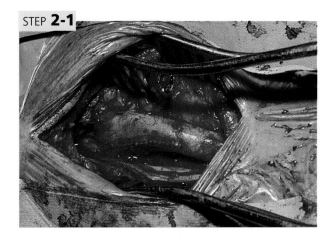

STEP **2-1**

3. With dissecting scissors the soft tissue is dissected and the carotid sheath opened for identification and exposure of the carotid artery and its bifurcation. Local anesthetic should be available for injecting the carotid body as needed.

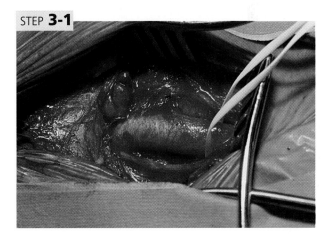

STEP **3-1**

4. Moistened umbilical tapes or vessel loops are passed around the common, internal, and external carotid arteries and double looped for control and ease of handling. The superior thyroid artery is temporarily controlled by placement of a silk tie or vessel loop.

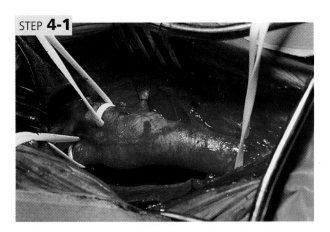

STEP **4-1**

STEP **4-2**

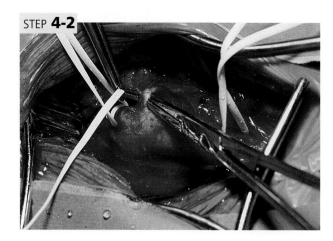

5. The patient is systemically heparinized. The external, common, and internal carotid arteries are occluded, either by vessel loops or vascular clamps.

CONSIDERATIONS As an optional step, the surgeon may choose to measure stump pressures (Box 11-5).

Box 11-5 **Stump Pressure Measurement**

Another means of monitoring cerebral blood flow is to measure the back pressure in the internal carotid artery or the pressure in the Circle of Willis. This is done by temporarily occluding the external and common carotid arteries. A needle that is connected to a pressure transducer is placed in the internal carotid artery (Figure 11-5). The patient's systemic blood pressure should be at baseline. The minimum acceptable reading of the carotid back pressure is debatable and dependent on the surgeon's assessment of the clinical situation. One acceptable minimum may be 25 mmHg (Gelabert & Moore, 1991). Stump pressure may be one factor in the decision to use a carotid shunt although it correlates poorly with EEG change and is considered the least reliable of cerebral blood flow measurements (Blume & Sharbrough, 1993).

---

6. With a #11 scalpel blade an arteriotomy is made over the stenotic area.

STEP **6-1**

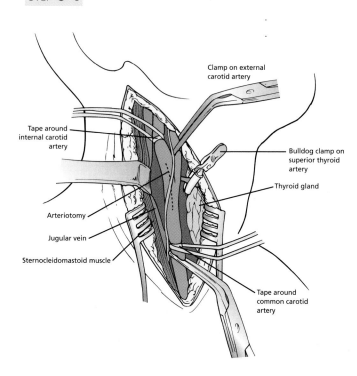

Clamp on external carotid artery

Tape around internal carotid artery

Bulldog clamp on superior thyroid artery

Thyroid gland

Arteriotomy

Jugular vein

Sternocleidomastoid muscle

Tape around common carotid artery

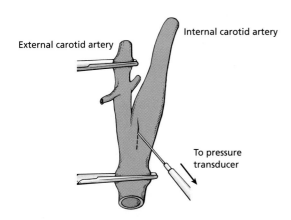

External carotid artery

Internal carotid artery

To pressure transducer

Fig. 11-5 The technique of carotid backpressure monitoring. Note the occlusion of the common carotid and the external carotid arteries (ECA). The needle is connected to a transducer to measure internal carotid artery (ICA) pressure.

With a blunt dissector (Freer elevator), the plaque is dissected from the arterial wall.

STEP **7-2**

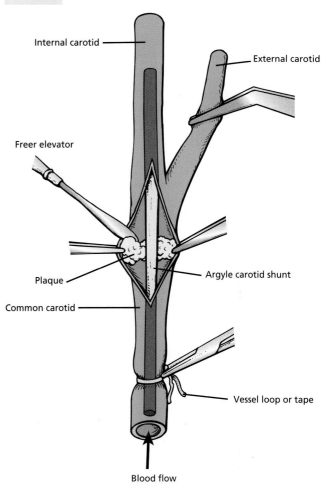

Internal carotid

External carotid

Freer elevator

Plaque

Argyle carotid shunt

Common carotid

Vessel loop or tape

Blood flow

7. The incision is lengthened with Potts angulated scissors to expose the full extent of the occluding plaque.

STEP **7-1**

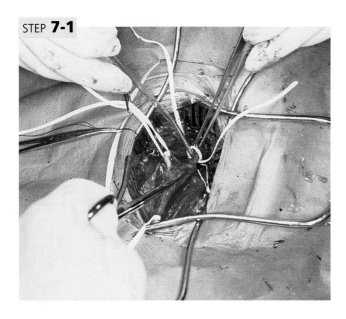

STEP **7-3**

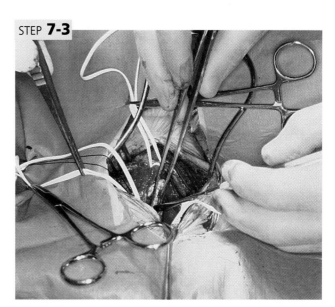

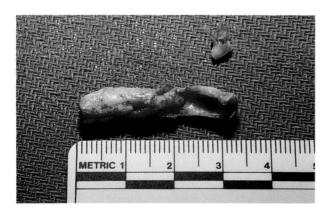

Example of carotid artery plaque.

Heparin solution in a syringe with a cannula on the tip is used as an irrigant to clean the intima and facilitate visualization of tissue fragments by lifting them. These fragments are removed to prevent blood flow disruption or embolization of the tissue fragment.

STEP **7-4**

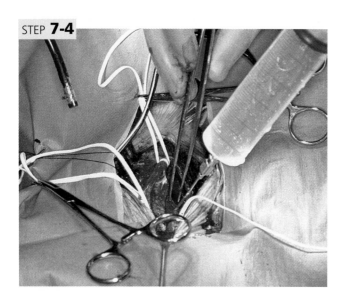

8. Before complete closure, blood flow is temporarily restored through the arteries to wash away any free plaque, air, or thrombi. To do this the occluding clamps are opened and closed individually, flushing any debris away from the internal carotid artery. The internal carotid artery is opened last.

9. The arteriotomy may be closed primarily with fine vascular sutures.

STEP **9-1**

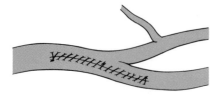

10. The blood flow and anatomy may be assessed intraoperatively by use of the duplex ultrasound scanner (the scanner probe is placed inside a sterile plastic sheath that has had gel loaded into the end of it).

STEP **10-1**

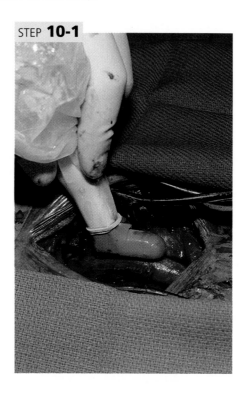

Closure of Arteriotomy with a Patch

A synthetic or autogenous (vein) patch graft may be used to restore the arterial lumen if the vessel is small (see Chapter 10). The closure of the arteriotomy is completed with the patch sewn in place using the same method of flushing the artery described in Step 6.

INTRO **1**

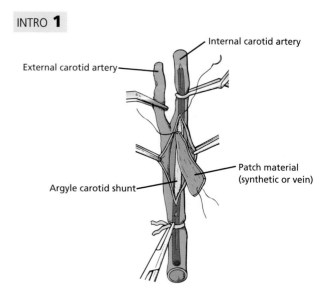

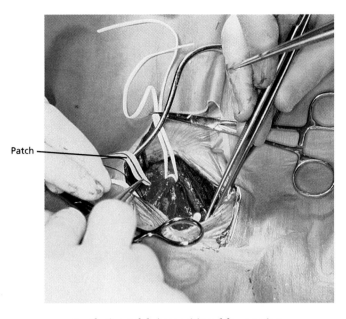

Patch

Synthetic patch being positioned for suturing.

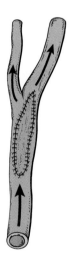

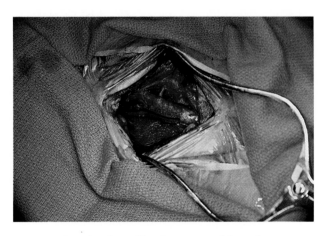

Completed carotid endarterectomy with patch.

11. Additional interrupted sutures may be needed to control leakage.

12. A drain is inserted via a separate stab incision (optional).

STEP **12-1**

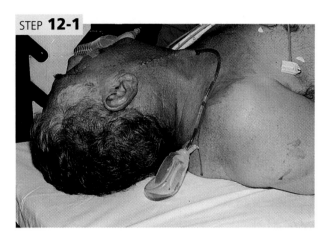

13. The wound closure is accomplished in the usual manner and dressings are applied.

STEP **13-1**

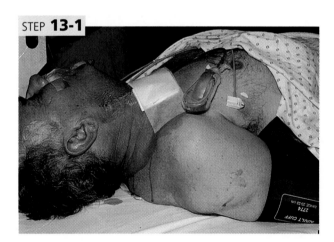

CAROTID ENDARTERECTOMY WITH SHUNT

If patient assessment by EEG or neurologic changes in the awake patient indicates reduced cerebral perfusion or if the patient has had a recent stroke or has known decreased collateral perfusion to the brain (based on preoperative testing), the surgeon may decide to use a temporary carotid artery shunt. Another means of assessing cerebral blood flow and determining the need to shunt may be based on measuring intraoperative stump pressures (see Box 11-5). The shunting device should always be available and sterile at the beginning of the procedure.

Intraoperative shunting remains an area of controversy. A shunt allows continuous blood flow through the carotid artery to the brain. Debate is based on research that has shown the majority of postoperative neurologic deficits to be from thromboembolism and not from decreased cerebral perfusion (Roizen & Ellis, 1992). Disadvantages in using this temporary device are the additional dissection necessary for its placement, the possibility of dislodging debris when inserting the shunt, difficult visualization of the endarterectomy endpoint, and increased difficulty in suturing a patch if used. Some surgeons shunt routinely, some never shunt, and others do so selectively. Carotid endarterectomy can be performed safely without shunting even in high risk patients with a contralateral carotid occlusion or stenosis (Redekop & Ferguson, 1992). When shunting is used selectively, EEG may be used to monitor cortical function. A minimum of 16 EEG leads are secured to the patient's head with collodion. A baseline EEG is done with the patient resting. At least 10 minutes of recording is required with the patient under general anesthesia in order to detect any changes that occur at the time of carotid clamping. Changes may be due to decreased cerebral perfusion from clamping, low BP, or anesthetic agents (Blume & Sharbrough, 1993).

Procedural Steps

The first five steps as described for carotid endarterectomy are followed.

6. The arteriotomy is lengthened as needed to permit direct visualization of the end of the plaque and insertion of a shunt.

7. A piece of tubing (polyethylene or Silastic) with a suture tied around its center or a commercially prepared shunt device is inserted in the common carotid artery and the internal carotid artery to maintain cerebral blood flow and is held in place with tourniquets or shunt clamps.

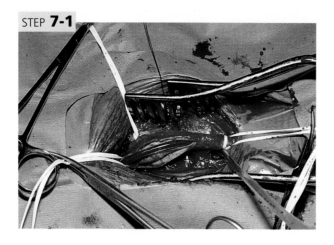

STEP **7-1**

8. The plaque is removed as described for carotid endarterectomy.

9. The arteriotomy is closed with or without a patch.

10. Before the arteriotomy closure is completed, the shunt clamp or tourniquet on the internal carotid artery is released, and the shunt is removed. The internal carotid artery is again-occluded. The arteriotomy closure is completed quickly to minimize cerebral ischemia time. The external carotid occluding clamp is removed, followed by the common carotid artery clamp, and lastly the internal carotid artery occluding clamp.

11. The wound is closed in the usual manner.

COMPLICATIONS

INTRAOPERATIVE

Damage to nerves (caused by retraction, compression, or electrocautery injury)

Facial (VII) lip droop on surgical side, drooling

Glossopharyngeal (IX) impaired swallowing

Recurrent pharyngeal-anterior vagus (X) vocal cord paralysis, hoarseness

Hypoglossal (XII) impairment of tongue movement on surgical side, impaired speech, and mastication

Greater auricular (a branch of brachial plexus) pain, paresthesia of earlobe

Stroke or TIA

Creation of intimal flap that obstructs cerebral blood flow

POSTOPERATIVE

Wound hematoma

Wound infection (rare)

Blood pressure anomalies

Stroke or TIA

Cerebral hyperperfusion leading to cerebral edema or hemorrhage and presenting with seizures, coma, or death

Reperfusion syndrome caused by revascularization of a previously ischemic area of the brain characterized by severe headache, which may progress to seizures if not treated

Imparato, 1996; Calne & Pollard, 1992; Anderson & Pearce, 1994; Donayre, Wilson, & Hobson, 1994; Kane & Wilson, 1993.

POSTOPERATIVE

Care and Discharge Planning

POSTANESTHESIA CARE UNIT

Monitor ECG, vital signs, and perform neurologic checks per routine

Maintain patient in normotensive state; avoid hypertension and hypotension (BP above patient's baseline places suture line at risk)

Avoid alterations in heart rate (bradycardia from vagal stimulation), which could alter cardiac output and decrease cerebral perfusion

Assess for signs of intracranial bleeding and cerebral ischemia

Observe dressing, neck, and posterior aspect of shoulder for drainage, swelling, (measure blood in drain reservoir if drain is used) or signs of bleeding; respiratory distress can develop from tracheal compression caused by hemorrhage

If a drain is placed, observe and measure output

Elevate head of bed 30 degrees to improve respirations and decrease neck swelling

PATIENT UNIT

Monitor telemetry for 24 hours

Monitor vital signs and perform neurologic checks every 2 hours for 24 hours, then every 4 hours for the next 24 hours, and then every 8 hours until patient is discharged

Discontinue bed rest on day of surgery, ambulate on postoperative day (POD) 1

Discontinue drain on POD 1 (if drain is used)

Turn, cough, deep breath (TCDB) every 2 hours after general anesthesia

Diet: clear liquids PO; advance to preoperative diet POD 1

Monitor intake and output (routine for postoperative patients and patients with IVs)

Assess for cranial nerve deficits every 2 hours

O_2 per nasal prongs, discontinue on POD 1 if SpO_2 is at baseline

If not previously done, perform duplex ultrasound exam on POD 1 or before discharge

MEDICATIONS

Antibiotics for 24 hours

ASA 325 mg qd

Resume patient's preoperative medications

POSTOPERATIVE TEACHING AND DISCHARGE PLANNING

The trend is toward patient discharge 24 hours after surgery; therefore discharge teaching must begin before surgery.

1. Educate the patient about reperfusion headaches, and advise the patient to call the surgeon to discuss treatment options. Mild headache and neck stiffness may be due to position during surgery, especially in patients with cervical arthritis.

2. The patient may return to baseline activity as tolerated. The patient may resume driving when neck discomfort no longer restricts range of motion (ROM) and after first postoperative visit to surgeon.

3. Explain that fatigue for 6 to 8 weeks after surgery is normal.

4. Incision care: keep incision clean and dry; the patient may shower with transparent dressing in place. Remove transparent dressing in 3 to 4 days, leaving wound open to the air. The patient may then wash the incision with soap and water, patting gently to dry. Until the incision is well healed, the patient should avoid powder, lotion, and shaving over it. Explain that numbness around the incision and extending to the ear and mid-chin is normal and should resolve in 2 to 3 months.

5. Teach the patient about any cranial nerve deficits they may have developed from manipulation of nerves during surgery. Assist the patient in understanding the difference between a stroke and cranial nerve deficit; that is, nerve injury or trauma from surgical manipulation occurs on the same side as surgery with the exception of eye symptoms. Stroke presents on the contralateral side, with the exception of eye symptoms as well. Use diagrams and pictures to review pertinent anatomy.

6. Encourage relevant lifestyle changes as indicated, e.g., low-cholesterol diet, review of diabetic diet, smoking cessation.

7. Teach the patient and family to observe and report any new symptoms, e.g., TIAs, mental status changes, personality changes, speech difficulties.

8. If the patient has a synthetic patch in place, he or she may need antibiotics before any dental work and all scope procedures. Instruct the patient to notify dentists and other health care providers of this.

Kane & Wilson, 1993.

References

Anderson, C. A., & Pearce, W. H. (1994). Extracranial cerebrovascular disease. In V. A. Fahey (Ed.), *Vascular nursing* (2nd ed., pp 325-345). Philadelphia: W. B. Saunders.

Berman, S. S., et al (1994). Critical carotid stenosis: Diagnosis, timing of surgery, and outcome. *Journal of Vascular Surgery, 20*(4): 499-510.

Blume, W. T., & Sharbrough, F. W. (1993). EEG monitoring during carotid endarterectomy and open heart surgery. In E. Niedermeyer, & F. Lopes da Silva (Eds.), *Electroencephalography: Basic principles. Clinical applications and related fields* (3rd ed., pp. 747-756). Philadelphia: Williams & Wilkins.

Chlebowski. S. (1996). Unpublished manuscript.

Calne, R., & Pollard, S. G. (1992). Extra-anatomic bypass. In R. Calne, & S. G. Pollard (Eds.), *Side atlas of operative surgery: Vascular surgery* (pp. 9.8-9.10). London: Gower Medical Publishing.

Donayre, C. E., Wilson, S. E., & Hobson, II, R. W. (1994). Extracranial carotid artery occlusive disease. In F. J. Veith, R. W. Hobson, R. A. Williams, & S. E. Wilson (Eds.), *Vascular surgery: Principles and practice* (2nd ed., pp. 649-664). New York: McGraw-Hill.

Gelabert, H. A., & Moore, W. S. (1991). Carotid endarterectomy: Current status. *Current Problems in Surgery, 28*(3): 187-262.

Glagov, S., & Zarins, C. K. (1989). What are the determinants of plaque instability and its consequences *Journal of Vascular Surgery, 9:* 202.

Executive Committee for ACAS Study (1995). Endarterectomy for asymptomatic carotid artery stenosis. *JAMA, 273*(18): 1421-1428.

Hobson, II, R. W. (1996). Asymptomatic carotid stenosis: Diagnosis and surgical management. In H. Haimovici, et al (Eds.), *Vascular surgery: Principles and techniques* (4th ed., pp. 938-947). Cambridge, MA: Blackwell Science.

Hollenhorst, R.W. (1961). Significance of bright plaques in the retinal arterioles. *Journal of the American Medical Association, 178*: 23.

Horn, M., et al (1994). Carotid endarterectomy without arteriography. *Annals of Vascular Surgery, 8*: 221-224.

Imparato, A. M. (1996). Carotid endarterectomy: Indications and techniques for carotid surgery. In H. Haimovici, et al, *Vascular surgery: Principles and techniques* (4th ed., pp. 913-937). Cambridge, MA: Blackwell Science.

Kane, H. L., & Wilson, L. B. (1993). Practical points in the care of the patient post-carotid endarterectomy. *Journal of Post Anesthesia Nursing, 8*(6): 403-405.

Redekop, G., & Ferguson, G. (1992). Correlation of contralateral stenosis and intraoperative electroencephalogram change with risk of stroke during carotid endarterectomy. *Neurosurgery, 30*: 191-194.

Roizen, M. F., & Ellis, J. E. (1992). Anesthesia for vascular surgery. In P. G. Barash, B. C. Cullen, & R. K. Stoelting (Eds.), *Clinical anesthesia* (2nd ed., pp. 1059-1094). Philadelphia: J.B. Lippincott.

Kyriazis, M. (1994). Developments in the treatment of stroke patients. *Nursing Times, 20*(90):30-32.

MacVittie, B. A. (1995). Vascular surgery. In M. H. Meeker, & J. C. Rothrock (Eds.), *Alexander's care of the patient in surgery* (10th ed., pp. 1032-1057) St. Louis: Mosby.

Skillman, J. J., Kent, K. C., & Anninos, E. (1994). Do neck incisions influence nerve deficits after carotid endarterectomy? *Archives of Surgery, 129*: 748-752.

Stoelting, R. K., & Dierdorf, S. F. (1993). Diseases of the nervous system. In R. K. Stoelting, & S. F. Dierdorf (Eds.), *Anesthesia and co-existing disease* (3rd ed., pp. 181-250). New York: Churchill Livingstone.

Zierler, R. E., & Sumner, D. S. (1995). Physiologic assessment of peripheral vascular arterial occlusive disease. In R. B. Rutherford (Ed.), *Vascular surgery* (4th ed., pp. 65-117). Philadelphia: W.B. Saunders.

12 Infrainguinal Bypass

INFRAINGUINAL BYPASS

Description

Infrainguinal bypass procedures are performed to restore arterial blood flow to the lower extremity. Procedures may be done to correct acute (thromboembolic) or chronic (atherosclerotic) conditions. Methods for bypassing an occluded segment of artery include the use of synthetic and autogenous materials. The decision to use autogenous vein graft (in situ versus reversed), synthetic graft (PTFE versus Dacron), or a combination depends on many factors. Long-term patency rates continue to be studied and techniques modified and refined (see Chapter 9)

Surgery to restore flow to the leg may include procedures to provide "inflow" to the femoral artery. This may require an aortofemoral bypass for aortoiliac occlusive disease (see Chapter 15) or a less invasive procedure such as an extraanatomic bypass (see Chapter 17). Lower extremity bypass may be combined with the varied techniques available for restoration other than bypass. These other techniques include endarterectomy, embolectomy, or a form of angioplasty (see Chapter 10).

Femoral-popliteal bypass is the restoration of blood flow to the leg with a graft bypassing the occluded section of the femoral artery. The bypass conduit may be a vein or straight synthetic graft. The patency of an outflow artery must be demonstrated for a successful bypass procedure. If popliteal patency is doubtful, artery exploration is necessary as the first procedure. Involvement of the popliteal artery may necessitate the exposure and use of the tibial vessels for the lower anastomosis. If this occurs, the procedure could require the use of microvascular instruments and techniques.

In situ femoral-popliteal bypass is the restoration of blood flow to the leg, bypassing an occluded portion of the femoral artery with a patient's saphenous vein, which remains in place. The procedure includes incising the venous valves and interrupting the venous tributaries. The adequacy of the patient's saphenous vein can be validated before the surgical procedure by an ultrasound duplex scan. Varicose veins or a previous saphenous vein ligation and stripping are contraindications to the procedure. The advantages of using vein graft for a bypass procedure include increased graft availability, favorable size match between vein and artery, decreased ischemia to vein (intima) because the vasavasorum remains intact, and improved patency (debated). Some argue that another advantage is vein distension by blood inflow rather than the potentially traumatic manual syringe method. A disadvantage is the time-consuming aspect of this technique and the potential intimal trauma from valve disruption, which could cause graft failure. Reoperation is more frequent with the in situ method because of missed valves and residual arteriovenous fistulae (Jacobs & Towne, 1996). Valves can be incised with microvascular scissors, a Mills valvulotome, or a Leather in situ valve cutter kit. An angioscope may be used to monitor the lysis of valve leaflets.

Nonreversed saphenous vein graft may be necessary when the vein is harvested at a point that does not allow close access to the anastomosis site. The valves must be disrupted in a nonreversed vein as described earlier.

Reversed saphenous vein graft (RSVG) may be used as the bypass conduit. Assessment of vein size by duplex ultrasound may be helpful (although not always accurate). This may assist in planning for an alternate vein harvest site, either the opposite leg or an arm.

Indications and pathophysiology

Indications for surgical intervention depend on the nature of the disease process (acute versus chronic), the general condition of the patient, and the surgeon's preference and skill in selected bypass techniques.

Acute arterial ischemia. A sudden loss of arterial flow to a leg requires immediate treatment. Although acute ischemia may occur in the presence of chronic occlusive disease, it is different because there may not be adequate time for the body to establish collateral circulation. Injury or a thromboembolic event are the primary causes of acute ischemia. The embolus is caused by the migration of material from another location that causes a blockage. Most emboli that arise from the heart are usually from atrial fibrillation or a recent myocardial infarction. Noncardiac sources include atheromatous plaque, debris from aneurysms, or foreign bodies. The major distal source of emboli causing lower extremity obstruction is the left heart (Brewster, Chin, & Fogarty, 1989) and the femoral artery as a proximal source (Fahey & McCarthy, 1994). Twenty-five percent of the time, no source is clearly differentiated (Holcroft & Blaisdell, 1994).

Symptoms of acute arterial ischemia are often referred to as the "six Ps." They include pain, pallor, pulselessness, paresthesia, paralysis, and poikilothermy (coolness). If allowed to progress, the limb swells, becomes waxen and cyanotic, and blisters. Tissue death results in infection or mummification. The patient usually presents with a history of sudden onset of unbearable pain and weakness in the effected leg (Pousti, Wilson, & Williams, 1994). Moderate obstruction results in delayed capillary refill. Severe obstruction produces a firm muscle and pain on dorsiflexion of the foot (Canobbio, 1990).

Diagnosis is based on history and physical examination. Laboratory tests are performed to evaluate the status of hydration, major organ function, and the extent of muscle damage. This includes basic blood work (complete blood count [CBC], blood-urea-nitrogen [BUN], CPK, creatine and glucose), prothrombin time/partial thromboplastin time [PT/PTT], ECG, chest x-ray, and arteriogram to define the extent of the obstruction (Holcroft & Blaisdell, 1994).

Treatment includes control of pain and anticoagulation with heparin to prevent further clot propagation. Antithrombolytic therapy may be indicated but must be used cautiously in severe obstruction because it takes 12 to 24 hours to restore patency. Embolectomy may be performed if the ischemia is less than 8 hours in duration. Beyond this time period, nonreversible muscle necrosis has occurred. Revascularization after this time will cause a washout of potentially organ damaging byproducts of ischemia. Tissue that does not blanch with pressure is considered to be beyond salvage. After 72 hours of anticoagulation, the limb will require either revascularization by bypass, amputation, or long-term anticoagulation (Holcroft & Blaisdell, 1994).

Chronic arterial insufficiency. Chronic arterial occlusive disease of the lower extremity is usually caused by atherosclerosis. Hypertension, diabetes, smoking, and elevated blood lipid levels are predisposing factors. A small percentage of patients present with occlusive disease as a result of inflammatory diseases. These include giant cell arteritis, Takayasu's arteritis, Buerger's disease (primarily young males who smoke) and systemic lupus erythematosus (Procter, et al, 1992).

Claudication (from the Latin word "claudicare," to limp) is the most common symptom of lower extremity occlusive disease (Procter, et al, 1992). In general claudication in the buttocks is due to bilateral iliac artery disease, thigh claudication is due to common femoral artery disease or iliac disease, and calf claudication is due to superficial femoral artery disease (Emma, 1992). Symptoms may vary in individuals, e.g., as many as 25% of patients with aortoiliac stenosis present with calf claudication (Perler, 1996). Claudication is the pain caused by muscle ischemia as a result of exercise. The increased metabolic demands of the exercising muscle are not met by the diseased arteries. The resultant anaerobic metabolism produces acidic byproducts. The acidosis causes a decrease in available adenosine triphosphate (ATP) leading to less flexibility of the red blood cells. Acidosis increases blood viscosity as a result of platelet aggregation. These factors contribute to the inability of the muscle to supply adequate oxygen (Emma, 1992). The discomfort subsides with rest. The majority of patients with intermittent claudication will remain stable and never require revascularization. Patients are counseled to begin a structured course of exercise for 6 months and are reassessed for the need for revascularization (Whittemore, 1995). Gradually increasing the distance walked and resting will promote collateral circulation. Walking for 20 minutes twice daily is recommended (Emma, 1992). However, some patients may be symptom free even with aggressive disease and medical treatment or exercise may not be appropriate at the onset of their symptoms. Approximately 20% to 25% will progress to severe claudication that severely limits their lifestyle or will develop ischemic ulcers or gangrene. These patients are candidates for revascularization within 5 years of the onset of symptoms (Dzsinich & Gloviczki, 1993; Whittemore, 1995). Cessation of smoking will also improve circulation.

Rest pain is a symptom of more severe arterial ischemia. Patients usually complain of severe, unrelenting foot pain that is not relieved by rest but may be alleviated by placing the foot in a dependent position. Gravity may increase arterial perfusion. Patients may describe awakening from foot pain and lowering their feet for relief (Table 12-1). *Critical leg ischemia* or *limb-threatening ischemia* generally refers to advanced disease with rest pain or tissue loss (ulcers) (Dormandy, 1993). These patients may require amputation unless revascularization is performed (Whittemore, 1995). Fontaine, et al (1954) developed a classification system for ischemic lower extremities (Sheperd, 1993). The stages are as follows:

Fontaine Stage 1: asymptomatic, demonstrable by noninvasive studies or arteriogram.
Fontaine Stage 2: intermittent claudication.
Fontaine Stage 3: intermittent claudication and/or constant rest pain.
Fontaine Stage 4: ischemic ulcers or gangrene (Dzsinich & Gloviczki, 1993).

There are three main indications for femoropopliteal bypass: intermittent claudication that restricts employment (after risk factor modification), unrelieved rest pain, and nonhealing ulcers or gangrene of heels or toes (Veith & Haimovici, 1996). Contraindications to revascularization include life-threatening sepsis or recent myocardial infarction, although an intervention such as an embolectomy performed under local anesthesia may be advisable for an acutely threatened limb. Age alone is not a contraindication. Adequate preoperative evaluation and preparation make revascularization procedures a viable option for preserving independent function in patients over the age of 75. The risk of MI is the same as in younger patients but the risk of death after MI increases in this population (70% versus 44%) (Nunnelee, Kurgan, & Auer, 1993).

Preoperative planning

Routine preoperative assessment is required with particular emphasis on the cardiac evaluation. Myocardial infarction is the primary cause of perioperative morbidity and mortality. Coronary artery bypass surgery may be a prerequisite to lower extremity bypass (Veith & Haimovici, 1996).

A tentative diagnosis of lower extremity arterial disease may be made on the basis of history and physical examination. Patients may have claudication of the buttocks, thigh, or calf; rest pain; diminished or absent peripheral pulses; dependent rubor; and atrophic skin changes and ulcers or gangrene. Some patients have peripheral neuropathy. A history of diabetes mellitus or alcoholism may cause foot neuropathies that mimic ischemic rest pain. Noninvasive studies are done to rule out ischemia. Nerve conduction studies may be helpful to differentiate a neuropathy from arterial occlusive disease. Once lower extremity ischemia has been ascertained, noninvasive studies (Doppler ultrasound and plethysmography) provide quantitative data and can localize the lesion or lesions. The ankle-brachial index (ABI) is an indicator of peripheral arterial blood supply. The value of the ABI is limited in severe disease, when no Doppler signal is audible, and

Table 12-1 **Comparison of Symptoms of Claudication and Rest Pain**

	CLAUDICATION	REST PAIN
Location	Distal to stenosis, in muscle	Distal to stenosis, usually in foot (especially toes)
Quality	Crampy, achy	Burning, throbbing
Quantity	Mild to severe	Severe, intolerable
Chronology	Increases/decreases with lifestyle changes	Increases over time
Aggravating factors	Muscle use	Lying down, elevating feet; pressure; any movement
Alleviating factors	Cessation of activity	Lowering foot, moving about, narcotics later
Setting	Ambulating	Resting, often waking from sleep
Associated activity	Increases with excess body weight or weight carrying; ambulating on an upward incline, walking faster	Any irritation may be constant

From Beare, P.G., and Myers, J.L. (1998). *Principles and practice of adult health nursing* (3rd ed.). St. Louis: Mosby.

in some diabetics with diffuse, calcified, or noncompressible vessels, which makes the index inaccurately high (see Chapter 5) (Porter, 1991).

An angiogram of the pelvis and both legs and feet is necessary to determine *inflow* (aorta and iliac arteries) and *outflow* (tibial and pedal vessels) of the arterial blood supply. Surgical intervention is based on multiple factors. Inadequate inflow (from the iliac artery) or bilateral iliac artery stenoses may be an indication for an aortobifemoral bypass (see Chapter 15). A patient who can not tolerate this may be a candidate for an extraanatomic bypass (see Chapter 17). In patients who have a short or isolated iliac lesion a balloon angioplasty with or without placement of a stent may be the most appropriate treatment. Angioplasty may be performed at the time of femoropopliteal bypass.

Patterns of lower extremity atherosclerotic lesions. Atherosclerotic lesions develop at vessel bifurcations and areas where the vessel curves or tapers. This is caused by the disruption of laminar flow that leads to turbulence and probable damage to the intima. Atherosclerotic lesions tend to be found in the distal superficial femoral artery (SFA), the entire SFA (20%), and rarely in the distal SFA alone. Lesions that are in the popliteal artery only are rare. The deep femoral artery (profunda femoris) is also usually diseased when the femoropopliteal artery is diseased but is generally stenotic and not totally occluded. The majority of popliteal lesions are in the distal segment. The tibial peroneal arteries are usually diseased in patients with femoropopliteal lesions. The peroneal artery is the least likely to be involved of the three distal vessels. Diabetic patients tend to have more diffuse patterns of atherosclerosis (Veith & Haimovici, 1996). Diabetics typically present with disease in the distal profunda, distal popliteal and tibial arteries, and digital arteries of the foot. The vessels also tend to be very calcified, which makes them difficult to compress (to obtain ABIs) and clamp (Green & Ouriel, 1994).

The blood flow rate in the legs varies a great deal. The SFA is a major vessel with few branches. The flow varies with leg activity and tends to be relatively slow. In contrast, the deep femoral artery is a smaller, muscular tributary that has many branches going to the lower leg. Its flow rate tends to be higher, which may account for it being less diseased than the SFA (Zarins & Glagov, 1994).

Equipment, instrumentation, medications, and solutions

Also refer to Chapter 8, Equipment, Supplies, and Instrumentation, and Chapter 4, Medications.

Basic OR furniture
Tourniquet box
Leg prep holder
ACT machine
In situ vein graft
Fluid infusion machine
Angioscopy
Angioscope
Video camera
Camera cover
Light source and fiberoptic cord
Irrigation pump and tubing
Video monitor and cassette recorder
Sterile Supplies
Contents of a custom pack for vascular surgery
For draping: add 2 large drape sheets
Clear plastic bag for foot
Vascular grafts
Foley catheter
Soft, round bolster (to support leg)
Sterile tourniquet cuffs
Extension tubing for tourniquet (optional)
Sterile cotton padding
Esmarch bandage for limb exsanguination
Fogarty inserts
Teflon pledgets
Radiopaque ruler
Valvulotomes (disposable)

Angioscopy: sterile pump tubing
Sterile camera cover
Instrumentation
Basic vascular instrument set
Vascular tunnelers
Deep self-retainers, small self-retainers, Darling popliteal retractor
Garrett dilators
In situ procedure instruments
In situ instruments
Vascular dilators
Microvascular scissors
Mills valvulotome
Leather in situ valve cutter kit
Endoscopic equipment
Doppler flow detector (amplifier)
Sterile Doppler probe
Gel (for Doppler detection over intact skin), sterile and unsterile
Duplex ultrasonography
Duplex machine
Intraoperative probe
Sterile probe covers with gel inside cover
Intraoperative medications and solutions
Saline
Heparinized saline
Vein graft solution: heparinized saline with or without papaverine HCl or heparinized blood.
Papaverine HCl (injected into artery or sprayed onto artery to mimic vasodilation of exercise for pressure gradient measurement)
Antibiotic irrigation (optional)
Hemostatic agents: Surgicel, Gelfoam, topical thrombin

Procedural Steps

The patient is placed in a supine position. Prepping and draping include the entire groin and leg. The foot may be included in the prep for distal anastomoses. It may be preferable to not

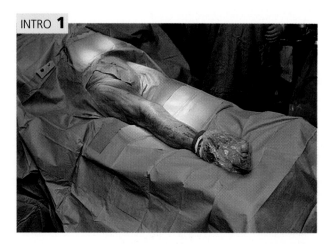

INTRO **1**

RNFA CONSIDERATIONS

Knowledge of anatomy of lower extremities and arms
Knowledge of incision choices for access to leg arteries and vein grafts
Ensure proper handling of vascular grafts

SYNTHETIC GRAFTS
Verify correct type and size
Protect graft from unnecessary handling, puncture, and contamination by contact with patient's skin
Use Fogarty clamps instead of DeBakey clamps on synthetic graft
Assist in use of graft tunneler

VEIN GRAFT (SAPHENOUS OR CEPHALIC)
Harvest vein graft or assist in harvest of vein graft; ligate branches of vein with ties and clips
Ensure availability of vein graft solution for storage and distension of graft; papaverine in solution and gentle handling of vein will decrease spasm and minimize endothelial damage
Avoid overdistension of vein graft, which also damages intima
Keep vein graft moist by spraying it with vein solution, covering it with moistened gauze sponge, or submerging graft in vein solution
Avoid damage to nerves by careful tissue dissection and placement of forceps
Protect patient's skin from pressure (especially prevent pressure on toes, avoid leaning on patient, prevent limb from lying on suction tubing or instruments)
In situ vein graft: assist in disruption of vein graft valve leaflets
Have knowledge of proper use and handling of angioscope, fluid pump, and accessories (assist in set-up as needed)

Cephalic vein graft
Protect patient's arm from venipunctures preoperatively by instructing patient in importance of plan
Check for physician's order in chart to prevent blood draws and IV insertion
Verbally communicate with perioperative caregivers
Suggest gauze to wrap arm with note in dressing to avoid venipuncture
Suggest sign on wall of inpatient room and patient's bed
Ensure availability of OR padded hand table and adequate sterile drapes for arm

Safe use of sterile tourniquet
Inspect condition of skin before and after application of tourniquet
Ensure adequate wrinkle-free padding of skin under cuff
Protect graft from inadvertently being caught in tourniquet cuff
Monitor inflation pressure and duration of inflation
Assess pulses and skin conditions before leaving OR
Cleanse skin and apply sterile dressings
Close wounds

Apyan, Schneider, & Andros, 1992; Jacobs & Towne, 1996.

discolor the foot with an iodophor solution and place it in a clear plastic bag. This isolates the toes, which have more areas to harbor bacteria and maintains the natural skin color for better assessment of perfusion.

INTRO **2**

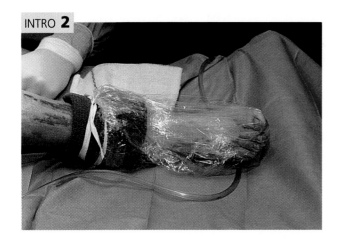

The hip is externally rotated and abducted with the knee flexed and the thigh supported on a soft bolster. The instrument set-up includes the basic minor and vascular sets plus the following: Gelpi retractors, Garrett or Weitlaner retractors, a tunneler, and supplies and equipment for operative arteriograms. Additional equipment and supplies for angioscopy and in situ bypass are added as needed.

INTRO **3**

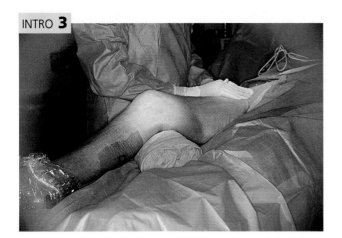

Exploration of common femoral artery

1. A vertical incision, extending downward about 3 to 5 inches along the medial aspect of the thigh, is made over the femoral artery below the inguinal area, and a self retaining retractor is inserted.

STEP **1-1**

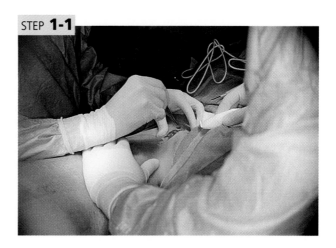

2. The common femoral artery is located, and the artery is dissected in both directions for complete exposure.

STEP **2-1**

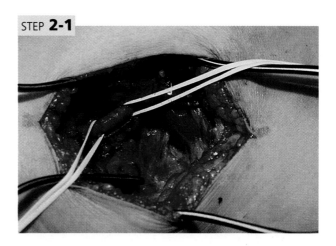

3. Moist umbilical tapes or vessel loops are passed around the common femoral, the superficial femoral, and the deep femoral arteries.

STEP **3-1**

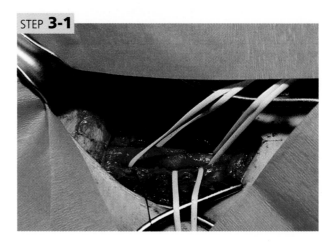

STEP **3-2**

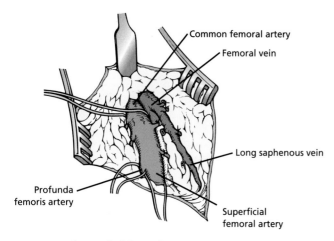

Exposure and control of femoral artery. (From Calne, R. Y., & Pollard, S. G. [1992]. *Operative surgery.* London: Gower.)

STEP **3-1**

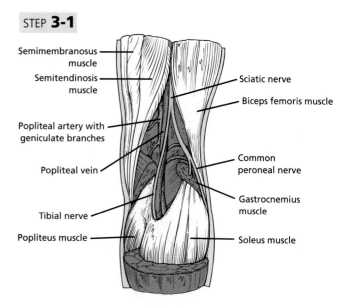

Relevant anatomy of the popliteal artery. (From Calne, R. Y., & Pollard, S. G. [1992]. *Operative surgery.* London: Gower.)

Exploration of above-knee popliteal artery

1. A vertical incision is made along the medial aspect of the lower thigh.

CONSIDERATIONS If the popliteal artery is diseased, an incision below the knee is necessary to expose the distal popliteal artery.

2. A self-retaining retractor is used to retract the muscles and expose the artery.

STEP **2-1**

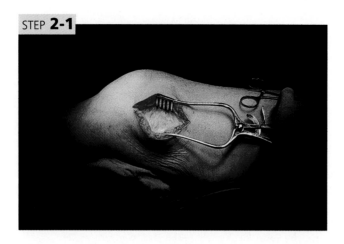

STEP **3-2**

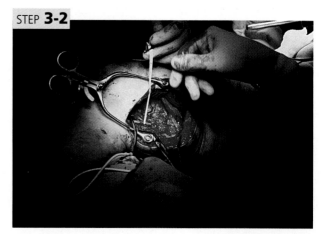

Saphenous vein graft

4. The saphenous vein is exposed by joining the femoral and popliteal incisions the length of the thigh or through multiple short incisions along the medial thigh. If the vein is suitable, the necessary length is resected *or* prepared for in situ grafting.

STEP **4-1**

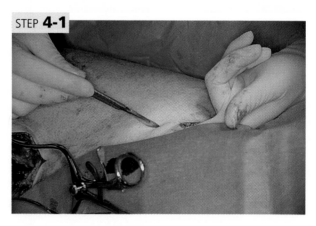

3. The popliteal artery is dissected free. A vessel loop is passed around the popliteal artery.

It may be desirable at this time to perform arteriograms if doubt exists about the patency of the popliteal artery or distal arterial tree.

5. The saphenous vein is prepared for use by carefully ligating side branches with fine silk and Hemoclips.

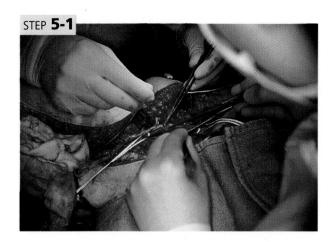

STEP **5-1**

6. The vein graft is removed from its bed (for reverse grafting), distended with the heparinized solution of choice, and assessed for size. The vein is gently occluded manually while it is distended to test for any leaks or holes. These may be due to injury or side branches. They are repaired with a fine silk tie or sewn with a fine polypropylene suture.

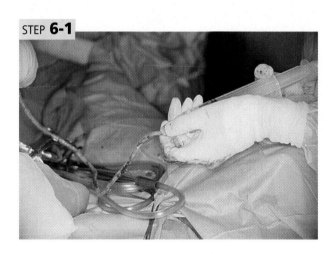

STEP **6-1**

7. The vein graft may be temporarily stored in the vein solution of choice. A mosquito clamp may be placed on one end to identify the orientation of the valves.

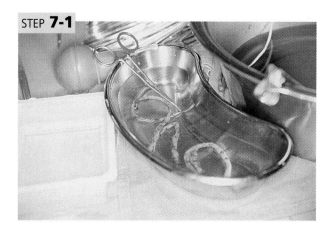

STEP **7-1**

CONSIDERATIONS The surgeon may elect to mark the vein graft with a skin marker or fine suture to ensure that it does not twist when relocated.

Finally, the vein is reversed (to permit flow past the valves) and the end originally in the groin is anastomosed to the popliteal artery and the end originally in the lower thigh is anastomosed to the femoral artery. Size discrepancies may be corrected by vein patch angioplasty (see Chapter 10).

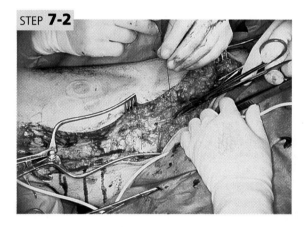

STEP **7-2**

8. The anastomoses are tested by releasing the arterial clamp and additional sutures placed as needed.

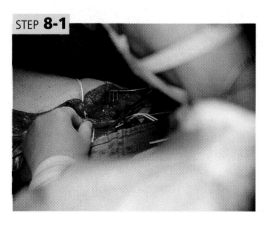

STEP **8-1**

Prosthetic grafting

1. The arteries are prepared as described for the placement of the vein graft.

2. The length and size of the prosthetic graft are determined. For a synthetic graft, the tunneler is passed (using the blunt end as the leading end to dissect the tissue) beneath the sartorius muscle from the popliteal fossa to the groin.

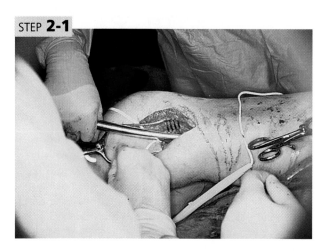

STEP **2-1**

3. The inner carrier of the tunneler is removed and reversed into the tunnel. The graft is sewn to the carrier and gently pulled through the tunnel and positioned to prevent kinks or twists. The graft is cut from the carrier after it reaches the distal anastomosis site.

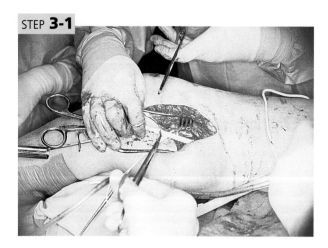

STEP **3-1**

4. The femoral artery is occluded and an incision is made into the femoral artery with a #11 knife blade and extended with a Potts angulated scissors.

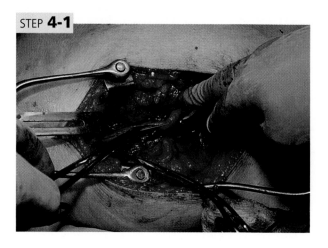

STEP **4-1**

9. The synthetic graft is trimmed with an S-shaped cut and anastomosed to the artery with fine vascular sutures.

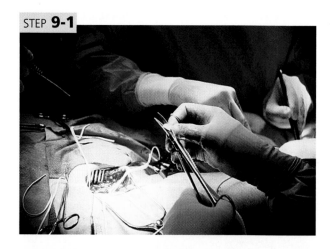

STEP **9-1**

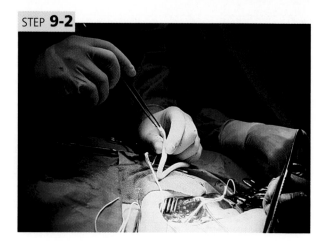

STEP **9-2**

10. Vascular clamps are placed on the popliteal artery at the site of the distal anastomosis.

Tourniquet application as an alternative to direct vessel occlusion

1. The leg is padded with cotton webril padding or several layers of x-ray sponges, and the tourniquet is wrapped around the leg.

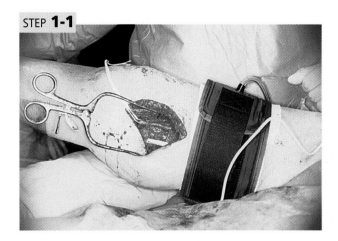

STEP **1-1**

2. The limb is exsanguinated by elevating it for 3 minutes or expressing the blood proximally by wrapping the limb with an elastic Esmarch bandage.

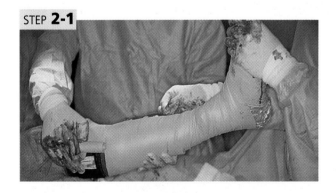

STEP **2-1**

3. The tourniquet is inflated by the circulating nurse, and inflation times, pressure, and duration are recorded.

11. An incision is made into the popliteal artery as for the femoral arteriotomy.

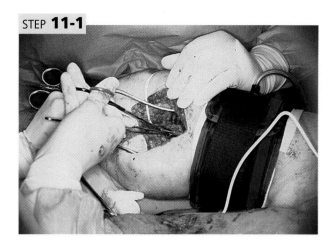

STEP **11-1**

12. The graft is cut, shaped, and sutured to the popliteal artery, and before completion the femoral occluding clamp is momentarily opened to eliminate air and debris ("flushed").

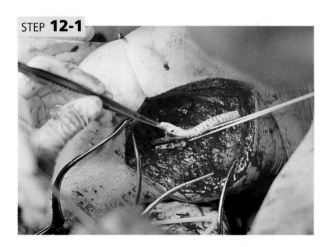

STEP **12-1**

13. All occluding clamps (or tourniquet) are removed and the graft is assessed for anastomotic leaks.

14. The incisions are closed and dressings applied.

FEMORAL-POPLITEAL BYPASS IN SITU

In situ femoral-popliteal bypass is the restoration of blood flow to the leg, bypassing an occluded portion of the femoral artery with a patient's saphenous vein, which remains in place. The procedure includes incising the venous valves and interrupting the venous tributaries. The adequacy of the patient's saphenous vein can be validated before the surgical procedure by an ultrasound duplex scan. Varicose veins or a previous saphenous vein ligation and stripping are contraindications to the procedure. The *advantages* of a vein bypass procedure include increased graft availability and improved patency (debated). The *disadvantages* are the time-consuming aspect of this technique and the potential intimal damage from valvulotomy. Valves can be incised with microvascular scissors, a Mills valvulotome, LeMaitre, or Leather (or other style) in situ valve cutter kit. An angioscope may be used to monitor the lysis of valve leaflets and locate remaining branches that require ligation. Branches must be ligated to prevent arteriovenous fistulae (a connection between the newly created artery and venous system), which can hamper adequate arterial flow.

Procedural Steps

1. The procedure is as for femoral-popliteal bypass. The groin incision is extended downward over the course of the saphenous vein. A skin bridge may be left between the groin and popliteal incisions.

2. The saphenous vein is exposed and divided at its proximal and distal ends. Venous tributaries are occluded with arterial clips, such as Hemoclips, or fine nonabsorbable sutures.

3. The valvulotome is passed from below to the top, usually through side branches. The valvulotome is used to incise the internal valve. In angioscopically assisted bypass, valve lysis is done under *indirect* vision.

STEP 3-1

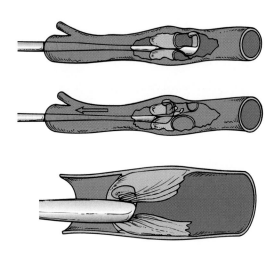

4. The saphenous vein is distended with heparinized saline, papaverine, or heparinized blood to identify any valvular obstruction or open venous tributary.

Another pass of the valve cutter alleviates any obstruction. Open branches of the saphenous vein can also be ligated with arterial clips or fine nonabsorbable sutures.

5. The **incompetent** saphenous vein is used to bypass the occluded segment of the femoral artery (see the femoral-popliteal bypass procedure).

Distal bypasses

The same basic steps are used. Vein graft or synthetic graft may be utilized.

1. Tibial arteries are exposed.

STEP 1-1

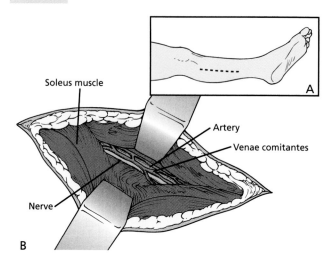

Exposure of posterior tibial artery. (From Calne, R. Y., & Pollard, S. G. [1992]. *Operative surgery.* London: Gower.)

STEP 1-2

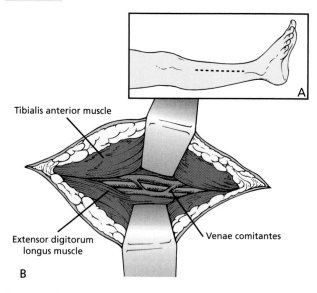

Exposure of anterior tibial artery. (From Calne, R. Y., & Pollard, S. G. [1992]. *Operative surgery.* London: Gower.)

STEP **1-3**

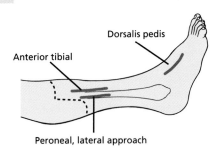

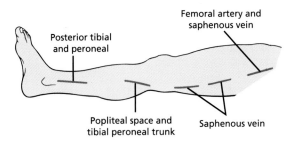

Placement of incision for femoropopliteal and femorotibial bypass and for saphenous vein harvest. These should avoid the incision lines for a below-knee amputation.

2. Vein graft harvest may begin near the ankle to obtain the maximum length of usable vein and continue the length of the leg using a continuous incision to follow the course of the saphenous vein or skin bridges may be created.

STEP **2-1**

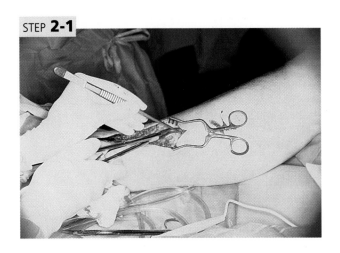

STEP **2-2**

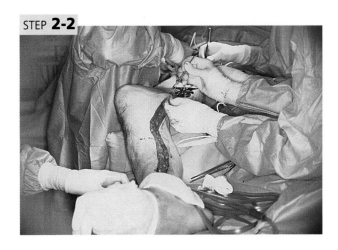

3. The tourniquet may be used for distal bypasses and placed below the knee or above the ankle.

COMPLICATIONS

INTRAOPERATIVE
Myocardial infarction
Damage to nerves
Damage to vein graft, leading to early graft failure
Blood loss

POSTOPERATIVE
Wound hematoma and infection
Poor wound healing, especially if a flap is created when
  harvesting saphenous vein graft
Anastomotic hemorrhage (increased risk in presence of
  infection)
Thrombosis of graft (because of technical error at anastomo-
  sis site, damage to vein graft, or hypercoagulable state)
Sudden loss of pulses, excruciating pain, and decreased
  motor-sensory function (require immediate intervention)
Mortality rate of 2% to 3%
Graft infection rate of 1% to 2%
Compartment syndrome (caused by muscle injury from
  ischemia-reperfusion syndrome; severe swelling leads to
  vascular compromise and requires an emergency
  fasciotomy)

Greatorex, 1992; Yeager, Taylor, & Porter, 1991; Emma, 1992.

POSTOPERATIVE

Care and Discharge Planning

POSTOPERATIVE CARE
Monitor vital signs, telemetry, intake and output

Postanesthesia care unit
ECG
Vascular assessment of limb
ABI

Patient unit
Check vital signs every 2 hours for the first 24 hours, every 4 hours for the next 24 hours, and then every 8 hours until discharged (this includes assessment of surgical incision and limb perfusion)
Maintain bedrest for patient
Ask patient to turn, cough, and deep breath every 2 hours
Telemetry and O_2 for 24 hours (D/C O_2 when oxygen saturation is at baseline)
Give patient sheepskin booties and cradle to keep bedding off limb
Use overhead trapeze bar (prevent trauma to opposite heel from "digging" in to move in bed)
Ambulate femoropopliteal bypass patients on POD 2 (ambulate femoral-distal bypass patients on POD 4)
No upright sitting; recliner chair is preferred
Weigh patient daily
Monitor intake and output
Diet: clear liquids and advance as tolerated
Convert IV to a Heplock when patient is taking adequate PO liquids
Discontinue Foley catheter when patient is ambulatory

Tests
ECG every day for 3 days
SMA-7, CBC, and platelet count on POD 1
ABI and Duplex scan on POD 2

Medications
ASA 325 mg qd (for antiplatelet effect)
Antibiotic IV for 24 hours or until all invasive lines are removed
Pain medication
Oral hypoglycemic agents or insulin sliding scale for diabetic patients
Resume maintenance medications (antihypertensive agents, etc.)

POSTOPERATIVE TEACHING AND DISCHARGE PLANNING
Patients who have undergone a lower extremity arterial bypass are most interested in information that will assist them in recognizing, preventing, and managing complications. They need instruction on incisional care and bathing to optimize incisional healing. Many have had experience with slow healing of wounds because of their arterial disease. Pain, sleep disturbances, and fatigue have been identified as important areas for instruction. One study to determine discharge teaching needs in this population showed that patients are capable of identifying their discharge learning needs in the preoperative period (Galloway, et al, 1995). Teach patients to manage the discomfort of incisions and leg swelling in order to prevent sleep disturbances. Emphasize the need to balance activity and rest. Patients in the immediate postoperative period are often receptive to counseling on risk factor modification. Cessation of smoking is an important step to improved wound healing and slowing the progression of the occlusive disease process. Assess the patient for learning needs about control of hypertension and diabetes. Stress and support lifestyle modifications that are attainable and individualized for each patient. Patients may be fearful of limb loss. Providing realistic goals without overwhelming demands will be most productive. Patients must *believe* that their efforts will make a difference in improving their quality of life for lifestyle changes to be sustained (Emma, 1992.)

Patient teaching
Pain management
Control of diabetes and hypertension
Smoking cessation
Signs and symptoms of graft failure
Teach patient and family to assess pulses

Foot care and protection
Daily inspection (teach use of mirror assistive methods)
Observe for cracks, ulcers, blisters, rashes, or discoloration
Teach proper nail trimming, prevention of ingrown toenails
Shoes must fit properly (discourage walking barefoot)
Teach to avoid tight socks or hose

Incisional care
Teach proper use and application of ace wraps for leg swelling (normal after surgery)
Provide written instructions of teaching, follow-up appointment, and phone numbers for questions or emergency needs
Discuss pain management, sleep disruption, fatigue
Driving with surgeon's approval after follow-up office visit (approximately 2 weeks postop)
No heavy lifting, vigorous exercise, or prolonged upright sitting; walking, stair climbing, and out of doors as able
Encourage gently ROM exercise of leg to prevent flexion contractures
Showering is permitted
Diet: resume previous diet, review special diets with patient (diabetic, low salt, low fat); reinforce role of adequate nutrition in wound healing

Notify surgeon of
Return of preoperative symptoms
Wound changes (redness, swelling, drainage)
Fever
Change in color, temperature, sensation, or use of leg, foot or toes
Antibiotics may be recommended before any dental or endoscopic procedures if a synthetic graft was implanted

References

Apyan, L., Schneider, P. A., & Andros, G. (1992). Preservation of arm veins for arterial reconstruction. *Journal of Vascular Nursing, 10*(2): 2-5.

Brewster, D. C., Chin, A. K., & Fogarty, T. J. (1989). Arterial thromboembolism.

Canobbio, M. M. (1990). Vascular diseases and disorders. In M. M. Canobbio (Ed.), *Cardiovascular disorders* (pp. 186-213). St. Louis: Mosby.

Dormandy, J. A. (1993). Critical leg ischemia. In D. L. Clement, & J. T. Shepherd (Eds.), *Vascular diseases in the limbs: Mechanisms and principles of treatment* (pp. 91-102). St. Louis: Mosby.

Dzsinich, C., & Gloviczki, P. (1993). Principles of vascular surgery. In D. L. Clement, & J. T. Shepherd (Eds.), *Vascular diseases in the limbs: Mechanisms and principles of treatment* (pp. 259-278). St. Louis: Mosby.

Emma, L. A. (1992). Chronic arterial occlusive disease. *Journal of Cardiovascular Nursing, 7*(1): 14-24.

Galloway, S., et al (1995). Symptom distress, anxiety, depression, and discharge information needs after peripheral arterial bypass. *Journal of Vascular Nursing, 13*(2): 35-40.

Greatorex, R. A. (1992). Femoropopliteal bypass. In *Operative surgery: Vascular surgery* (pp. 948-951). New York: Gower.

Green, R. M., & Ouriel, K. (1994). Peripheral arterial disease. In S. I. Schwarz, G. T. Shires, & F. C. Spencer (Eds.). *Principles of surgery* (pp. 925-987). New York: McGraw-Hill.

Holcroft, J. W., & Blaisdell, G. W. (1994). Acute arterial insufficiency. In F. J. Veith, R. W. Hobson, II, R. A. Williams, & S. E. Wilson (Eds.), *Vascular surgery: Principles and practice* (2nd ed., pp. 381-387). New York: McGraw-Hill.

Jacobs, D. L., & Towne, J. B. (1996). Femoropopliteal bypass. In K. Ouriel (Ed.), *Lower extremity vascular disease* (pp. 187-194). Philadelphia: W. B. Saunders.

Nunnelee, J. D., Kurgan, A., & Auer, A. I. (1993). Distal bypasses in patients over age 75. *Geriatric Nursing, 14*(5): 252-254.

Pousti, T. J., Wilson, S. E., & Williams, R. A. (1994). Clinical examination of the vascular system. In F. J. Veith, R. W. Hobson, II, R. A. Williams, S. E. Wilson (Eds.), *Vascular surgery: Principles and practice* (2nd ed., pp. 74-89). New York: McGraw-Hill.

Procter, C. D., Sr., Kazmier, F. J., Hollier, L. H., & Ramee, S. R. (1992). Selection of patients for peripheral revascularization surgery. *The Medical Clinics of North America, 76*(5), 1159-1168.

Shepard, J. T. (1993). Historical aspects. In D. L. Clement & J. T. Shepherd (Eds.), *Vascular diseases in the limbs: Mechanisms and principles of treatment* (pp. 1-10). St. Louis: Mosby.

Veith, F. J., & Haimovici, H. (1996). Femoropopliteal arteriosclerotic occlusive disease. In H. Haimovici, et al (Eds.), *Vascular surgery: Principles and techniques* (4th ed., pp. 605-631). Cambridge, MA: Blackwell Science.

Whittemore, A. D. (1995). Infrainguinal bypass. In R. B. Rutherford (Ed.), *Vascular surgery* (4th ed., pp. 794-814). Philadelphia: W. B. Saunders.

Yeager, R. A., Taylor, L. M., & Porter, J. M (1991). The present status of infrainguinal arterial reconstructive surgery for chronic lower-extremity ischemia. *Current Problems in Surgery, 25*(2): 125-139.

Zarins, C. K., & Glagov, S. (1994). Pathophysiology of human atherosclerosis. In F. J. Veith, R. W. Hobson, II, R. A. Williams, & S. E. Wilson (Eds.) *Vascular surgery: Principles and practice* (2nd ed., pp. 21-39). New York: McGraw-Hill.

13 Thoracic Outlet Surgery

FIRST RIB RESECTION

Description

A first rib resection is performed to relieve neurovascular compression that has not responded to physical therapy. In approximately 10% of surgical candidates, venous or arterial compression is involved. The three primary approaches include resection of the first rib, scalenectomy, or a combination. The combination of scalenectomy, and rib resection may reduce recurrence and improve results (Cina, et al, 1994). The surgical approach may be either transaxillary or supraclavicular. This is a technically demanding surgery. The anatomy is complicated, the incision is small, and exposure and lighting are difficult. For these reasons, there is a trend toward utilizing thoracoscopic equipment to improve the visibility with lighting and image magnification (Urschel, 1993).

Indications and pathophysiology

The area described as the **thoracic outlet** has the following borders: the manubrium is anterior, the first rib is anterolateral, and the first thoracic vertebra is posterior. The major vessels and nerves of the head and upper extremity pass through this area (Atkinson & Fortunato, 1996). Resection of the first rib removes the "floor" of the thoracic outlet (Figure 13-1) (Ouriel, et al, 1994). **Thoracic outlet syndrome (TOS)** is a compression disorder that may involve the brachial plexus, subclavian vein, or subclavian artery. The etiology may be from a congenital cervical rib, abnormal fibrous band, or a callus from a clavicular fracture (Graham & Ford, 1994). The scalenus anticus muscle lies over the brachial plexus. The muscle has fibrous attachments to the plexus and attaches to the first rib (Machleder, 1994). Abnormal fibrous bands may be fairly common but asymptomatic unless stressors or injury lead to a narrowing of the outlet (Juvonen, et al, 1995).

Neurologic. The vast majority of patients present with neurologic symptoms caused by compression of the brachial plexus. Only occasionally is the artery or vein compressed. The predominant complaint is dull or aching pain involving the neck, shoulder, forearm, or hand. The pain may be constant, intermittent, or associated with particular activities, especially those that involve overhead lifting and may therefore necessitate lifestyle restriction. Numbness and paresthesia may be described and in severe, chronic cases, muscle wasting of the upper arm is seen (Williams, Lee, & Ekers, 1994).

The differential diagnosis of TOS for patients presenting with pain, pallor or cyanosis, numbness, and cold intolerance must include carpal tunnel syndrome, ulnar and median nerve entrapment, cervical arthritis or cervical nerve entrapment, tumor, and cervical disc compression. (Ouriel & DeWeese, 1991; Machleder, 1994). The diagnosis of TOS is then often made only after the patient has endured multiple tests, consultations, and the passage of time. Patients are often discouraged, may have been treated as if their condition is psychosomatic, and are in need of emotional support. Underlying anxiety may make these patients difficult to manage although psychosocial history often reveals a well-adjusted individual before the onset of symptoms. Explanations of chronic pain syndromes and the diagnostic difficulties along with clear descriptions of anatomy and the proposed surgery or other treatment plans are most reassuring and helpful to both patient and family. It may be relieving for them also to learn that they do not have a systemic disorder (Machleder, 1994).

Venous. Subclavian vein compression at the thoracic outlet, although very rare, may cause arm pain, edema, and superficial vein distension. First rib resection must be combined with decompression of other compressing structures (medial clavicle, muscle, ligaments). Venous angioplasty may be required to repair any stenotic lesion of the vein (Ouriel, et al, 1994).

Arterial. Arterial compression is an infrequent but serious problem demanding prompt attention. If a subclavian aneurysm is present, it is excised and bypassed. Compression usually occurs at the point where the subclavian artery crosses the first rib. This can cause poststenotic dilatation, embolization, and acute claudication (Ouriel & DeWeese, 1991). Treatment is aimed at restoration of arterial flow to the limb by decompression, with arterial repair and embolectomy as indicated. Occasionally, cervicothoracic sympathectomy is indicated to denervate the forearm (Haimovici, 1996). This relieves the vasospasm that may contribute to pain and hand ischemia and may be performed with or without resection of the first rib (Urschel, 1993) (see Chapter 14).

Treatment is controversial and surgery is not always helpful. The majority of patients who are without arterial or venous compromise may benefit from a conservative approach. Physical therapy, including cervical traction and heat application, may provide relief in 70% of patients. Activity restriction and use of muscle relaxants can be of benefit also. Patients should be instructed to avoid sleeping with arms elevated and under the head. A course of exercise designed to elevate the shoulder girdle and relieve compression may be effective and prevent unneeded surgery (Ouriel & DeWeese, 1991).

Preoperative planning

Patients may be evaluated by neurologists, orthopedic specialists, and vascular surgeons. Multiple diagnostic studies are

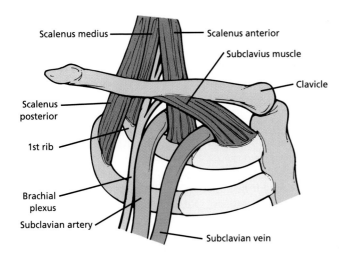

Fig. 13-1 Schematic drawing of the right thoracic outlet. The subclavian artery and brachial plexus exit through the scalene triangle, bordered by the anterior and middle scalene muscles and the first rib. The subclavian vein crosses the first rib between the anterior scalene and subclavius muscles anteriorly. *(From Young, R. J., Jr., Olin, J. W., & Bartholomew, J. R. [1996].* **Peripheral vascular diseases.** *St. Louis: Mosby.)*

usually required to differentiate the diagnosis and assess for arterial and venous compromise. Testing is ordered to address the specific symptoms. The full range of tests are not necessary for every patient.

- X-ray of chest and cervical spine (cervical rib, abnormal transverse process of C7, anomalous first rib, clavicular callus, abnormal vertebrae)
- Plethysmographic recording to determine arterial patency
- Arteriogram and MRI
- Areterial and venous duplex scanning with patient in neutral and aggravating positions
- Duplex scan (Haimovici, 1996)
- Venography with venous pressure measurements
- Nerve conduction studies (although a negative test does not rule out TOS)
- Routine blood work and urinalysis as indicated for preoperative work-up

Anesthetic considerations. General endotracheal anesthesia is required. An IV is inserted in the nonsurgical side arm or hand. These patients do not have the typical vascular patient profile of systemic disease or advanced age. They are often in their 20s or 30s and generally healthy. Routine blood work and urinalysis are performed before admission. Chest x-rays are available from their diagnostic work-up.

Patients are instructed about the procedure, recovery from general anesthesia with emphasis on deep breathing and coughing, and discharge information.

Equipment, instrumentation, medications, and solutions

Also refer to Chapter 8 Equipment, Supplies, and Instrumentation, and Chapter 4, Medications.

Positioning for transaxillary approach
Bean bag positioner
Axillary roll and variety of gel pads
3 pillows
Safety belt and wide adhesive tape
Soft support for head and neck (no pressure on eyes or dependent ear)
Standing platforms for the assistant who retracts patient's arm

Sterile supplies
Custom pack (all supplies needed except suture boots; vessel loops are optional)

Supraclavicular
Minor soft tissue set and bone instrumentation
No vascular instrumentation is needed
Electrocautery pencil
Suction set-up
Kittner dissector
Vessel clips
Silk or absorbable ties and vessel loops
A deep self-retaining retractor, such as a Travers, is adequate for the initial exposure
Small ribbon retractors may be helpful
Basic soft tissue instruments

First rib
Instrumentation set (see Figure 8-53) plus:
Long scissors
Long DeBakey forceps
Hemoclips
Kittners (blunt dissection)
Hook Bovie tip
Periosteal elevator
Long right-angled clamp
Retractors: self-retaining, Deavers, narrow ribbons
Long instruments for transaxillary approach only

Thoracoscopic assistance with transaxillary approach
10 mm 0 degree lens
Video cart
In-line video (to scope)
27 inch color TV screen
Xenon light
VCR
FRED (fog reduction liquid)
light carrier

Intraoperative medications
Saline to instill in wound to check for pleural leak (evidenced by bubbling)

Procedural Steps

Supraclavicular approach
The patient is positioned supine with the operative side arm secured at side or both arms secured at sides, and the head is in a head-up tilt and turned away from the operative side. A roll under the shoulders may be helpful for some patients.

RNFA CONSIDERATIONS

Knowledge of selected surgical approach (supraclavicular versus transaxillary).

Knowledge of relevant anatomy

Assist in set-up of thoracoscope and video equipment as needed.

Assist in positioning patient intraoperatively: adequate padding for all potential pressure areas; (thoracotomy position): especially check bean bag and pad with gel pad before positioning pillows between legs.

Assist in retraction of arm (transaxillary approach), prevent hyperabduction or hyperextension of greater than 90 degrees (brachial plexus injury), retraction of wound.

Provide adequate lighting of wound (through use of scope, lighted retractor, or disposable light).

5. Identify the brachial plexus

6. Identify and place a loop around the subclavian artery. Gently retract it.

7. Remove the entire lower attachment of the scalene muscle to the first rib, being careful to gently remove any attachments to the brachial plexus.

8. Remove the periosteum from the first rib with an elevator, and free it from any fibrous bands.

9. Remove the first rib with first rib cutters, bone cutters, and Rongeurs as far posterior as possible.

10. Smooth the bone with a rasp.

11. Check for hemostasis, and fill the wound with saline to check for pneumothorax. (Repair the pleura as needed).

12. Close the wound in two layers.

Transaxillary approach

Position the patient in the lateral decubitus position.

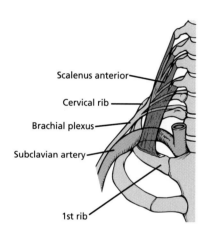

Anatomy for supraclavicular approach. (From Young, R., Jr., Olin, J. W., & Bartholomew, J. R. [1996]. *Peripheral vascular diseases.* St. Louis: Mosby.)

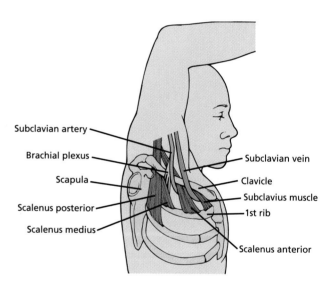

Anatomy for transaxillary approach. (From Young, R., Jr., Olin, J. W., & Bartholomew, J. R. [1996]. *Peripheral vascular diseases.* St. Louis: Mosby.)

1. Make a 6 cm incision above the clavicle, over the sternocleidomastoid muscle.

2. Incise through the sternocleidomastoid muscle and insert the self-retaining retractor.

3. Identify the phrenic nerve.

CONSIDERATIONS On the left side, the thoracic duct arises from the mediastinum behind the jugular vein and enters the subclavian. *If it is injured, it must be ligated to prevent a chylous fistula.*

4. Insert the self-retaining retractor and divide the anterior scalene muscle.

1. Make the incision between the lateral border of the pectoralis major and medial border of the latissimus dorsi muscle.

2. Divide the insertion of the scalenus anticus and the subclavius muscle tendon.

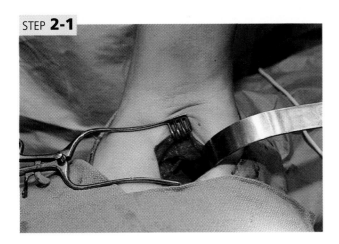

STEP **2-1**

3. Divide the periosteum from the first rib and remove the *middle section* of the first rib and its superior periosteum (the more posterior the removal of the rib, the better the outcome).

STEP **3-1**

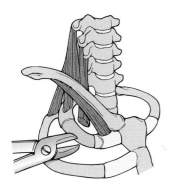

4. Cut the costoclavicular ligament and divide the anterior section of the first rib at the sternum.

5. The posterior section of the first rib is grasped with a Kocher clamp to stabilize it. It is separated from the subclavian artery and brachial plexus. The scalenus medius muscle is stripped from the rib by a subperiosteal dissection (to avoid the long thoracic nerve). The rib is removed at its articulation to the transverse process of the vertebra. (Complete rib resection and removal of periosteum will prevent recurrence).

6. If a cervical rib is present it is also removed at this time.

STEP **6-1**

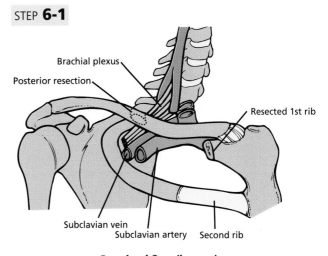

Completed first rib resection.

7 . Ensure hemostasis. Assess for pneumothorax by filling the wound with saline and observing for air bubbles with respiration. (A pneumothorax can be corrected by inserting a tube drain, which is withdrawn when the wound is closed.)

STEP **7-1**

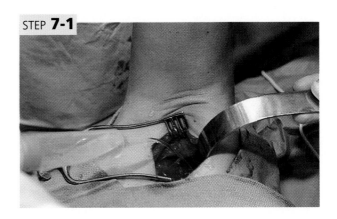

8. Close the wound in 2 layers (subcutaneous and skin) and apply a dressing.

STEP **8-1**

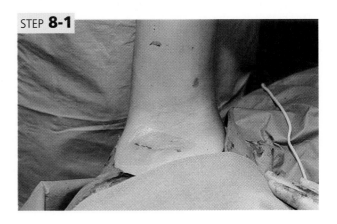

COMPLICATIONS

SUPRACLAVICULAR APPROACH

Damage to any of the vessels can cause bleeding (subclavian, vertebral).

Damage to the phrenic nerve can cause paralysis of the hemidiaphragm.

Damage to the apical pleura can cause a pneumothorax.

TRANSAXILLARY APPROACH

Pneumothorax.

Injury to the long thoracic nerve (results in winging of the scapula).

Injury to the brachial plexus (results in paresis of arm) from instrumentation or overzealous hyperextension or hyperabduction of the arm.

(See Chapter 14 if sympathectomy is performed.)

POSTOPERATIVE

Care and Discharge Planning

POSTOPERATIVE CARE (POD 1 & 2)

Upright chest x-ray to check for residual pneumothorax

Pain management (transaxillary approach involves continuous and rigorous retraction of muscles and ipsilateral arm intraoperatively).

Routine vital signs including CMS checks of surgical arm and hand.

Avoid hyperabduction or hyperextension of surgical arm greater than 90 degrees until physical therapy regimen is instituted.

Postoperative care is focused on assisting the recovery from general anesthesia: deep breathing and coughing to prevent respiratory complications

Regular diet and early ambulation may be resumed as tolerated.

Discharge on POD 2 or 3.

POSTOPERATIVE TEACHING AND DISCHARGE PLANNING

The patient may remove transparent dressing after 3 to 4 days or sooner if it becomes wet from showering or operative drainage. The incision site may then be left open to the air.

The patient should avoid powder, lotion, deodorant, and shaving over transaxillary incision until it is well healed.

The patient may shower, ambulate, and be out of doors as desired. No driving until the surgeon gives permission.

The patient may return to other activity as able but the arm may only be used passively for 3 weeks, with avoidance of hyperabduction and hyperextension greater than 90 degrees.

The patient may make a gradual progression to normal activity with active and full ROM at 6 weeks or later based on the judgment of the surgeon. Physical therapy is reinstituted in a like manner.

Provide emotional support and reassurance as needed with respect to surgical procedure, anatomic changes, and recovery.

References

Atkinson, L. J., & Fortunato, N. (1996). Thoracic surgery. In L. J. Atkinson, N. Fortunato (Eds.), *Berry & Kohn's operating room technique* (8th ed., pp. 783-795). St. Louis: Mosby.

Beven, E. G. (1996). Thoracic outlet syndromes. In Jr. R. Young, J. W. Olin, & J. R. Bartholemew (Eds.), *Peripheral vascular diseases* (pp. 553-552). St. Louis: Mosby.

Cina, C., Whitacre, L., Edwards, R., & Maggisano, R. (1994). Treatment of thoracic outlet syndrome with combined scalenectomy and transaxillary first rib resection. *Cardiovascular Surgery, 2*(4): 515-518.

Graham, L. M., & Gord, M. B. (1994). Arterial disease. In V. A. Fahey (Ed.), *Vascular nursing* (2nd ed., pp. 3-20). Philadelphia: W.B. Saunders.

Haimovici, H. (1996). Arterial thoracic outlet syndrome. In H. Haimovici, et al (Eds.), *Vascular surgery: Principles and techniques* (4th ed., pp. 1082-1091). Cambridge, MA: Blackwell Science.

Juvonen, T., et al. (1995). Anomalies at the thoracic outlet are frequent in general population. *American Journal of Surgery, 170*(1): 33-37.

Machleder, H.I. (1994). Thoracic outlet disorders: Thoracic outlet compression syndrome and axillary vein thrombosis. In F. J. Veith, R. W. Hobson, R. A. Williams, & S. E. Wilson (Eds.), *Vascular surgery: Principles and practice* (2nd ed., pp. 797-808). New York: McGraw-Hill.

Ouriel, K., & DeWeese, J. A. (1991). Nonoperative management of thoracic outlet syndrome. In C. B. Ernst, & J. C. Stanley (Eds.), *Current therapy in vascular surgery* (2nd ed., pp. 224-227). St. Louis: Mosby.

Ouriel, K., et al (1994). First rib resection for symptomatic venous stenosis at the thoracic inlet. Unpublished manuscript.

Urschel, H. C. (1993). Dorsal sympathectomy and management of thoracic outlet syndrome with VATS. *Annals of Thoracic Surgery, 56*(3): 717-720.

Urschel, H. C. (1985). Thoracic outlet syndrome. In J. A. DeWeese (Ed.), *Rob and Smith's operative surgery: Vascular surgery* (4th ed.) Boston: Butterworth's

Williams, L. R., Lee, J. F., & Ekers, M. A. (1994). Upper extremity arterial problems. In V. A. Fahey (Ed.), *Vascular nursing* (2nd ed., pp. 346-367). Philadelphia: W. B. Saunders.

14   Sympathectomy

SYMPATHECTOMY

Description

A sympathectomy is the interruption of the sympathetic nerve chain and can be of the cervical, thoracic, or lumbar region. The means of accomplishing this include radio frequency ablation, electrocautery, chemical injection, or dissection and excision of a segment of the sympathetic nerve chain.

Indications and pathophysiology

Sympathectomies for reflex sympathetic dystrophy, causalgia, Raynaud's disease, hyperhydrosis, and arterial occlusive disease gained popularity in the 1930s. In the 1940s and early 1950s surgical sympathectomy was the standard treatment for arterial occlusive diseases of the limbs. This was generally replaced by arterial reconstruction procedures in the 1950s and 1960s. The idea of sympathectomy was based on studies of normal individuals given sympathetic nerve blocks, which resulted in increased blood flow. The effect of increased sympathetic tone is a significant decrease of blood flow to the cutaneous tissue and a smaller decrease in flow to the muscle. Injection of a local anesthetic into the stellate ganglion blocks the sympathetic effects, resulting in increased flow to the cutaneous tissue. The decreased flow to the muscle is less significant because exercise can overcome this localized response (Rutherford, 1993). Good results were usually short lived and some patients were found to have reestablished nerve pathways to both blood vessels and sweat glands (Sheperd, 1993). More recent research has dispelled the earlier belief that sympathectomy improves the circulation to the muscles; blood flow is primarily diverted to the cutaneous tissue. Sympathectomy can actually cause harm in patients with distal arterial occlusive disease by lowering the cutaneous vascular resistance and disrupting the minimal arterial flow the patient had previously (Rutherford & Shannon, 1995). Diabetic patients are not usually considered candidates for sympathectomy because their preexisting neuropathy reduces any benefit the procedure may offer. This neuropathy is sometimes referred to as "autosympathectomy" (Dzsinich & Gloviczki, 1993).

The sympathetic nerves have three basic functions. Stimulation causes direct constriction of the arteries and arterioles. Secondly, sympathetic stimulation stimulates secretion of sweat from the sweat glands. Sympathetic nerves perform a role in pain transmission, but the exact mechanism is not well understood (Barnes, 1994). The afferent (sensory) nerves conduct painful stimuli of vascular insufficiency and the efferent sympathetic nerve fibers are the motor pathways that cause vasoconstriction, which increases pain (Fahey & McCarthy, 1994).

Pain relief is one indication for sympathectomy in arterial occlusive disease. One theory of its effect is that lumbar sympathectomy alters the pain perception by lowering tissue norepinephrine levels and altering the pain transmission to the brain. For this reason, patients treated for rest pain have a fair response to this, while foot ulcer healing is less successful. This may be true because less oxygen is needed to relieve rest pain than to heal ulcers. Patient selection criteria for sympathectomy include an ABI greater than 0.3, absence of neuropathy, and minimal tissue loss (Rutherford & Shannon, 1995).

Although today's OR personnel may rarely see a sympathectomy performed, there are patients who may benefit from this surgery. Box 14-1 summarizes indications for surgical sympathectomy.

Cervical and cervicothoracic sympathectomy involves excision of the lower portion of the stellate ganglion (a fusion of the inferior cervical and first thoracic ganglion) and T2 and T3 ganglion. Sympathectomy in this region affects the upper extremity. However, it may also cause **Horner's syndrome**, which is ptosis (eyelid droop) and miosis (constriction of the pupil of the eye) and reduced sweat production of the side of the face (Haimovici, 1996; Calne & Pollard, 1992). In 1988 Raynaud described the phenomenon of well-demarcated ischemia and pallor of the digits. Some patients also exhibited pallor, cyanosis, and reactive hyperemia. It has since been differentiated into primary and secondary Raynaud's. Primary Raynaud's is idiopathic, occurs mostly in females, and is a hyperactive response to local cold exposure or emotional stress. Secondary Raynaud's has multiple causes (connective tissue diseases, neurovascular compression, toxins, drugs, and others). Cervical sympathectomy is probably no better than conservative treatment for primary Raynaud's and is of no value in secondary Raynaud's (Duprez, 1993).

Lumbar sympathectomy usually involves the sympathetic ganglion from L2 to L4 and sometimes L1. L1 affects the buttocks, thigh, and parts of the leg but also interferes with male ejaculation. L2 and L3 innervate the leg below mid-thigh, including the foot (Haimovici, 1996; Calne & Pollard, 1992).

Hyperhydrosis, or excessive sweating, has been amenable to sympathectomy. Sweating that exceeds the needs of normal thermoregulation can be extremely embarrassing. Some individuals cannot shake hands without sweat dripping from them. This condition can become very limiting for those who must work with papers or must wear gloves or rubber boots (Harris, Satchell, & May, 1995). Hyperhydrosis may resolve after puberty (McFadden & Hollier, 1996).

> **Box 14-1   Indications for Surgical Sympathectomy**
>
> Vasospastic disease of the leg or foot (relieves pain, assists
>   ulcer healing)
> Pain relief from peripheral vascular disease (especially blue
>   toe syndrome)
>   Nonreconstructible arterial disease
>   Cold injuries
> Hyperhydrosis
> Posttraumatic pain syndromes
>   Causalgia
>   Reflex sympathetic dystrophy
>   Phantom limb pain

Data from Haimovici, 1996; Beare & Meyers, 1994; Dzsinich &
Gloviczki, 1993; Fahey & McCarthy, 1994; Harris, Satchel, & May, 1995.

Causalgia and **reflex sympathetic dystrophy (RSD)** are considered to be separate entities but are difficult to differentiate clinically. Causalgia is described as a severe burning pain of the foot or hand after an injury to the nerve or a nerve branch. Patients usually describe the sensations as constant burning that is aggravated by light touch, stress, temperature change, or emotional reactions. A series of nerve blocks may be effective to break the pain cycle. If not, surgery is indicated. RSD is another syndrome that is characterized by continuous pain in a distal extremity after mild trauma. The difference is that no major nerve is involved. This is sometimes seen after a fracture. Nerve blocks and physical therapy may relieve the pain but surgery is necessary when blocks do not provide long-term pain relief. The International Association for the Study of Pain endorses sympathetic blocks and surgical sympathectomy for both causalgia and RSD (Drott, Gothberg, & Claes, 1995). The choice of cervical or lumbar sympathectomy would depend on the anatomic location of the problem.

Preoperative planning

Sympathectomies are usually performed under general anesthesia. An IV is needed. An arterial line for monitoring may be required if the patient has advanced cardiovascular disease. Arterial monitoring may be needed in the patients having lumbar sympathectomy for phantom limb pain, those with nonreconstructible lower extremity arterial disease, and those with blue toe syndrome. Causalgia must be treated promptly with sympathectomy for it to be helpful but it often goes untreated (Rutherford & Shannon, 1995).

An adequate preoperative nerve block is a predictive test for the success of surgery for chronic pain syndromes. Most patients will have had trial nerve blocks performed to determine the potential for effective results. Hyperhydrosis usually responds to sympathectomy and these patients do not need a trial nerve block. In patients with vascular occlusive disease, collateral reserve must be present, i.e. a capillary refill time of 20 seconds or less, an ABI of greater than 0.3 and distal thigh-brachial index of greater than 0.7. Plethysmography and skin temperature tests can provide objective measurement of effective blocks (Barnes,

1994). Preoperative x-rays of the neck and thoracic outlet may be required to rule out a first rib or thoracic outlet obstruction (Calne & Pollard, 1992).

Patient teaching includes the routine care of the surgical wound and dressing, pulmonary toilet after general anesthesia, and activity and diet as tolerated. The cervical sympathectomy patients should have the complication of Horner's syndrome reviewed by their surgeon. Male lumbar sympathectomy patients should have the potential for ejaculatory dysfunction explained since it is a potential complication.

Equipment and instrumentation
Supraclavicular
Minor soft tissue set
Electrocautery pencil
Suction set up
Kittner dissector
Vessel clips
Silk or absorbable ties
Vessel loops
A deep self-retaining retractor, such as a Travers, is adequate
    for the initial exposure
Small ribbon retractors may be helpful
No special or vascular instrumentation is needed
Transaxillary thoracic sympathectomy
A major basic instrument set is needed for a variety of
    retractors (Travers retractor, Deavers, and long malleable
    retractors)
Rib spreader
Long forceps
Long right-angled clamps
Long tissue clamps
Cervicothoracic sympathectomy (endoscopic)
and lumbar sympathectomy (laparotomy)
A major basic set-up is needed with long instruments because
    the incision is small and the wound deep
Long dissecting scissors
Long Debakey forceps
A variety of sizes of Hemoclips
Long right-angled clamps and cystic duct clamps
The only unique instrument is the Smithwick sympathec-
    tomy dissector and nerve hook (Figure 14-1).
A headlight is helpful for illumination of the surgical area,
    particularly for lumbar sympathectomy, which entails a
    small incision and deep structures; an alternative would
    be a disposble light on a long flexible wand
Lumbar sympathectomy (endoscopic)
Appropriate endoscope (0 degree lens)
Fiberoptic light cord
Light source
Video monitor
Disposable or reusable 10 mm trocars
Electrocautery tip
Endoscopic clip applier
Blunt dissector
Nerve hook
Endoscopic graspers and coagulating scissors
Laparoscopic fan retractors may be helpful

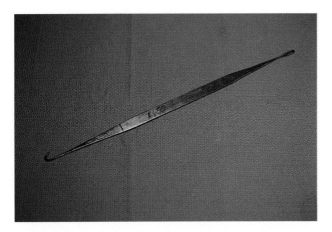

Fig. 14-1 Smithwick sympathectomy dissector and nerve hook.

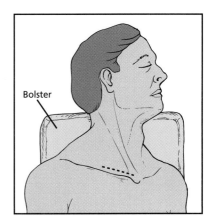

Fig. 14-2 Position of the patient and line of skin incision.

RNFA CONSIDERATIONS

1. Discuss the intended approach for the surgical procedure with a surgeon. Reinforce the explanations of the procedure with the patient.
2. Communicate the approach to the OR staff and assist in obtaining the necessary positioning devices, headlights or video equipment as needed. Check the equipment for completeness and function (scopes and TV monitor).
3. Review anatomy to ensure careful handling of tissue and recognition of relevant nerves.
4. For video-assisted approach, assist with insertion of ports and provide illumination by directing the light at the surgical area.
5. Close incisions. Insert chest tube as needed and connect to closed chest drain. Cleanse skin and apply dressings.
6. Assess patient's skin for any problems from positioning devices.
7. Assist in patient transfer.
8. Follow up on any needed chest x-ray.

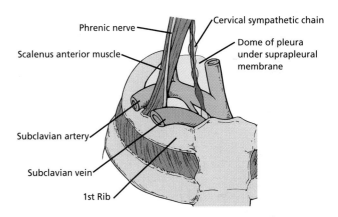

Fig. 14-3 Relevant anatomy of cervical sympathectomy. *(From Calne, R., & Pollard, S. G. [1992]. Operative surgery. London: Gower.)*

1. Make a 6 cm incision above the clavicle, running to the lateral border of sternocleidomastoid muscle.

As with any endoscopic procedure, full instrumentation for an open procedure should be available in case of an emergent complication (McFadden & Hollier, 1996; Sardi & Hollier, 1996).

Procedural Steps
Supraclavicular

Cervical sympathectomy by way of a **supraclavicular incision** is performed with the patient supine. The arm on the operative side or both arms are secured at the patient's sides. The head is in a head-up tilt and turned away from the operative side. A roll under the shoulders may be helpful for some patients (Figures 14-2 and 14-3).

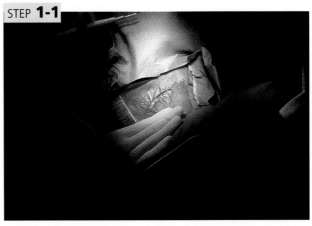

STEP **1-1**

2. Incise through the sternocleidomastoid muscle and ligate or retract the external jugular vein.

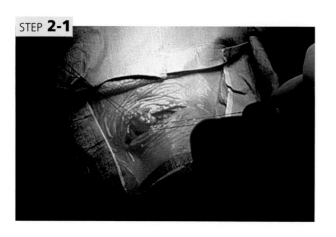

3. Insert the self-retaining retractor.

4. Identify the phrenic nerve, free it, and gently retract it with a vessel loop.

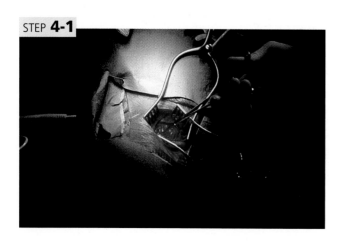

CONSIDERATIONS On the left side, the thoracic duct arises from the mediastinum behind the jugular vein and enters the subclavian. *If it is injured, it must be ligated to prevent a chylous fistula.*

5. Divide the scalenus anterior muscle, identify the subclavian artery, and place a vessel loop around it. Identify and loop the vertebral artery.

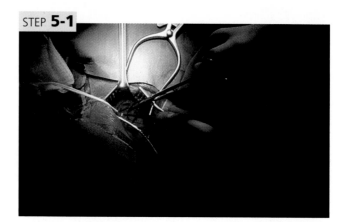

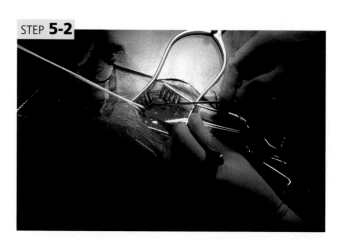

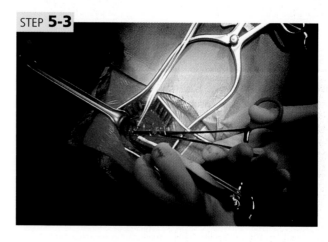

6. Free up the pleural membrane and retract the lung apex downward with a ribbon retractor. *If the pleura is opened, it must be repaired with a fine, absorbable suture.*

STEP **6-1**

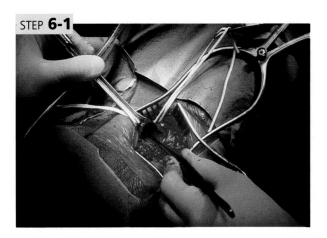

STEP **7-3**

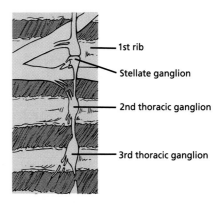

(From Calne, R., & Pollard, S. G. [1992]. *Operative surgery.* London: Gower.)

7. Identify the stellate nerve ganglion; excise the 2nd and 3rd ganglion.

STEP **7-1**

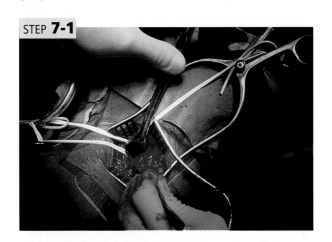

STEP **7-2**

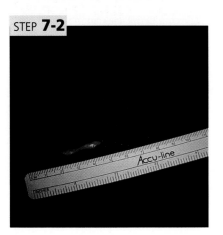

8. Close the skin and platysma together; apply a dressing. A drain is inserted as needed.

STEP **8-1**

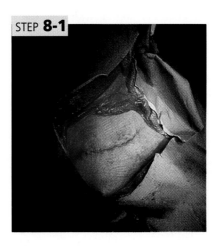

COMPLICATIONS

Supraclavicular Sympathectomy

Damage to the stellate ganglion causes Horner's syndrome.
Phrenic nerve damage causes paralysis of the hemi-diaphragm.
Damage to the thoracic duct can cause a fistula.
Damage to the pleura can cause a pneumothorax, requiring a chest tube.
Damage to any of the vessels can cause bleeding.
Damage to the first thoracic nerve can cause impaired functioning of hand muscles.

POSTOPERATIVE

Care and Discharge Planning for Supraclavicular Sympathectomy

A chest x-ray is taken to rule out a pneumothorax.
The need for a chest tube and closed water seal drain would increase the patient length of stay and require assessment of fluid intake and output.
Postoperative care is focused on assisting the recovery from general anesthesia: coughing and deep breathing to prevent respiratory complications.
Early ambulation is encouraged.
Regular diet and activity may be resumed as tolerated.
The patient may be discharged the day of surgery.

Calne & Pollard, 1992; Haimovici, 1996.

Procedural Steps
Transaxillary Thoracic Sympathectomy

A transaxillary approach to the thoracic ganglion requires the patient to be in a lateral or semilateral position with support for the arm on the operative side (Figure 14-4). Appropriate arm supports for both arms, an axillary roll, pillows under the head and between the legs, and any other padding of bony prominences is required. A safety belt or wide tape is used across the hips to stabilize the position.

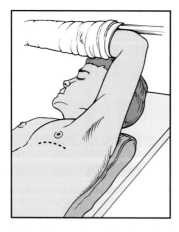

Fig. 14-4 Position of the patient, showing the line of incision in the third intercostal space. Left upper extremity is in marked abduction with the forearm supported by a crossbar in a sling.

1. Make a transverse incision in the midaxillary area, over the third rib.
2. Incise through the serratus anterior muscle. Identify the long thoracic and thoracodorsal nerves.
3. Insert a rib spreader to retract the third rib and divided muscle.
4. Incise the anterior parietal pleura and expose the lung.
5. Incise the posterior parietal pleura to expose the sympathetic chain. (Note the esophagus, superior vena cava, superior intercostal vein, trachea, and azygos vein.)
6. Excise the sympathetic chain.
7. Insert a chest tube, suture it in place with a heavy silk suture on a cutting needle.
8. Close the thoracotomy with pericostal sutures, close the muscle layers, and close the skin.
9. Connect the chest to to the closed suction drain (pleurovac); apply an occlusive dressing.

COMPLICATIONS

Transaxillary Thoracic Sympathectomy

Horner's syndrome
Bleeding from damage to any of the vessels
Pneumothorax or pleural effusion
Traction injury to the nerves of the arm

POSTOPERATIVE

Care and Discharge Planning for Transaxillary Thoracic Sympathectomy

A chest x-ray is taken to check for a pleural effusion or pneumothorax.
Intercostal pain is controlled with narcotics or other analgesics.
An arm sling may provide comfort by relieving movement on the incision line.
The chest drainage is observed and recorded.
The patient remains in the hospital until the drainage subsides and the chest tube is removed.
Coughing and deep breathing and early ambulation are encouraged.
Analgesics are timed to optimize activity.

Procedural Steps
Endoscopic Cervicothoracic Sympathectomy

Endoscopic sympathectomy has become an acceptable approach to sympathectomy (Box 14-2). For an endoscopic cervicothoracic sympathectomy the patient is placed in thoracotomy position requiring a beanbag positioner, pillows, padding, and tape across the hips for stabilization. The chest is prepped and draped.

> **Box 14-2** **Endoscopic Sympathectomy**
>
> Patients treated with bilateral endoscopic transthoracic sympathectomy showed no life-threatening complications; 2% of patients failed to have symptoms resolve, and 98% reported satisfaction at 31-month follow-up for hyperhydrosis of the axillary, palmar, and facial areas.

From Drott, 1995.

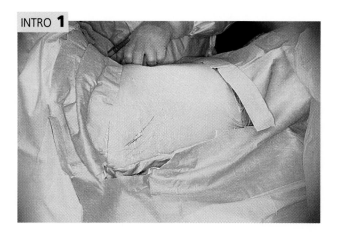

1. Three to four ports are inserted for the lighted scope (connected to the camera), a suction-irrigator-coagulation device, and the retractors and/or scissors or clip appliers. The location is confirmed by retracting the lung and identifying the ribs.

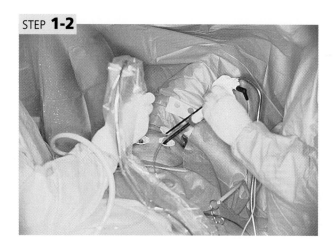

2. The graspers and cup forceps are used to dissect down to the sympathetic chain. The forcep stabilizes the sympathetic ganglion and a clip is applied.

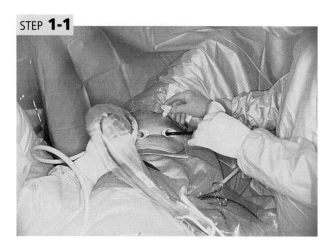

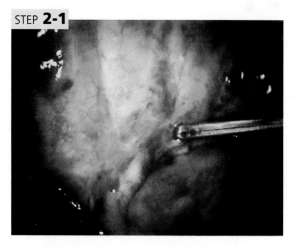

Cup forcep dissecting.

STEP **2-2**

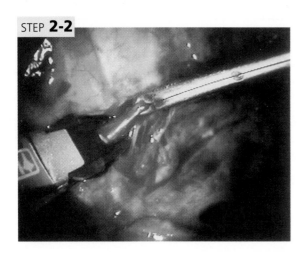

Clipping the nerve.

3. The nerve is cut. The nerve is dissected further, clipped, cut, and removed.

STEP **3-1**

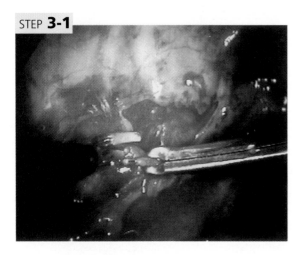

Cutting the nerve.

STEP **3-2**

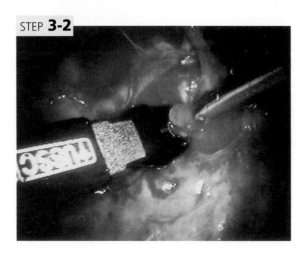

Nerve clipped at anterior end.

Procedural Steps
Lumbar Sympathectomy (Laparotomy)

Lumbar sympathectomy is performed with the patient supine, arms abducted less than 90 degrees (to prevent brachial plexus injury) on padded armrests, and a sandbag or folded towels placed either under the buttock or flank of the operative side. The goal is to elevate the flank by 30 degrees. A pillow under the knees will relax the psoas muscles. The lumbar sympathetic trunk consists of four or five ganglia. The first lumbar ganglion is usually anterior to the L1 vertebra, the second is anterior to the L2 vertebra, and the fourth ganglion is found behind the iliac vessels at the level of the sacral promontory. The left trunk is along the lateral border of the aorta and the right lies behind the inferior vena cava.

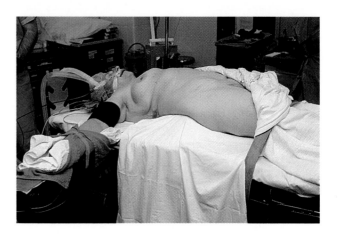

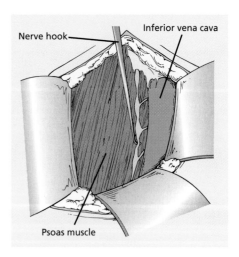

(From Calne, R., & Pollard, S. G. [1992]. *Operative surgery.* London: Gower.)

1. Make a transverse incision lateral to the umbilicus to the anterior axillary line.

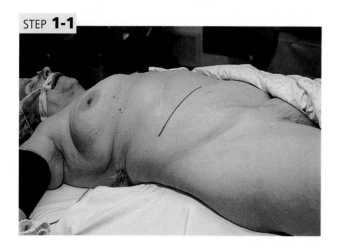

2. Divide the external oblique and lateral portion of the rectus sheath.

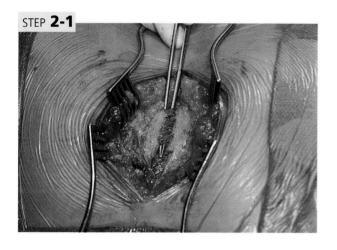

3. Open the lateral margin of the posterior rectus sheath and enter the extra peritoneal space. Move the peritoneum, using a blunt finger sweep, and use the electrocautery to divide the internal oblique and transversus abdominus muscles.

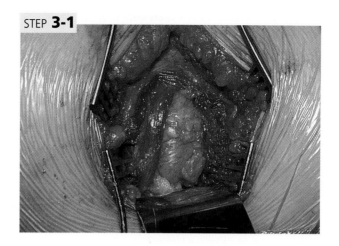

4. Identify the psoas muscle and the ureter (pinch and observe for peristalsis).

5. Identify the sympathetic trunk as a thick cord that "snaps" when plucked. Insert Deaver retractors (avoid trauma to vena cava on the right and the aorta on the left).

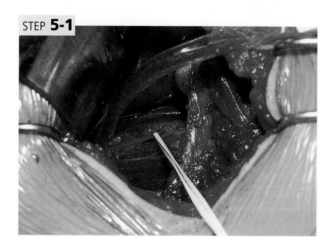

6. Mobilize and excise the sympathetic chain.

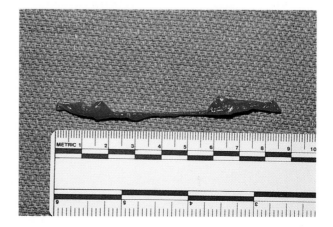

7. Close the muscles in two layers and close the skin.

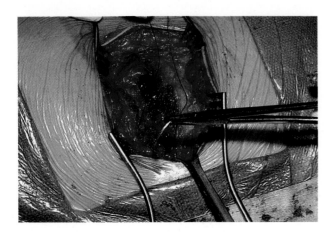

COMPLICATIONS

Cervicothoracic Sympathectomy (Endoscopic) and Lumbar Sympathectomy (Laparotomy)

If the peritoneum is entered it should be closed immediately
Damage to the vena cava
Damage to ureter or genitofemoral nerve
Paralytic ileus usually resolves quickly and is managed with a nasogastric tube
Postsympathectomy neuralgia (most common of complications)

Rutherford & Shannon, 1995; Calne & Pollard, 1993; Haimovici, 1996.

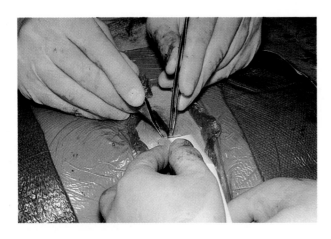

Apply a dressing.

POSTOPERATIVE

Care and Discharge Planning for Cervicothoracic Sympathectomy (Endoscopic) and Lumbar Sympathectomy (Laparotomy)

Routine care after any general anesthetic: Coughing, deep breathing, ambulation, pain management, and adequate intake and output.

The patient should be instructed about the possibility of a return of pain, known as postsympathectomy neuralgia. It is described as an ache in the anterior and lateral aspects of the thigh that increases at night and is not related to any activity. The cause is not understood but it can be managed by mild analgesics and resolves in 2 to 4 months. Patients who are forewarned of this possibility manage better (Rutherford & Shannon, 1995).

A warm, dry lower extremity usually is evident within hours as well as relief of ulcer or rest pain.

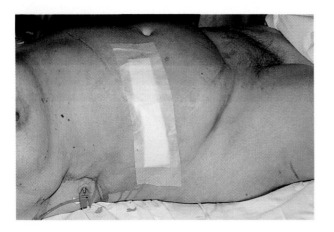

Procedural Steps
Endoscopic Lumbar Sympathectomy

The patient is placed in a semilateral position with Trendelenburg. Three ports are used for one side and five ports for a bilateral procedure (Figure 14-5). The operative technique for the left side is as follows (Figure 14-6).

1. Insert an umbilical port, a port in the lower abdominal quadrant lateral to the rectus abdominus muscle, and a port in the upper quadrant 2 cm below the costal margin.

2. Retract the small bowel upward with the fan retractors.

3. Incise the peritoneum to the left of the aorta above the inferior mesenteric artery.

4. Identify the sympathetic ganglion and excise.

The operative technique for the right side is as follows (Figure 14-7)

1. Insert the ports and fan retractor.

2. Incise the peritoneum superior and lateral to the bifurcation of the inferior vena cava.

3. Retract the vena cava, identify the sympathetic chain, and excise it.

4. Close the muscle at the umbilical port and approximate the skin of all port sites with subcuticular absorbable sutures and adhesive strips. (An umbilical port and two lateral ports are used for a unilateral procedure and five ports for bilateral procedure).

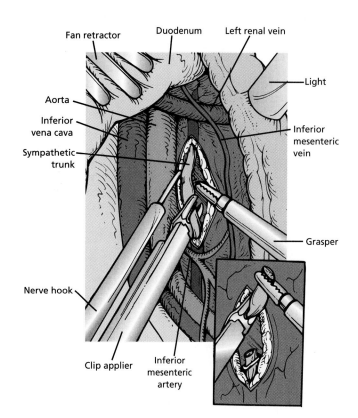

Fig. 14-6 Left side sympathectomy.

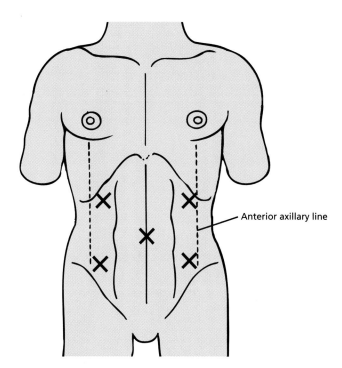

Fig. 14-5 Trocar placement. All trocars should be 10 mm to allow instruments to be placed from different angles depending on the desired exposure.

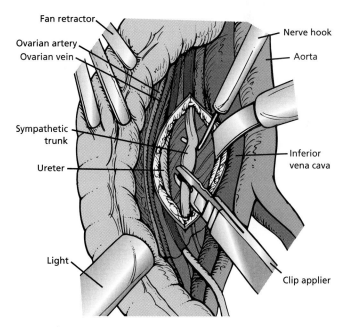

Fig. 14-7 Right side sympathectomy.

COMPLICATIONS

Endoscopic Lumbar Sympathectomy

Injury to bowel from trocar placement
Bleeding from vessel injury
Emboli to lower extremities from retraction of the aorta

POSTOPERATIVE

Care and Discharge Planning for Endoscopic Lumbar Sympathectomy

Routine postoperative care is provided.
Mild analgesics are recommended.
Patients usually resume all activities and regular diet.
Patients are discharged on POD 1.

Sardi & Hollier, 1996.

References

Atkinson, L. J., & Fortunato, N. (1996). Neurosurgery. In L. J. Atkinson, & N. Fortunato (Eds.), *Berry & Kohn's operating room technique* (8th ed., pp. 763-782). St. Louis: Mosby.

Barnes, R. W. (1994). Sympathectomy: Quo vadis? *Cardiovascular Surgery, 2*(1); 9-15.

Calne, R, & Pollard, S. G. (1992). Lumbar sympathectomy. In R. Calne, & S.G. Pollard (Eds.), *Slide atlas of operative surgery: Vascular surgery* (pp. 9.14-9.16). London: Gower.

Drott, C., Rothberg, G., & Claes, G. (1995). Endoscopic transthoracic sympathectomy: An efficient and safe method for the treatment of hyperhidrosis. *Journal of the American Academy of Dermatology, 33*(1): 78-81.

Duprez, D. A. (1993). Secondary vasospastic disorders. In D. L. Clement, & J. T. Sheperd (Eds.) *Vascular diseases in the limbs: Mechanisms and principles of treatment* (pp. 169-186). St. Louis: Mosby.

Dzsinich, C., & Gloviczki, P. (1993). Principles of vascular surgery. In D.L. Clement, & J.T. Sheperd (Eds.) *Vascular diseases in the limbs: Mechanisms and principles of treatment* (pp. 259-278). St. Louis: Mosby.

Fahey, V. A., & McCarthy, W. J. (1994). Arterial reconstruction of the lower extremity. In V. A. Fahey (Ed.), *Vascular nursing* (2nd ed., pp. 291-324). Philadelphia: W.B. Saunders.

Haimovici, H. (1996). Lumbar sympathectomy: Conventional technique. In H. Haimovici (Ed.), *Haimovici's vascular surgery: Principles and techniques* (pp. 1127-1133). Cambridge, MA: Blackwell Science.

Harris, J. P., Satchell, P. M., & May, J. (1995). Upper extremity sympathectomy. In R. B. Rutherford (Ed.), *Vascular surgery* (pp. 1008-1016). Philadelphia: W. B. Saunders.

McFadden, P. M., & Hollier, L. H. (1996). Thoracoscopic sympathectomy. In H. Haimovici (Ed.), *Haimovici's vascular surgery: Principles and techniques* (pp. 1116-1126). Cambridge, MA: Blackwell Science.

McGuire, L. (1998). Pain. In P. G. Beare, & J. L. Myers (Eds.)., *Adult health nursing* (3rd ed., pp. 62-89). St. Louis: Mosby.

Rutherford, R. B., & Shannon, F. L. (1995). Lumbar sympathectomy: Indications and technique. In R. B. Rutherford (Ed.), *Vascular surgery* (pp. 874-883). Philadelphia: W. B. Saunders.

Sardi, A., & Hollier, L. H. (1996). Laparoscopic lumbar sympathectomy. In H. Haimovici (Ed.), *Haimovici's vascular surgery: Principles and techniques* (pp. 1134-1136). Cambridge, MA: Blackwell Science.

Sheperd, J. T. (1993). Historical aspects. In D. L. Clement, & J. T. Sheperd (Eds.), *Vascular diseases in the limbs: Mechanisms and principles of treatment* (pp. 1-10). St. Louis: Mosby.

15

Surgery on the Abdominal Aorta

ABDOMINAL AORTIC ANEURYSM (AAA): TRANSPERITONEAL AND RETROPERITONEAL APPROACHES

Description

Abdominal aortic resection is surgical obliteration of the aneurysm, which may or may not include the iliac arteries, with insertion of a synthetic prosthesis to reestablish functional continuity. The majority of abdominal aortic aneurysms begin below the renal arteries and many extend to involve the bifurcation and common iliac arteries (Atkinson, 1992).

Indications and pathophysiology

Symptoms. Abdominal aortic aneurysms (AAA) are usually *asymptomatic* and found on routine physical examination. They occur four times more frequently in men than women. Severe back pain, along with symptoms of hypotension, shock, and distal vascular insufficiency (diminished pulses, cool, mottled skin), usually indicates rupture and represents a true emergency. However, hypotension is often absent when a leaking or ruptured aneurysm has been contained in the retroperitoneum. Pain the is most consistent finding in impending rupture and although back pain is most common, pain in the abdomen or flank or pain radiating to the chest, groin, or legs may be described by the patient. Less common presentations occur when the aorta ruptures into the duodenum (GI bleeding) or inferior vena cava (congestive heart failure and lower extremity edema). Symptoms may mimic more common disorders, e. g., myocardial infarction, acute abdomen, renal colic, or disc disease (Bessen, 1993). The prime surgical consideration when a rupture occurs is the control of hemorrhage by occluding the aorta proximal to the point of rupture.

Pathophysiology. Aneurysms occur most often in the abdominal aorta, thoracic aorta, and the popliteal arteries (Atkinson, 1992). Two percent of the population over age 50 have an abdominal aneurysm (Bessen, 1993). For years the etiology of aortic aneurysms was attributed to atherosclerosis. Currently, atherosclerosis in patients with aortic aneurysm is described as "coincidental" (Mitchell, Rutherford, & Krupski, 1995). However, many differences can be found in aneurysmal versus occlusive diseases in terms of epidemiology, biochemistry, and genetics (Norman, Wysocki, & Lamawansa, 1995). In a review of the literature, Anderson (1994) describes some of the differences. Aneurysmal disease exhibits a loss of tensile strength in the vessel wall primarily of the tunica media.

Atherosclerosis involves the intima. Atherosclerosis generally affects men and women in the fifth decade of life but aneurysms are found more often in the sixth decade with a preponderance of men being affected. Aneurysmal disease is caused by a disruption of the media, which structurally weakens the aortic wall. There is mounting evidence that altered genetic expression, chronic inflammatory cells in the vessel wall, and an immunologic response may be contributing factors in causing aneurysms (Mitchell, Rutherford, & Krupski, 1995). There is recognition of a possible familial tendency. Patients with family members with known AAAs, especially siblings, may benefit by screening so that they may followed if an AAA is detected (Anderson, 1994). Smoking is considered a risk factor associated with aneurysmal disease. Smoking may contribute to the accelerated expansion rate of small aortic aneurysms (MacSweeney, et al 1994).

Diagnosis. Diagnosis is based on physical examination that reveals a pulsatile abdominal mass. This finding prompts further work-up. Ultrasonography is used to confirm the presence of an aortic aneurysm and to follow it for enlargement. CT scan may be used as a screening tool and to detect factors that may contribute to the planning of AAA surgery (Box 15-1) (Silva & Hobson, 1996). Contrast enhanced CT scan is considered the best preoperative study and contributes to surgical safety (Mitchell, Rutherford, & Krupski, 1995). MRI and MRA (magnetic resonance angiography) may provide superior information about

---

Box 15-1 **Indications for Transperitoneal versus Retroperitoneal Approach**

TRANSPERITONEAL
Permits full abdominal exploration
Fastest and easiest approach
Right renal artery, celiac, or mesenteric bypass
Access to distal leg arteries

RETROPERITONEAL
Easier access in obese patients
To avoid entering hostile abdomen or to avoid an ostomy
For suprarenal aortic control, endarterectomy of visceral vessels
For patients with high cardiac/pulmonary risk, may permit patient to cough and deep breath more readily
To bypass left renal artery

From Silva & Hobson, 1996; Brewster, 1995.

renal and mesenteric involvement but this technology is not universally available or cost effective (Silva & Hobson, 1996). In cases of suspected or impending rupture, diagnosis is based on history and physical examination and other diagnostic tests are deferred.

Indications for surgery. Patients with an aneurysm that enlarges to 6 cm and high-risk patients with an aorta of less than 5 cm should be observed (Mitchell, Rutherford, & Krupski, 1995). Patients with an aneurysm that measures 6 cm or more have a greater risk of death from rupture than from elective surgery (Silva & Hobson, 1996). The natural progression of abdominal aneurysms is enlargement to eventual rupture (O'Hara, 1996). Rupture is the greatest risk that indicates a need for surgery although thrombosis and distal embolization may also be an indication (Silva & Hobson, 1996). When rupture is diagnosed or suspected, the patient is taken directly and emergently to the operating room.

Risks of rupture. Factors that place a patient at greater risk of rupture include an aneurysm diameter of 6 cm or more, chronic obstructive pulmonary disease (COPD), pain, an aneurysm that is a source of distal emboli, one that is associated with sepsis, or one that is enlarging (Hollier & Rutherford, 1989). Hypertension and COPD as predictors of rupture are disputed. The aneurysm size is the most consistent finding that relates to rupture. However, small aneurysms can rupture and the expansion rate of aneurysms is often unpredictable (Mitchell, Rutherford, & Krupski, 1995). Ouriel et al (1992) presented another means of determining risk of rupture based on the size of the aorta and the size of the spine. They derived a ratio or index for the normal aortic size based on age and sex. They compared aneurysm diameters with the diameter of the third lumbar vertebral body. In a retrospective review, they found that no aneurysms ruptured below an index of 1. For patients who rup-

ture an aneurysm outside the hospital setting, 60% die before reaching the hospital and only 50% of those who do reach the hospital survive. Those who become severely hypotensive before surgery have a poor survival rate (Bessen, 1993).

Aortic dissection. Although the etiology of aortic dissection differs from that of aneurysmal disease, the surgery and care are similar. Dissection is the tearing of the intimal layer, permitting bleeding between the layers. Aortic dissection may be caused by blunt trauma deceleration accidents, e.g., a motor vehicle accident with or without the use of seatbelts. It is seen in pregnant women, patients with Marfan's syndrome, and cocaine users. More often the patients are 50 to 70 years old with hypertension. It occurs in men two to three times more frequently than in women. Dissection usually involves the thoracoabdominal aorta to the left subclavian artery but this may also occur in the abdominal aorta. Laboratory tests, x-rays, and ECG will not rule out an aortic dissection. CT scan is the quickest way to diagnose dissection. But transesophageal echocardiography and MRI are also sensitive to detecting dissection (Bessen, 1993). Some surgeons may require aortography (Figure 15-1). These patients typically present after trauma with bleeding, hematoma, and pulse deficits. They may describe a sense of "impending doom." Their blood pressure must be controlled in the 90 to 110 range and their pain controlled with narcotics. An abrupt onset of severe pain in the upper back or anterior chest and occasionally in the abdomen may be described. Patients may be symptomatic for hours or days before eventually rupturing. Of those who are untreated, 48% will die within 48 hours. Reports of increasing pain should be heeded as a probable sign of progression of the dissection. Rupture of the dissecting aorta may result in exsanguination but the most common cause of death is cardiac tamponade when the ascending aorta bleeds into the pericardium (Bessen, 1993).

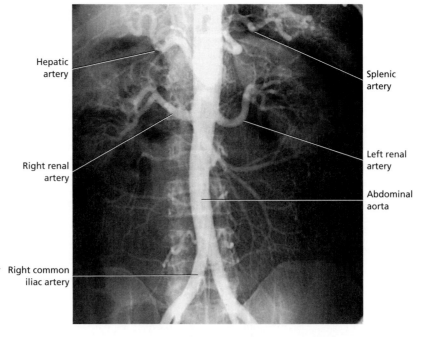

Fig. 15-1 Abdominal aortogram of normal aorta and iliac arteries. *(From Ballinger, P. W. [1995]. Merrill's atlas of radiographic positions and radiologic procedures [8th ed.]. St. Louis: Mosby.)*

Preoperative planning
Preoperative testing
Routine preoperative labs (SMA-7, platelet count, PT, PTT, BUN, type and cross-match for blood)

ECG

Chest x-ray

Creatinine levels for renal disease, which may be elevated after an angiogram (Parthum, 1996)

CT scan

Cardiac work-up:

Noninvasive evaluation of cardiac status through dipyridamole-thallium stress testing is indicated in patients with two or more of the following: advanced age, diabetes mellitus, history of MI, congestive heart failure (CHF), angina, or abnormal ECG; these patients may be candidates for cardiac catheterization.

Percutaneous transluminal coronary angioplasty (PTCA) or coronary artery bypass grafting (CABG) may be indicated before elective repair of an AAA

Segmental Doppler and ABIs should be done in legs in order to identify patients who develop complications from embolization from surgery (Silva & Hobson, 1996)

Physiologic age overrides physical age (Mitchell, Rutherford, & Krupski, 1995)

Bowel prep

Nasogastric tube

Anesthetic considerations
Ensure adequate cardiac work-up (cardiac complications constitute >50% of perioperative morbidity)

Adequate hydration, especially if patient has impaired renal function and underwent angiogram with injected contrast

IVs, large bore to accommodate massive fluid/blood replacement intraoperatively, arterial line for constant BP, pulse, and drawing arterial blood gases

Instruct patient to take antihypertensive medications as usual (except diuretics)

Assess for extent of diabetes mellitus

Anxiety: assess and medicate as needed because stress and anxiety can alter the oxygen demands of the heart and initiate ischemia

Pulmonary function tests may be ordered for patients with COPD

Room air arterial blood gas may help guide anesthetic management

Epidural catheter for postoperative analgesia

Intraoperative monitoring:

Basic ASA monitoring (see Chapter 7), ECG with ST-T segment analysis

Central venous pressure

Pulmonary artery catheter (more accurate measurement of left ventricular [LV] filling pressures, cardiac output, and systemic vascular resistance [SVR])

Transesophageal echocardiography (TEE).

Hypothermia.
Prevention of hypothermia is critical and requires a team effort. Shivering can increase the oxygen demands of the myocardium, cause arrhythmias, coagulopathy and prolong neuromuscular blockade. When the body core temperature falls below 35° C, the patient is at risk for decreased cardiac output, metabolic acidosis, altered drug metabolism, electrolyte imbalance, and pulmonary edema (Piatkowski, 1994). Forced air heating blankets, warm ambient temperature of the OR, keeping the patient covered, and warming fluids and inspired gases will assist in preventing heat loss. Forced air heating blankets are manufactured in a variety of forms and sizes. Upper body and lower body blankets may be used. If a lower body warmer is used, it should be off when the aorta is clamped to decrease the metabolic demands of the lower extremity tissues and possible injury when perfusion is minimal. Some blanket manufacturers print this warning on the blanket. Blood should be immediately available, from banked blood and blood salvage. A rapid infusion system is helpful in maintaining adequate fluid volume.

Equipment, instrumentation, medications, and solutions
Also refer to Chapter 8, Equipment, Supplies, and Instrumentation, and Chapter 4, Medications.

Basic OR furniture

Water coil warming blanket and radiant forced air warmer unit

Cell saver machine

Rapid fluid infuser

I-Med

ACT machine

TEE and probe

Major basic set

Basic vascular pan

Abdominal self-retaining retractor

Vascular custom pack

Assorted vascular prosthetic grafts (straight and bifurcated, sizes from 14 mm to 20 mm)

Vascular suture

Pledget material

Dual lumen suction tubing for blood salvage

Occlusion catheter or large Foley/large balloon

Kittner dissectors

Hemoclips in 3 sizes

Umbilical tapes

Fogarty inserts of varying sizes

Magnetic pad to hold instruments on field (optional, helpful for semilateral position)

Positioning devices
Supine for transperitoneal approach to AAA and aortoiliac occlusive disease:

Gel mattress

Padded arm rests

Safety belt

Semi-recumbent or thoracotomy position for retroperitoneal approach:

Bean bag positioner, gel pad, suction

Axillary roll

Pillows, gel pads

3 inch wide adhesive tape

Mayo stand, ether screen, or pillows to support left arm

Intraoperative medications and solutions
Saline

Heparinized saline

Heparin (1 mg/kg) to systemically anticoagulate patient (may be injected by surgeon)

Heparin may or may not be given in case of ruptured AAA

Cold IV solution (surgeon's choice) to perfuse kidneys when aorta is clamped suprarenal

Mannitol may be given by the anesthesiologist before aortic clamping (this raises serum osmotic pressure, intravascular volume, and glomerular filtration rate, which may serve to keep the renal tubules open) (Hatswell, 1994, Part 1).

Procedural Steps
Elective Repair of Infrarenal Abdominal Aortic Aneurysm (Transperitoneal, Midline Incision)
(Figure 15-2)

The patient is placed in the supine position. A Foley catheter is inserted for measurement of intake and output and assessment of renal function. The pedal pulses should be marked before the beginning of the procedure so they may be located immediately if the surgeon requests a check of the pulses. This assessment of pulses can be done manually or with an ultrasonic instrument

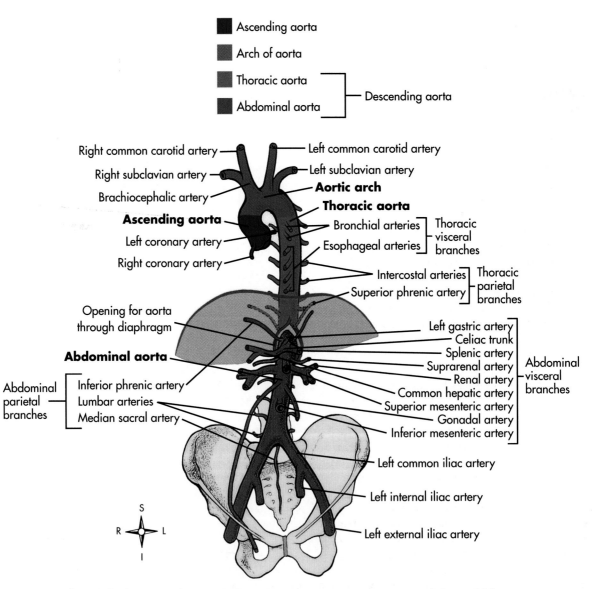

Fig. 15-2 The aorta. The aorta is the main system artery, serving as a trunk from which other arteries branch. Blood is conducted from the heart first through the ascending aorta, then through the thoracic and abdominal segments of the descending aorta. *(From Thibodeau G. A., & Patton, K. P. [1996]. Anatomy and physiology [3rd ed.]. St. Louis: Mosby.)*

RNFA CONSIDERATIONS

Knowledge of anatomy and specific surgical intervention.

Assist in patient preparation: teaching, positioning, placement of Foley catheter, placement of electrocautery ground pad, skin prep, draping.

Communicate with anesthesia and nursing team members when crucial steps are to occur: clamping of aorta, release of clamps, uncontrolled bleeding, irrigation, need for additional supplies or hemostatic agents.

Provide teaching and emotional support to patient and family during all phases of care.

STEP 1-2

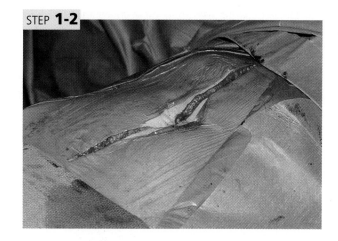

(Doppler). The skin is prepped from the nipple line to knees for a midline abdominal incision. Alternatively, patients at high risk for distal embolization may have both legs prepped circumferentially for the possibility of lower extremity arterial exploration and bypass. Draping is performed to permit access to the groin region for possible exploration of femoral arteries.

1. The abdomen is opened through a midline incision from the xiphoid process to the symphysis pubis. Hemostasis is accomplished, and exploration of the abdominal and pelvic cavities is performed to assess the condition of the organs, detect any other pathology, and confirm the extent of the aneurysm.

STEP 1-1

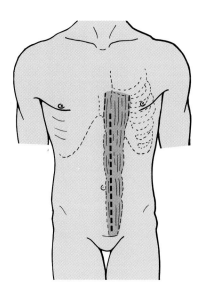

2. The transverse colon is eviscerated, packed in moist towels, and placed on abdomen. Ligament of Treitz is incised, permitting lateral mobilization of the duodenum.

STEP 2-1

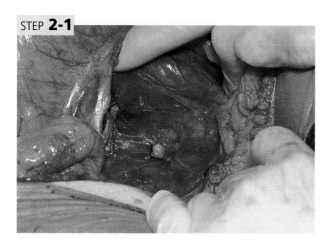

Incise the small bowel peritoneum where it attaches to the posterior abdominal wall. An abdominal self-retaining retractor is inserted into the wound. If necessary for exposure, a portion of the small bowel can be placed outside the abdomen, covered with moist laparotomy packs, and enclosed in a sterile plastic bag (retains heat and moisture). Free the duodenum from the aneurysm as needed.

3. The parietal peritoneum is incised over the aorta and extended superiorly to expose the aneurysm and also inferiorly over the bifurcation and beyond the iliac arteries. Scissors, DeBakey forceps, and hemostats are used.

STEP **3-1**

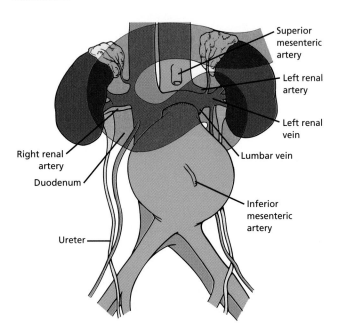

Relevant anatomy of infrarenal abdominal aortic aneurysm. (From Calne, R. Y., & Pollard, S. G. [1992]. *Operative surgery.* London: Gower.)

4. Careful blunt and sharp dissection is continued to expose the aorta above the aneurysm to permit placement of an aortic clamp.

STEP **4-1**

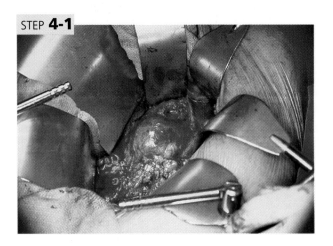

The renal artery and ureters are identified and avoided. The iliac vessels and bifurcation are inspected for evidence of aneurysms, thrombosis, and calcification. The patient is given systemic heparin by the anesthesiologist or the surgeon and the drug is allowed to circulate for 3 minutes before clamping. Clamps are applied to a *normal* segment of the distal aorta or iliac arteries (this minimizes the risk of sending atheromatous debris to the lower extremities).

STEP **4-2**

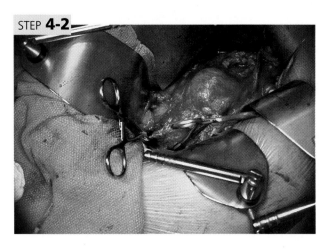

5. An aortic clamp such as a DeBakey, Fogarty, or Satinsky is applied to the aorta just above the aneurysm and closed. Opening of the aneurysm is undertaken with a scalpel or electrosurgical blade and heavy scissors.

STEP **5-1**

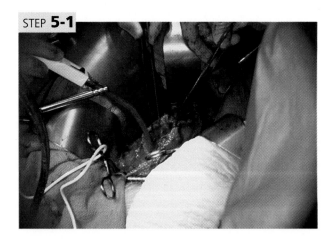

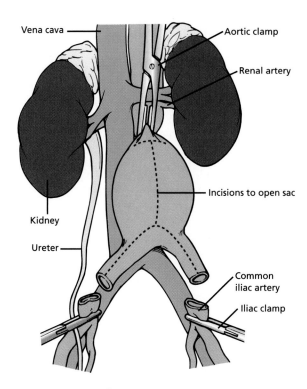

Aneurysm sac is opened. (From Meeker, J. M., & Rothrock, M. H. [1995]. *Alexander's care of the patient in surgery* [10th ed.]. St. Louis: Mosby.)

7. Bleeding is controlled, especially from the lumbar vessels that enter posteriorly. The scrub nurse has 2-0 or 3-0 Prolene sutures on long needle holders ready for this task. The medial sacral and inferior mesenteric arteries may be suture ligated at this time if not done so earlier.

STEP **7-1**

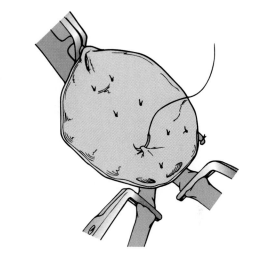

Oversew lumbar artery orifices. (From Calne, R. Y., & Pollard, S. G. [1992]. *Operative surgery.* London: Gower.)

6. The aneurysm is completely opened, and all atheromatous and thrombotic material is removed.

STEP **6-1**

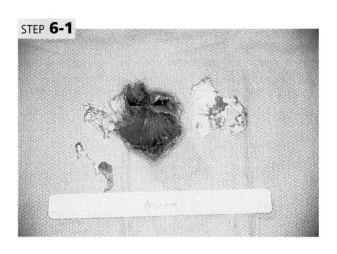

STEP **7-2**

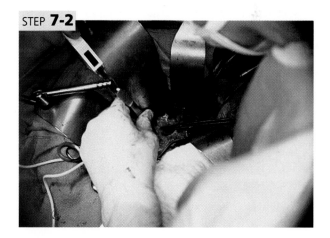

The aneurysm walls may be excised but usually are left in place for eventual coverage of the prosthesis. In either case the posterior aspect of the aorta is left intact.

8. A prosthetic graft of appropriate size is prepared for insertion. Graft size may be determined by visual estimate or by direct measurement. If the aneurysm does not involve the aortic bifurcation, a straight tubular graft is used; otherwise a bifurcated or Y-shaped graft is necessary. Preclotting of a knitted graft may be accomplished by immersing the graft in a small quantity of the patient's own blood before systemic heparinization (see Chapter 9).

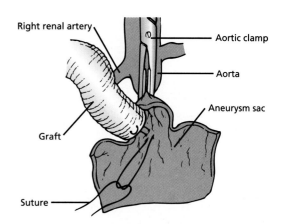

Prosthetic graft is sewn to back wall of aorta, creating a cuff. (From Meeker, J. M., & Rothrock, M. H. [1995]. *Alexander's care of the patient in surgery* [10th ed.]. St. Louis: Mosby.)

STEP 8-1

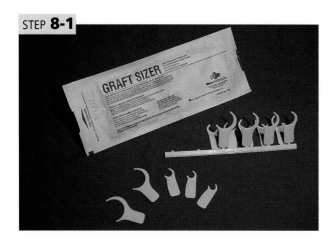

Graft sizer.

The graft is parachuted down into position.

STEP 9-2

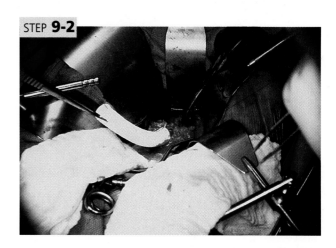

9. The aortic cuff is prepared for anastomosis by irrigating it with heparinized saline solution and by removing all fibrotic plaques. Several vascular stitches (double armed) are placed through the aortic cuff and the graft (this creates the posterior anastomosis).

STEP 9-1

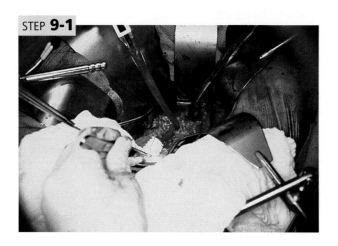

STEP 9-3

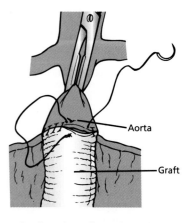

Completion of proximal aortic graft anastomosis. (From Meeker, J. M., & Rothrock, M. H. [1995]. *Alexander's care of the patient in surgery* [10th ed.]. St. Louis: Mosby.)

10. Communicate to the anesthesiologist that the proximal clamp is to be released. A giant Fogarty clamp is placed on the proximal portion of the *graft* and the initial aortic clamp is released to test the anastomosis. Additional interrupted sutures may be needed if the anastomosis leaks on completion. Pledgeted suture may also be used to contain leaks. The distal aorta is opened and inspected for back bleeding. Heparinized saline solution may be injected to prevent clotting. It is reclamped and the distal end of the graft sewn in place.

STEP **10-3**

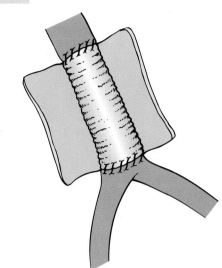

Both anastomoses completed. (From Calne, R. Y., & Pollard, S. G., [1992]. *Operative surgery.* London: Gower.)

STEP **10-1**

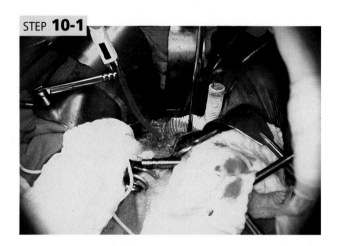

STEP **10-2**

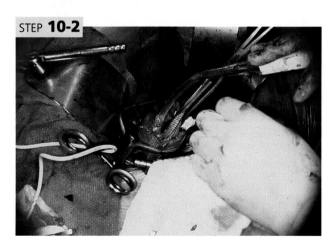

Distal end of graft sewn in place.

STEP **10-4**

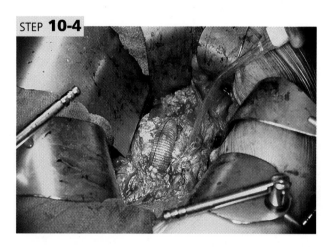

Graft completed.

CONSIDERATIONS A bifurcated graft may be used as needed. If a bifurcated graft is used, the iliac vessels are opened, inspected for back bleeding, and injected with heparinized saline solution to prevent clotting.

11. Each limb of the graft is anastomosed to the iliac artery using a smaller vascular suture and similar technique. After the first side of the anastomosis has been completed, communicate with the anesthesiologist that a distal graft limb is to be released. Blood is permitted to circulate, and the remaining limb of the graft is clamped to prevent leaking during the last part of the anastomosis.

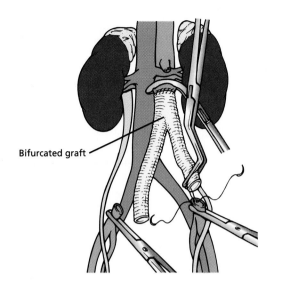

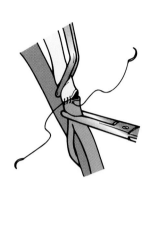

Iliac artery anastomosis. (From Meeker, J. M., & Rothrock, M. H. [1995]. *Alexander's care of the patient in surgery* [10th ed.]. St. Louis: Mosby.)

12. The aneurysm is closed over the graft.

STEP **12-1**

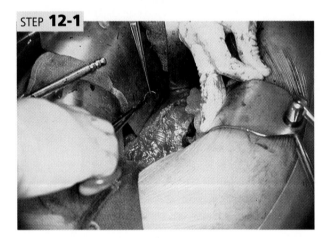

Assess perfusion to bowel, check for femoral pulses, assess perfusion to feet by inspection and palpation of pulses (by circulating nurse). Use a Doppler if they are not palpable.

13. The abdominal wound is closed and dressings applied.

Procedural Steps
Elective Repair of Infrarenal Abdominal Aortic Aneurysm (Retroperitoneal, Oblique Incision)

1. An oblique incision is made from the left margin of the rectus muscle, inferior to umbilicus, to the eleventh intercostal space (tenth space for suprarenal control of aorta). Divide abdominal muscles, left kidney, ureter and peritoneum are bluntly mobilized anteromedially. The lymphatics over the aorta are divided. This gives exposure of the aorta from the left renal artery to the bifurcation.

STEP **1-1**

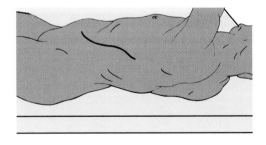

2. Tunneling is done bluntly superficial to iliac arteries and deep to the crossing ureters.

Femoral arteries are clamped first, then the aortic is clamped just distal to the renal arteries.

3. End-to-end graft placement is selected when aortic dilatation is present. End-to-side is selected to preserve the inferior mesenteric artery (IMA), accessory renal arteries, or to preserve antegrade flow to the hypogastrics (choice is debated). Note that the graft is cut at a 45-degree angle to prevent a kink that could impede blood flow.

STEP **3-1**

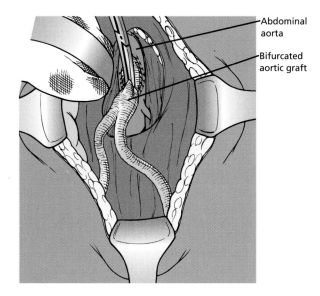

Example of an end-to-side anastomosis of a bifurcated graft to the abdominal aorta. The graft has been cut at a 45-degree angle to prevent kinking.

Complications

Risks from AAA surgery include massive hemorrhage, injury to the ureters, renal failure, spinal cord ischemia, and death. Patients with aneurysms often have concomitant coronary artery disease. Myocardial infarction is the leading cause of death after AAA repair. Therefore it is imperative that a patient with cardiac symptoms or ECG abnormalities have a thorough preoperative cardiac assessment (Golden, Whittemore, & Mannick, 1990). Mortality is 2% for elective repair of AAA in an otherwise healthy patient. Death as a result of rupture is 70% for 7 cm aneurysms, 40% for 6 cm aneurysms, and 20% for 5 cm aneurysms. Death from surgical repair of a ruptured aneurysm is still greater than 50% (DeWeese, 1989). This statistic has not altered significantly in 40 years despite improved surgical and anesthetic techniques. However, the survival rate for elective AAA patients has improved dramatically as a result of improved detection, intraoperative management, graft materials, and postoperative care (Mitchell, Rutherford, & Krupski, 1995). In instances where the bowel is inadvertently entered before vascular graft insertion, the bowel is repaired and the repair of the AAA is postponed to a later date to prevent graft contamination (Silva & Hobson, 1996).

Declamping shock. The nurse must be alert to the fact that at the time the aortic clamp is released to permit distal flow, "declamping shock" or severe hypotension may occur. This may be due to inadequate volume replacement, the sudden reestablishment of flow to vasodilated distal vessels, increased potassium, or the release of acidic metabolites. These metabolites, decreased afterload from distal vasodilation, and hypotension may contribute to cardiac complications (Mitchell, Rutherford, & Krupski, 1995). Hemorrhage and the release of acidic metabolites have been proposed as a cause of renal failure from acute tubular necrosis (Hollier & Rutherford, 1989). Contrast angiography within 24 hours of surgery may also contribute to renal toxicity. Delaying surgery for a day or two after angiography is recommended (Mitchell, Rutherford, & Krupski, 1995). In aortic surgery that requires clamping above the renal arteries, there is increased risk of renal failure. If the clamp is on for more than 60 minutes, renal failure occurs in about 80% of patients. Coselli (1995) advocates cold fluid perfusion of the kidney despite a lack of conclusive research.

Injury to the ureters occurs more often in the emergency aortic repair but may occur in the presence of inflammation and fibrosis. Immediate repair is required with insertion of ureteral stents, copious wound irrigation, and placement of an encircling omental flap for protection (Mitchell, Rutherford, & Krupski, 1995).

Procedural Steps
Ruptured AAA

Speed is critical to the patient's survival. Rapid transport has been cited as a major factor in decreasing patient mortality. When a ruptured AAA is diagnosed, the patient will bypass x-ray, CT scan, and blood work and go emergently to the operating room (Parthum, 1996). The patient may be brought to the OR with little or no warning to the operating room staff. The nursing team must be able to work with utmost speed under pressure, prioritize their activities, delegate appropriately, and make sound judgments. Depending on the time of day, the availability of operating rooms, staff,

COMPLICATIONS ▆▆▆▆▆

AAA Surgery

INTRAOPERATIVE

Injury to vena cava
Injury to left renal vein
Hemorrhage (from anastomoses or from torn lumbar vessel)
Injury to ureter
Occlusion of renal arteries
Embolization to lower extremities
Trash foot
Myocardial infarction
Impotence (neurogenic or vasculogenic)
DIC
Pancreatitis (uncommon, caused by retraction injury)
Ischemic bowel
Renal failure
Paraplegia (rare, not predictable or preventable)
Death

LATE COMPLICATIONS

Infection (1% of patients)
Anastomotic aneurysms
Aortoenteric fistula

RUPTURED AAA PATIENTS ARE AT GREATER RISK OF:

Hemorrhage
Damage to ureter
DIC
Transfusion reaction (because of greater number of
   transfusions)
Acute renal failure from episodes of hypotension
Paraplegia
Death

POSTOPERATIVE

Hemorrhage
Myocardial infarction
Ileus
Renal failure
Paraplegia
Graft infection
Bowel ischemia
Pneumonia
Adult respiratory distress syndrome (ARDS)

Silva & Hobson, 1996.

equipment, and supplies will vary. An experienced team can make a difference in patient outcomes. Extra staff may be helpful to perform counts, provide supplies, or run for equipment and supplies. Alerting ancillary staff to the emergent nature of the surgery will assist in obtaining maximum cooperation and rapid responses to requests. The patient will need large bore IV access and a Foley catheter. Transfer the patient to the OR bed, position them safely, and ensure they have a Foley catheter to drainage. A skin prep may or may not be performed. If the patient's condition warrants, either an immediate incision

will be made or the patient may need fluids and further resuscitation before the incision. In a stable patient, additional monitoring lines could be placed at this time. The patient may be prepped and draped *before induction* so that an immediate incision may be made if needed. Induction of general anesthesia may cause a relaxation of the abdominal wall that could cause severe hypotension from release of tamponade or the incision could have a similar effect. Systemic heparin may or may not be given. The urgency of the surgery generally precludes the insertion of an epidural catheter for postoperative pain management.

Surgical priorities include the ability to make an incision (knife blade), clear the operative site of blood (two suction setups, ideally with cell saver as one; counted laparotomy sponges), and control of the hemorrhage (manually, with aortic clamp, or with intraluminal occlusion device). Intraluminal devices may be a commercially available device, e.g., occlusion catheter (see Figure 8-32) or a Foley catheter with a 30 or 75 cc balloon. Either device can be placed into the aortic lumen, inflated, and the inflation maintained by a stopcock or clamp. The occlusion device can sometimes be threaded through the selected vascular graft before placing the balloon into the aorta.

1. A midline incision is made from the xiphoid to the symphysis pubis. If the rupture is intraperitoneal, the bleeding will be immediate. Suctioning and packs are used to enable control of the aorta. For a retroperitoneal rupture the blood will be confined behind the peritoneum, elevating the small bowel and sigmoid colon. The aorta is clamped below the renal arteries, compressed with downward pressure with a sponge on a stick (the aorta is compressed against the spine), or an intraluminal occlusion device is inserted. The common iliac arteries are clamped (without dissecting behind them or encircling them).

2. The surgery proceeds as for an elective repair. If a balloon tamponade is used and threaded through the graft, the device is deflated and removed after the completion of the proximal anastomosis. A clamp is placed on the graft and the suture line inspected and reinforced as needed.

SURGERY FOR AORTOILIAC OCCLUSIVE DISEASE

Description

A bifurcated graft is inserted to bypass the diseased segment of the aorta and iliac arteries. The graft is sewn to the infrarenal aorta and bilateral common femoral arteries. Midline abdominal and bilateral vertical groin incisions are made for a transperitoneal approach. The two graft limbs are tunneled retroperitoneally.

Indications and pathophysiology

Symptoms. Symptoms include absent femoral pulses, proximal leg claudication, and male impotence. Symptoms vary a great deal. Impotence may or may not be a problem. Claudication may be described anywhere from the buttocks, thighs, or calves (25%). Neurogenic causes from spinal canal narrowing or herniated lumbar disc must be ruled out. Symptoms may be similar but symptoms caused by spinal disorders usually are relieved by a change in position and occur at inconsistent walking distances. Occlusive disease usually results in very consistent claudication walking distances.

Pathophysiology. Atherosclerosis is the primary cause of aortoiliac occlusive disease (see Chapter 3). Most of these patients have a history of smoking and the ratio of men to women is 2:1. The atherosclerosis tends to start distal to the renal arteries and is more extensive on the posterior wall of the vessels. There is better development of collateral circulation in aortoiliac disease than in the lower extremity vessels (Johnston, Kalman, & Baird, 1994). The majority of patients will have multi-level occlusive disease. Patients with aortoiliac occlusive disease tend to have a lower incidence of diabetes mellitus and hypertension and are 10 years younger than patients who present primarily with infrainguinal disease (Perler, 1996).

Indications. The atherosclerotic disease process that results in symptoms of ischemic rest pain, tissue necrosis, and ulcers or gangrene are indications for reconstructive surgery. Claudication is controversial but if it restricts or interferes with employment or lifestyle it is a relative indication to operate (Brewster, 1996).

Diagnosis. Diagnosis is made primarily on history and physical examination. However, since about one third of patients present with only calf claudication, further work-up is needed for confirmation. Noninvasive studies, including Duplex ultrasonography and measurement of ABIs clarify the level of involvement (Johnston, Kalman, & Baird, 1994). Preoperative evaluation of the hemodynamics will assist in the determination of the need for correction of the inflow (aorta and iliacs) versus outflow (infrainguinal) revascularization (Perler, 1996). Arteriography is ordered when the symptoms indicate a need for intervention, e.g., percutaneous balloon angioplasty or surgery. Angiograms remain the "gold standard" for planning reconstructive procedures.

Endarterectomy. In a small percentage of patients (5% to 10%) an endarterectomy may be adequate. Theoretically, endarterectomy has the advantages of drastically reducing the risk of infection by avoiding groin dissection and prosthetic graft material. It may provide better flow to the hypogastrics and reverse ischemic male impotence. However, endarterectomy is contraindicated for extensive disease or in the presence of any aneurysmal changes in the vessels. For most patients, bypass is simpler, faster, and carries a lower risk of occlusion (Brewster, 1996).

The selected anastomosis technique of end-to-end versus end-to-side depends on the patterns of occlusion. End-to-side may allow preservation of flow to the inferior mesenteric artery and the pelvis. End-to-end at the proximal anastomosis will eliminate flow to the pelvis when there is no retrograde flow from the iliacs (Brewster, 1996).

Preoperative planning
Epidural catheter for postoperative analgesia
General anesthesia
Arterial line
IVs

Since many patients with aortoiliac occlusive disease are heavy smokers, it may be advisable to perform pulmonary functions tests. The patient needs to be counseled to refrain from smoking and any suspected pulmonary infection should be treated with antibiotics. Antibiotics and local control of any ischemic lesions is indicated. Blood salvage may be preferable to banked blood to prevent the potential of pulmonary damage from miccroaggregates in stored blood (Johnston, Kalman, & Baird, 1994).

Equipment, instrumentation, intraoperative medications, and solutions
Same instrumentation sets and supplies as for elective repair of infrarenal AAA
Supplies and equipment for the cell saver (optional because of less blood loss)

Procedural Steps

1. The patient is positioned supine with arms abducted at less than 90 degrees on armrests. Positioning, prepping, and draping are the same as for elective repair of AAA, transperitoneal approach.

2. The midline abdominal incision is the same as for AAA.

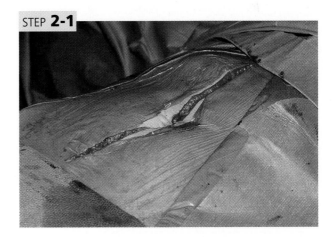

STEP **2-1**

3. The groin incisions and dissection and preparation of the femoral arteries are the same as for femoropopliteal bypass (see Chapter 12). The groin dissections may be performed first, second, or simultaneous to the abdominal incision.

STEP **3-1**

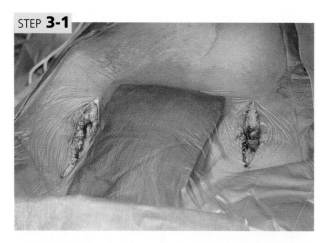

STEP **3-2**

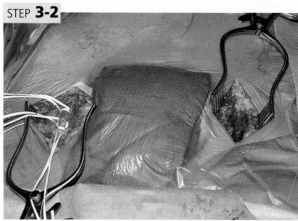

4. After the aorta and femoral arteries are prepared for clamping and subsequent anastomoses, the bifurcated graft is placed in position. The plane for tunneling the graft limbs is prepared by manual dissection.

STEP **4-1**

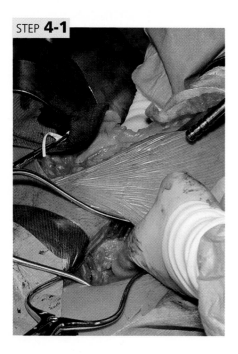

5. A large clamp, such as a DeBakey aortic clamp, may be used to pass through the created tunnel.

STEP **5-1**

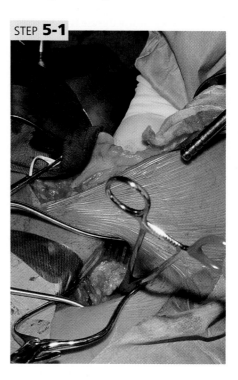

6. The limb of the graft is grasped by the clamp.

STEP **6-1**

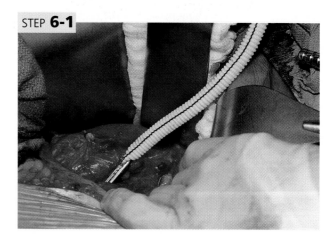

7. The graft limbs are both pulled into place over the femoral arteries.

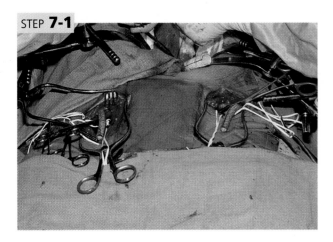

STEP **7-1**

8. The iliac arteries are clamped. The aorta is clamped and opened and the proximal anastomosis is completed. The Step 8-2 photo shows an end-to-end anastomosis, but an end-to-side anastomosis may be preferable (see Step 3-1 illustration, p. 183).

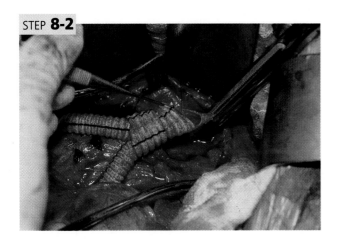

STEP **8-2**

9. The aortic clamp is released to flush any air and debris out of the graft. The graft is clamped to test the proximal anastomosis. Additional sutures are applied as needed.

10. The graft limbs are clamped. The graft is cut at a bevel (note the cut on the scrap of graft at the left of Step 10-1 photo). The graft is anastomosed to the femoral artery. Air and debris are flushed just before the final stitch. The clamp is released and the anastomosis tested. Additional sutures are placed as needed.

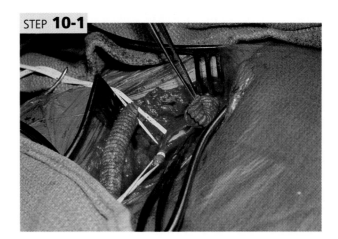

STEP **10-1**

11. Perfusion to the feet is assessed. If perfusion is adequate and hemostasis achieved, the wounds are closed and dressings applied.

COMPLICATIONS

Aorto-Bifemoral Bypass

INTRAOPERATIVE
Damage to vena cava or iliac veins during dissection or clamping
Embolization to lower extremities ("trash foot" or blue toe syndrome)
Damage to ureters or blood supply to colon when tunneling the graft

POSTOPERATIVE
Thrombosis of graft
Aortoenteric fistula
Pneumonia
Ileus
Infection (risk increased by groin incisions)
(Additional complications as in AAA surgery are possible but rare)

POSTOPERATIVE

Care and Discharge Planning

POSTOPERATIVE CARE

Intubated and ventilated for 12 hours (varies with setting and surgeon preference).

Monitor cardiac, respiratory, and renal function.

ECG on admission to ICU and then every day for 3 days.

Blood work: CBC, SMA-12, platelet count, PT, PTT on admission to ICU and POD 1.

Maintain normothermia.

NPO and nasogastric tube until patient displays bowel signs and flatus; advance as tolerated.

Prophylactic antibiotics for 24 hours.

Monitor for signs of bleeding, including tachycardia, hypotension, increased abdominal girth, decreased urine output, restlessness, anxiety, and altered mental status.

Check dressings.

Assess lower extremity perfusion hourly.

Assess pain and provide relief and periods of rest.

Provide oral care as needed.

Have patient turn, deep breath, and cough every 2 hours.

Bedrest, out of bed on POD 2, ambulate on POD 3.

Provide emotional support to patient and family, explain purpose of procedures (Fellows, 1995; Hatswell, 1994).

DISCHARGE PATIENT TEACHING

Provide written instructions; include phone number of physician, emergency numbers, and follow-up appointment.

Reassure patient that feelings of fatigue are normal and take weeks to resolve.

Incision care: showering is permitted. Use soap and water only and pat dry. Protect incision from oils, lotions, and powder. If steri-strips are in place, showering is permitted. The strips will peel away in about 5 days.

Activity: specific restrictions per surgeon.

Avoid lifting more than 5 to 10 pounds for 6 weeks to allow abdominal healing.

Walk to increase strength and improve circulation; progress gradually.

Stair climbing and out of doors as desired.

Avoid sitting for more than 1 to 2 hours.

Avoid crossing legs.

Driving requires permission from surgeon, usually after first office visit and when no longer taking pain medication.

Smokers should be counseled about the impact of smoking on vascular disease and wound healing.

Review all medications and any dietary recommendations.

Antibiotics may be prescribed before any scopes, surgery, or dental procedures.

Instruct patient in foot care.

Notify surgeon of the following: changes in wounds, e.g., redness, swelling, increased tenderness, bleeding, drainage; fever; change in bowel habits.

References

Anderson, L. A. (1994). An update on the cause of abdominal aortic aneurysms. *Journal of Vascular Nursing, 12*(4):95-100.

Bessen, H. (1993). Averting aortic catastrophes. *Emergency Medicine, 25*(5):57-74.

Brewster, D. C. (1995). Transabdominal versus retroperitoneal approach for abdominal aortic aneurysm repair: Current status of the controversy. *Seminars in Vascular Surgery, 8*(2): 144-154.

Brewster, D. C. (1996). Aortoiliac, aortofemoral, and iliofemoral arteriosclerotic occlusive diseases. In H. Haimovici, et al (Eds.) *Vascular surgery: Principles and techniques* (4th ed., pp. 581-604). Cambridge, MA: Blackwell Science.

Coselli, J. S. (1995). Thorocoabdominal aortic aneurysms. In R. B. Rutherford (Ed.), *Vascular Surgery* (4th ed.) (pp. 1069-1087) Philadelphia: W.B. Saunders.

Eaton, M. Anesthesia for aortic surgery (unpublished manuscript).

Fellows, E. (1995). Abdominal aortic aneurysms: Warnings flags to watch for. *American Journal of Nursing, 95*(5): 26-33.

Greatorex, R. A. (1992). Elective repair of infrarenal abdominal aortic aneurysm. In R. Calne, & S. G. Pollard (Eds.), *Slide atlas of operative surgery* (pp. 9.26-9.31). New York: Gower.

Hatswell, E. M. (1994). Abdominal aortic aneurysm surgery. Part 1: An overview and discussion of immediate perioperative complications. *Heart & Lung, Journal of Critical Care, 23*(6): 228-239.

Johnston, K. W., Kalman, P. G., & Baird, R. J. (1994). Aortofemoral occlusive disease. In F. J. Veith, R. W. Hobson, R. A. Williams, & S. E. Wilson (Eds.), *Vascular surgery: Principles and practice* (2nd ed., pp. 409-420). New York: McGraw-Hill.

MacSweeney, S. T., et al (1994). Smoking and growth rate of small abdominal aortic aneurysms. *Lancet, 344*(8923): 651-652.

Mitchell, M. B., Rutherford, R. B., & Krupski, W. C. (1995). Infrarenal abdominal aortic aneurysms. In R. B. Rutherford (Ed.), *Vascular surgery* (4th ed., pp. 1032-1060). Philadelphia: W. B. Saunders.

Normal, P. E., Wysocki, S. J. & Lamawansa, M. D. (1995). The role of vitamin D_3 in the aetiology of abdominal aortic aneurysms. *Medical Hypotheses, 45*(1):17-20.

O'Hara, P. J. (1996). Arterial aneurysms. In J. R. Young, J. W. Olin, & J. R. Bartholomew (Eds.), *Peripheral vascular diseases* (2nd ed., pp. 343-357). St. Louis: Mosby.

Ouriel, K., et al (1992). An evaluation of new methods of expressing aortic aneurysm size: Relationship to rupture. *Journal of Vascular Surgery, 15*(1): 12-18.

Parthum, J. (1996). Vascular emergencies. In J. M. Clochesy, et al (Eds.), *Critical care nursing* (2nd ed., pp. 535-557). Philadelphia: W. B. Saunders.

Perler, B. A. (1996). Aortoiliac reconstruction. In K. Ouriel (Ed.), *Lower extremity vascular disease* (pp. 157-185). Philadelphia: W. B. Saunders.

Piatkowski, C. A. (1994). Emergency abdominal aortic aneurysm: Maintaining normovolemia. *Today's OR Nurse, 16*(1): 13-17.

Silva, M. B., & Hobson, R. W., II (1996). Infrarenal aortic aneurysms. In K. Ouriel (Ed.), *Lower extremity vascular disease* (pp. 71-85). Philadelphia: W. B. Saunders.

16 Arteriovenous Fistula

ARTERIOVENOUS FISTULA

Description

Arteriovenous fistulas are the standard means of vascular access for long-term renal dialysis (Doyle, 1994). The best access is achieved by using the patient's own vessels and creating a subcutaneous connection between the artery and vein. Other choices include using a bovine carotid artery, human umbilical vein graft, or a synthetic vascular graft, usually PTFE (polytetrafluoroethylene) (Bennion, Williams, & Wilson, 1994). Eighty percent of all fistulas placed (including revisions) use PTFE (Lazarus, Denker, & Owen, 1996). Anastomoses between the artery and vein may be created to be end-to-side, end-to-end, or side-to-side (McEwen, 1994) (Figure 16-1). The Brescia-Cimino fistula is a connection between the radial artery and cephalic vein at the wrist (Figure 16-2). A basic principle of creating a fistula is to start in the distal arm and move proximally with subsequent fistulas. These include ulnar artery to basilic vein and brachial artery to brachial or cephalic vein (Doyle, 1994) (Figure 16-3).

Indications and pathophysiology

Arteriovenous fistulae are indicated for long-term renal dialysis access. Patients with end stage renal disease have their creatinine clearance levels followed. When the creatinine clearance falls to 10 ml/minute, a Cimino fistula may be created in anticipation of the need for dialysis (Bennion, Williams, & Wilson, 1994).

A **Cimino** (or **Brescia-Cimino**) type of fistula has proven to have the longest patency and lowest infection rate. It is created to connect the patient's artery to a vein that will "arterialize" or dilate and become thick walled (muscle layer hypertrophies). This occurs from the high rate of blood flow delivered by the connection to the artery. The arterialization, or maturation process, necessary to allow the fistula to withstand the repeated needle punctures of dialysis takes about 3 to 5 weeks (Bennion, Williams, & Wilson, 1994).

Despite the favorable track record of the Cimino fistula, this is a relative success and may not be the best choice for all patients. Leapman, et al (1996) did a retrospective review of fistula patency rates. They found patency rates of 42% at 1 year and 18% at 5 years for the diabetic population. Patients aged 70 years and older had a patency of 40% at 1 year. The conclusion was that elderly diabetic patients might have better success with synthetic conduits or permanent indwelling venous catheters.

When renal failure is imminent it may be possible to create the fistula and allow maturation time in anticipation of the need for long-term dialysis. Alternatively, patients must use a percutaneous centrally placed venous hemodialysis catheter in the interim (Bennion, Williams, & Wilson, 1994). When the Cimino fistula fails and cannot be revised or when the patient does not have a suitable vein and artery in close proximity, the next choice of fistula is called a **bridge**.

A bridge fistula is an alternative to the Cimino fistula. It is constructed by placing a *graft* between an artery and vein. Bridge fistulas do not need to mature and therefore are available for immediate dialysis use. For connections between an artery and vein that are in close proximity, a U-shaped graft is placed. Grafts that are far apart require a straight or slightly curved graft. Patency rates for bridge grafts using PTFE grafts are reported to be 70% to 80% at 1 year, which is comparable to the Cimino fistula in comparable patients. Although saphenous vein, umbilical vein graft, and bovine carotid artery are used, the PTFE grafts work the best and are most commonly used for bridge fistulas (Bennion, Williams, & Wilson, 1994). Some surgeons prefer to use a specially designed PTFE step graft, or tapered graft. These have a short segment of 4 mm in diameter at one end and the majority of the graft with a 7 mm diameter (Figure 16-4). This graft may avoid steal or an output or flow rate that is so high it causes cardiac overload (Wilson, 1996). Primary sites for bridge fistulas include the upper arm between the brachial artery and axillary vein and the forearm between the brachial artery and antecubital vein (Figure 16-5). Other choices are the axillary artery to axillary vein, either on the upper arm or across the chest. The axillary artery can be connected to the jugular vein or the superficial femoral artery to the proximal saphenous vein (Schanzer & Skladany, 1996) (see Chapter 17). The axillofemoral graft for dialysis is reserved for those patients who have exhausted other fistula sites. A regular walled (versus a thin-walled) graft is placed from the axillary artery to the common femoral vein. PTFE grafts may be used immediately but it may be better to wait 2 weeks for anastomotic healing to occur. These grafts may cause a slight steal phenomenon in the ipsilateral arm, which will have a BP 10 to 20 mmHg lower than the contralateral arm. Some patients have reported an increased sense of well being from the fact that dialysis flows are higher and more efficient (Rueckmann, Berry, Ouriel, & Hoffart, 1991).

The **side-to-side** was the original subcutaneous method introduced by Brescia in 1966 (see Figure 16-2). Side-to-side is technically the easiest to perform and creates the highest flow rate. The **arterial end to vein side** decreases the incidence of

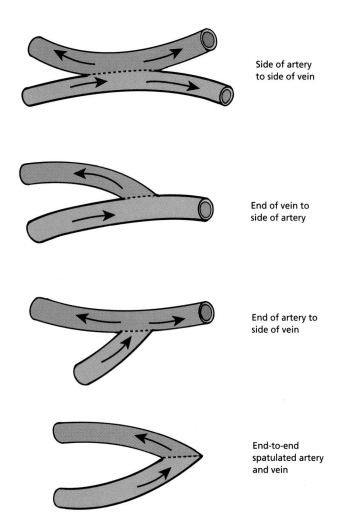

Side of artery
to side of vein

End of vein to
side of artery

End of artery to
side of vein

End-to-end
spatulated artery
and vein

Fig. 16-1 Four anastomoses between radial artery and cephalic vein. *(From Wilson, S. E. [1996]. Vascular access [3rd ed.]. St. Louis: Mosby.)*

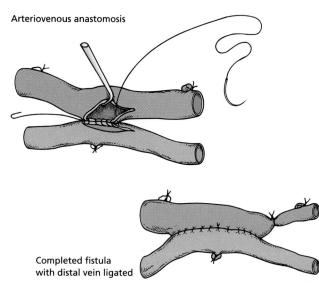

Arteriovenous anastomosis

Completed fistula
with distal vein ligated

Fig. 16-2 Arteriovenous fistula. *(From Calne, R., & Pollard, S. G. [1992]. Operative surgery. London: Gower.)*

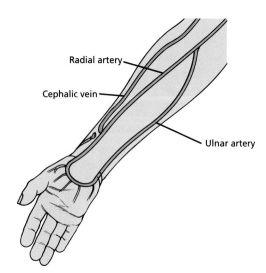

Radial artery

Cephalic vein

Ulnar artery

Fig. 16-3 Radiocephalic fistula. *(From Wilson, S. E. [1996]. Vascular access [3rd ed.]. St. Louis: Mosby.)*

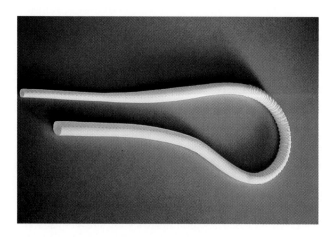

Fig. 16-4 Tapered PTFE graft. *(Courtesy W. L. Gore & Associates.)*

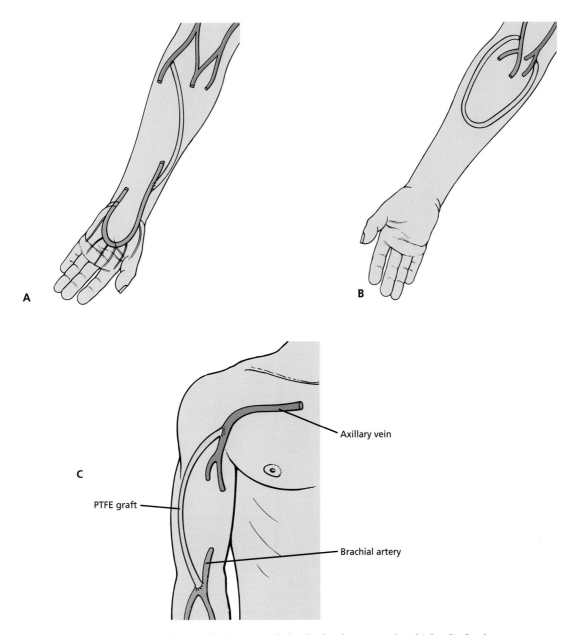

Fig. 16-5 Examples of bridge fistulas. **A,** Radiobasilic fistula. **B,** Loop brachiobasilic fistula. **C,** Brachioaxillary fistula. *(From Wilson, S. E. [1996]. Vascular access [3rd ed.]. St. Louis: Mosby.)*

distal arterial steal but has a lower flow rate. The **arterial side to vein end** is technically more difficult to create but has a lower incidence of venous hypertension. The **end-to-end** construction has the lowest rate of either venous hypertension or steal but also has the lowest flow rate (Bennion, Williams, & Wilson, 1994). There is a trend toward performing fewer side-to-side fistulas and more artery to vein side-to-end fistulas (McEwen, 1994).

Fistula revision. Because the patency of fistulas is limited, dialysis patients return for revision or embolectomy in attempts to salvage their function (see Chapter 10). Unfortunately the success rate for salvage is low and it may be better managed by

the creation of another site or a bridge fistula (Bennion, Williams, & Wilson, 1994). Risk factors for complications include being female, black, over 65 years old, and diabetic (Lazarus, Denker, & Owen, 1996; Rocco, Bleyer, & Burkart, 1996). Treatment for the most common complication, stenosis, is surgery. Stenosis usually results in thrombosis and these are considered a single problem. It is estimated that the majority of dialysis patients will have at least one hospital admission for access complications within 2 years (Beathard, Welch, & Maidment, 1996). Duplex scanning of fistulas may prove to be a cost-effective surveillance tool by allowing intervention before thrombosis, thereby possibly improving the success rate

(Lazarus, Denker, & Owen, 1996). But even before this, nephrology or dialysis nurses who cannulate the fistulas may observe signs of impending fistula stenosis. They may notice changes in the extremity, e.g. pain, pallor, or swelling, and altered dialysis flow, a decreased bruit, or clots in the cannulation needle (Berry & Cestero, 1992). Some stenotic fistulas respond to percutaneous transluminal angioplasty (PTA) performed in the radiology suite. PTA in conjunction with urokinase is an option if the stenosis is less than 4 cm in length. Stenosis may be treated with a patch angioplasty at the venous anastomosis if the area involved is short. If the area is long, then a jump graft is used. Stents have been used to maintain patency, but no controlled studies have been done to permit assessment of this technique. PTFE grafts for dialysis also thrombose most frequently at the venous anastomosis site. Intimal fibromuscular hyperplasia at the stenotic site may be caused by shear forces, high turbulence, and repeated injury from cannulation for dialysis (Lazarus, Denker, & Owen, 1996). Occasionally, the high flows that develop during dialysis, may lead to vein enlargement in the area around the failing fistula. As a result, some patients develop suitable sites for native vessel fistulas that were not present initially (White, 1996).

Preoperative planning

Site assessment. The arm pulses are assessed and an Allen's test is performed (see Chapter 5) to ensure that the ulnar artery will provide adequate blood flow to the hand when the radial flow is diverted in a fistula. Doppler systolic pressures may be needed to determine the adequacy of the arteries (Doyle, 1994). It is technically difficult to construct a fistula in obese patients and it may be impossible to construct a fistula in patients with tiny or fragile veins or those with a history of thrombophlebitis from multiple intravenous injections (Bennion, Williams, & Wilson, 1994). Chemotherapy or recreational drug abuse may contribute to this difficulty.

Placement of a sphygmomanometer on the upper arm allows visualization of the venous anatomy. The veins are then marked preoperatively by the surgeon with an indelible marker. The most distal site of the nondominant arm is the preferred site for surgery (Bennion, Williams, & Wilson, 1994). Fistula site selection is determined by the need for an artery to provide adequate blood flow and a vein large enough to provide venous drainage. Fistula site selection is also based on ease of cannulation and patient comfort during dialysis. It should be placed to avoid problems with joint movement and away from major structures that could be injured by needle puncture attempts (White, 1996).

The surgical arm must be protected from trauma or venipuncture. The nurse can ensure this protection by instructing the patient of the plan, placing a sign near the patient's bed or stretcher, and wrapping the arm with a loose bandage with a warning written on it (Apyan, Schneider, & Andros, 1992).

Anesthetic considerations. The majority of patients for fistula surgery have chronic renal failure. These patients tend to have anemia, platelet dysfunction, hypertension, metabolic acidosis, and delayed stomach emptying. They often present with cardiac risk factors and may be at risk for congestive heart failure, pulmonary edema, pericarditis, or pericardial effusion. Their predialysis and postdialysis weights may be helpful in assessing

intravascular fluid status. Preoperative transfusion of packed red cells may be needed for severe anemia (less than 6 g/dl). Drugs that are primarily excreted by the kidneys are avoided (Ezekiel, Alkire, & Barker, 1996).

The creation of an AV fistula may be performed under local anesthesia, regional (brachial or axillary) nerve block, monitored anesthesia care, or general anesthesia. Regional block has the advantage of causing vasodilation, which may assist the surgeon in creating the fistula. General anesthesia may be necessary for fistula revisions that make use of areas other than the arm. Potassium levels in chronic dialysis patients may be as high as 6 mEq/L but this should not deter surgery (Stein, 1995). Basic intraoperative monitoring is used. Because of the possibility of both upper extremities having fistulas, a thigh may be used for blood pressure monitoring. IV access is desirable but may be very difficult to obtain.

Nursing assessment. Nursing assessment must incorporate a sensitivity to the level of the patient's acceptance of their disease process. This information will assist the nurse in planning appropriate interventions. Patients who are recently diagnosed with renal failure may have very different reactions and informational needs than patients who have been on dialysis for years and return for a fistula revision. A new dialysis patient may be in a phase of denial and prefer to know as little as possible or need frequent repetition of instructions. Patients who are chronically returning for fistula revision may be more appreciative of efficient care that returns them to their home and routine quickly. Encouragement and support are essential to assisting the patient and family in coping with the chronic nature of their health care needs.

The majority of these procedures are performed under local anesthesia with monitored anesthesia care. Because the patient may be aware for much of the surgery the nurse assists the patient by describing the sights, sounds, and sensations that will be experienced. The position, safety belt and grounding pad placement, monitors, prepping, draping, and injection of local anesthesia are included in this discussion (see Chapter 7).

Equipment, instrumentation, medications, and solutions

Also refer to Chapter 8, Equipment, Supplies, and Instrumentation.

Basic OR furniture
Hand table with padding
Sitting stools
Doppler probe and amplifier
Sterile supplies
Custom vascular pack
Balloon embolectomy catheters
Syringes for balloon inflation
Penrose drain (as a tourniquet to plan incision site)
Vascular suture (5-0, 6-0, 7-0 nonabsorbable monofilament) and absorbable suture for subcuticular or nonabsorbable monofilament suture for subcutaneous closure
Vascular grafts (including tapered) and patch grafts (usually PTFE) used in bridge fistulas or revision procedures
Instrumentation
Basic vascular instrument set
Microvascular instruments

Minor soft tissue set (mosquito clamps, knife handles, heavy scissors)
Arterial dilators
Medications and solutions
Local anesthesia
Saline
Heparinized saline
Papaverine HCl
Topical hemostatic agents
Antibiotic irrigation

Procedural Steps
Creation of a Cimino Arteriovenous Fistula

1. The patient is positioned supine with the axilla of the surgical arm at the edge of the OR bed and the arm abducted less than 90 degrees on a padded hand table.
A pillow under the knees and warm blankets may increase the patient's comfort.

RNFA CONSIDERATIONS

Assist in positioning, prepping, and draping.
Ensure that the patient's arm is not abducted more than 90 degrees during the surgery to prevent brachial plexus injury.
Gently apply a Penrose drain to dilate veins for marking before the incision.
Apply gentle retraction with skin hooks (steroid use places the patient at higher risk for altered skin integrity).
Avoid placing forceps on the vein.
Protect intima of vessels from injury from forcep placement or vigorously irrigating.
Observe for vascular spasm and apply papaverine topically as needed.
Hemostasis is achieved at the anastomosis site by gentle pressure or the application of topical hemostatic agents.
Reinforce patient and family teaching of purpose and care of dialysis fistula.

STEP **1-1**

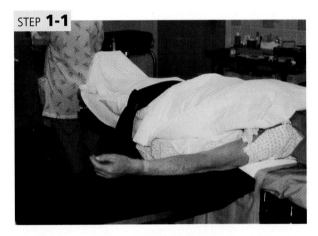

(Courtesy Gratia Nagle.)

A Penrose drain (or manual compression) is gently applied around the distal arm to permit visualization of the venous anatomy and a marking pen is used to delineate the vessels (if this was not previously marked by the surgeon).

STEP **1-2**

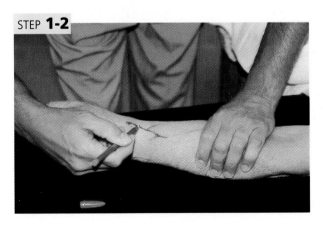

(Courtesy Gratia Nagle.)

The hand, arm, axilla, and shoulder are prepped and draped.

STEP **1-3**

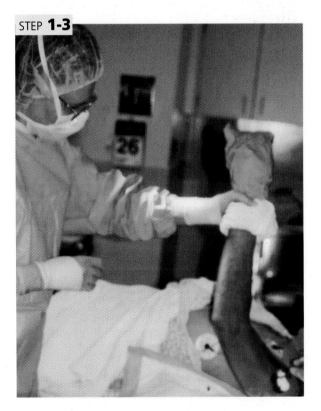

(Courtesy Gratia Nagle.)

2. Local anesthesia is infiltrated at this time if needed.

STEP **2-1**

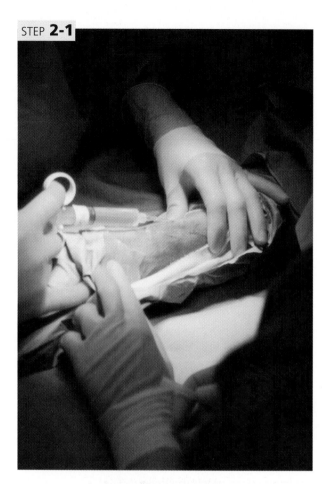

(Courtesy Gratia Nagle.)

3. A 3 cm longitudinal skin incision is made between the radial artery and cephalic vein (or a transverse incision is made over the vessels).

STEP **3-1**

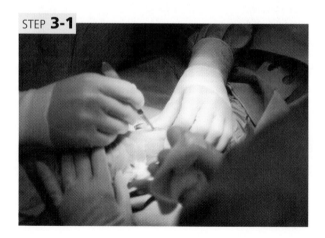

(Courtesy Gratia Nagle.)

STEP **3-2**

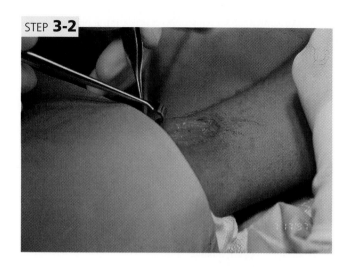

4. Skin hooks or a small self-retaining retractor hold the wound open while the cephalic vein is mobilized and branches ligated and divided.

STEP **4-1**

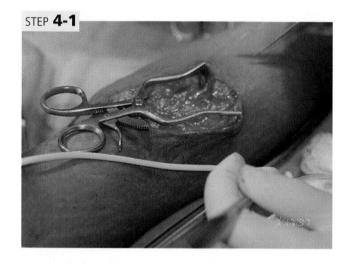

STEP **4-2**

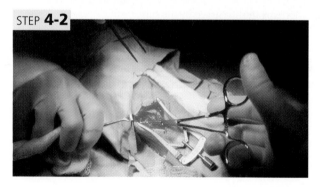

(Courtesy Gratia Nagle.)

5. The radial artery is mobilized and branches ligated and divided. Vessel loops are placed proximally and distally around both vessels.

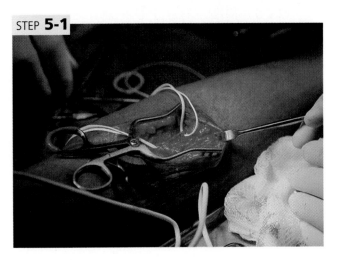

STEP **5-1**

(Courtesy Gratia Nagle.)

6. The vein and artery are pulled together without tension, twisting, or kinking.

7. A venotomy is performed and heparinized saline is injected to dilate the vein and confirm patency.

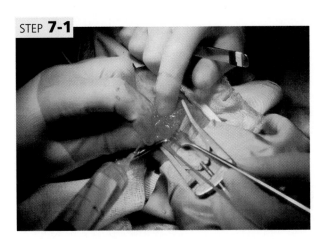

STEP **7-1**

(Courtesy Gratia Nagle.)

8. Papaverine may be injected or sprayed onto the vessel to prevent spasm and allow maximal dilation without injury to the intima. Any visible valve is carefully resected.

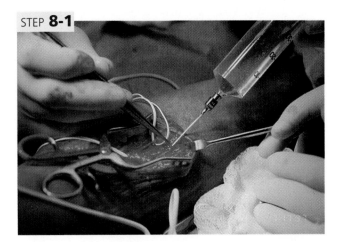

STEP **8-1**

9. The vein is ligated distally and a bulldog clamp is placed on the vein proximally to control bleeding. (This creates a side-to-side anastomosis but the vein ligation makes it a vein-to-artery end-to-side in function.)

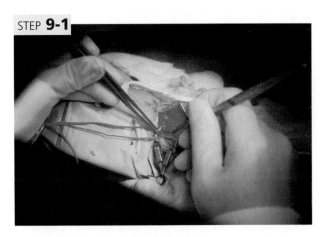

STEP **9-1**

(Courtesy Gratia Nagle.)

10. Further dilation may be achieved by passage of a balloon embolectomy catheter or Garrett dilator.

11. Bulldog clamps are placed on the artery; an arteriotomy is performed with a #11 blade and enlarged with a Potts scissors. The lumen is flushed with heparinized saline.

STEP **11-1**

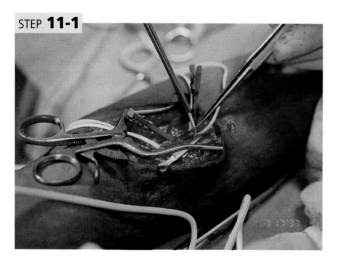

(Courtesy Gratia Nagle.)

12. (Stay sutures may be placed to facilitate the anastomosis.) The anastomosis of the vein to the artery begins with the suturing at the center of the posterior wall using a 6-0 or 7-0 continuous monofilament suture and is completed on the anterior wall.

STEP **12-1**

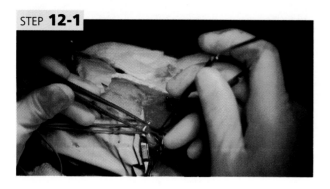

(Courtesy Gratia Nagle.)

STEP **12-2**

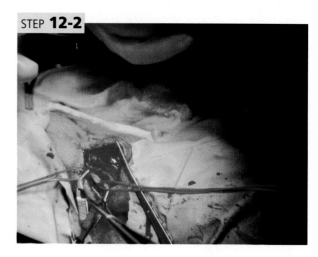

(Courtesy Gratia Nagle.)

13. The venous clamp is removed followed by the distal arterial clamp and then the proximal arterial clamp.

14. The patency is evaluated; a thrill should be palpable. Hemostasis is achieved by gentle pressure or the application of topical hemostatic agents.

15. The wound is closed with a single layer.

16. The bruit is assessed using a sterile Doppler probe. A loose (noncircumferential) gauze or transparent dressing is applied (Bennion, Williams, & Wilson, 1994; McEwen, 1994; Pollard, 1992).

COMPLICATIONS

Bleeding
Kinking of the vessel
Thrombosis (the most common complication [early and late])
Arterial steal and hand ischemia
Venous hypertension of the hand (discomfort and swelling); rare, responds to arm elevation and resolves in 1 to 2 weeks
Infection (rare), usually caused by Staphylococcus
Massive output can cause congestive heart failure and require ligation of the fistula
Aneurysm and pseudo-aneurysm formation (late)
Sclerosis of the vein after repeated dialysis punctures
Stenosis (usually of the vein)
Early cannulation of fistulas (before maturation) may lead to hemorrhage, hematoma, or pseudoaneurysm formation
PTFE grafts may leak if used before the graft is incorporated into the surrounding tissue

POSTOPERATIVE

Care and Discharge Planning

POSTOPERATIVE CARE

Assess surgical site for signs of bleeding.

Assess circulation, motor function, and sensation to affected hand.

Assess fistula for patency by palpation and auscultation.

DISCHARGE PLANNING AND PATIENT TEACHING

Protect site from pressure or constriction.

Instruct and observe return demonstration of hand-washing technique, dressing change, palpation of fistula for thrill.

Teach the patient signs and symptoms of infection.

Keep the dressing in place for the 24 hours.

Teach the patient care of the surgical arm including elevating the arm for 1 to 2 days, keeping the arm straight, and keeping the incision clean and dry for 2 days.

Tight clothing, jewelry, or watch bands should not be worn on the fistula arm.

Patient should avoid carrying heavy objects that could restrict blood flow to the arm.

Encourage the patient to obtain an identification bracelet that identifies the wearer as having an AVF for hemodialysis.

Teach the patient to remind others that venipuncture and blood pressure cuffs are not premitted on the fistula arm.

McEwen, 1994; Vogel, 1996.

Rocco, M. V., Bleyer, A. J., & Burkart, J. M. (1996). Utilization of inpatient and outpatient resources for the management of hemodialysis access complications. *American Journal of Kidney Diseases, 28*(2): 250-256.

Reuckmann, I., Berry, C., Ouriel, K, & Hoffart, N. (1991). The synthetic axillofemoral graft for hemodialysis access. *ANNA Journal, 18*(6):567-571.

Schanzer, H., & Sklandany, M. (1996). Vascular access for dialysis. In H. Haimovici, et al (Eds.), *Vascular surgery: Principles and techniques* (4th ed., pp. 1029-1041). Cambridge, MA: Blackwell Science.

Stein, P. (1995). Perioperative considerations of vascular access for dialysis. *AORN Journal, 60*(6): 947-956.

Vogel, S. C. (1996). Care and use of vascular access devices. In S. E. Wilson (Ed.), *Vascular access: Principles and practice* (3rd ed., pp. 271-283). St. Louis: Mosby.

White, G. H. (1996). Planning and patient assessment for vascular access surgery. In S. E. Wilson (Ed.), *Vascular access: Principles and practice* (3rd ed., pp. 6-11). St. Louis: Mosby.

Wilson, S. E. (1996). Vascular interposition (bridge fistulas) for hemodialysis. In S. E. Wilson (Ed.), *Vascular access: Principles and practice* (3rd ed., pp. 157-169). St. Louis: Mosby.

References

Apyan, L., Schneider, P. A., & Andros, G. (1992). Preservation of arm veins for arterial reconstruction. *Journal of Vascular Nursing, 10*(2): 2-5.

Bennion, R. S., Williams, R. A., & Wilson, S. E. (1994). Principles of vascular access surgery. In F. J. Veith, R. W. Hobson, R. A. Williams, & S. E. Wilson (Eds.), *Vascular surgery: Principles and practice* (2nd ed., pp. 1025-1038). New York: McGraw-Hill.

Berry, C., & Cestero, R. V. M. (1992). Indications of hemodialysis access demise related to clotting and possible associated vessel stenosis: What to look for. *ANNA Journal, 19*(2); 162.

Doyle, J. E. (1994). Vascular access surgery. In V. A. Fahey (Ed.), *Vascular nursing* (2nd ed., pp. 491-508). Philadelphia: W. B. Saunders.

Ezekiel, M. R., Alkire, M. T., & Barker, S. J. (1996). Anesthesia for vascular access surgery. In S. E. Wilson (Ed.), *Vascular access: Principles and practice* (3rd ed., pp. 12-18). St. Louis: Mosby.

Lazarus, J. M., Denker, B. M., & Owen, W. F. (1996). Hemodialysis. In B. M. Brenner (Ed.), *The kidney* (5th ed., pp. 2424-2506). Philadelphia: W. B. Saunders.

Leapman, S. B., et al (1966). The arteriovenous fistula for hemodialysis access: Gold standard or archaic relic? *The American Surgeon, 62*(8); 652-656.

McEwen, D. R. (1994). Arteriovenous fistula: Vascular access for long-term hemodialysis. *AORN Journal, 59*(1): 225-237.

Pollard, S. G. (1992). Techniques of Vascular Access. In R. Calne, & S. G. Pollard (Eds.), *Slide atlas of operative surgery: Vascular surgery* (pp. 9.2-9.7). London: Gower.

17

Extraanatomic Bypasses

The usual approach to revascularization surgery is direct, either by bypass, endarterectomy, balloon angioplasty, or a combination of interventions. These interventions restore arterial flow by following the normal anatomical route. There are times when a different route is needed that does not follow this normal path and this is called **extraanatomic**. The most common indication for these procedures is the need for revascularization of the lower extremity in patients who are poor candidates for more invasive procedures. Extensive scarring or localized infection in a graft may also require revascularization by an extraanatomic route (Brener, Brief, & Veith, 1994). The extraanatomic bypasses most commonly performed are the **femorofemoral** and **axillofemoral bypasses**.

FEMORAL TO FEMORAL ARTERIAL BYPASS

Description

A **femoral to femoral** arterial bypass or **crossover femorofemoral** graft is the placement of a synthetic graft from one femoral artery to the other in order to provide blood flow to both lower extremities from one iliac artery. The procedure requires two groin incisions and two anastomoses to sew a short segment of graft into the right and left common femoral arteries. A short segment of graft is sewn into the right and left common femoral arteries. It is performed in patients with unilateral iliac artery obstruction or those with occlusion on one side and minor obstruction on the other. It is usually an easy surgical procedure to perform.

It may be necessary to perform a concomitant iliac endarterectomy or balloon angioplasty on the better side to provide adequate blood flow. Direct arterial blood pressures may be measured in the OR to determine the existence of pressure gradients, before the procedure or immediately following, to verify adequacy of inflow to both extremities. Gradients of 10 to 15 mmHg are considered critical values indicating a hemodynamically significant stenosis (Ascer & Veith, 1996).

Indications and pathophysiology

Femorofemoral crossover grafts are indicated for patients who have unilateral common or internal iliac artery atherosclerotic occlusions. Symptoms may include disabling claudication, rest pain, and nonhealing ischemic ulcers. Axillofemoral bypass, aortofemoral bypass, iliac endarterectomy, or iliac balloon angioplasty are alternatives that may accomplish the same goal in selected patients. However, a fem-fem bypass may be the preferred procedure in those patients who could not tolerate a major abdominal surgery such as an aortofemoral bypass. Patients with kidney transplant complications that cause injury to the iliac artery may also be candidates. The procedure may be useful in patients with an iliac artery obstruction caused by an intraaortic balloon pump (Brief & Alpert, 1992). Femorofemoral bypass may also be performed in patients who have had a unilateral aortofemoral graft and now have an ischemic limb on the opposite side. Patients who have had an axillofemoral bypass may need a fem-fem bypass to provide flow to their opposite leg (Ascer & Veith, 1996).

Preoperative planning

Angiography and ultrasonography are used to define the extent of the lesions. Hemodynamic measurements are important to determine if a pressure gradient exists from the abdominal aorta to the femoral artery on the "good" side. If no gradient exists, that side will be an appropriate donor site for flow to both legs. If a significant gradient does exist, plans can be made for an endarterectomy or balloon angioplasty to improve the donor iliac artery flow. Once the surgery is planned, meticulous attention to groin hygiene is recommended to prevent postoperative infections. Patients with ischemic ulcers or gangrene probably have bacteria in the inguinal lymphatics. A broad-spectrum antibiotic is suggested immediately before surgery and for 48 hours postoperatively (Brief & Alpert, 1992).

Equipment, instrumentation, medications, and solutions

The majority of vascular surgeries should be performed on a radiopaque bed. Patients who are to undergo a femorofemoral bypass should be on the bed so that the iliac arteries can be visualized by x-ray if needed. The appropriate supplies for angiography should be available (x-ray contrast, syringe, sterile cover for x-ray machine, lead protection for patient and staff as needed).

If direct pressure measurements are taken, the following should be available: transducer and monitor screen, butterfly needle, and sterile pressure tubing to connect the butterfly needle to the transducer. Local arterial injection of papaverine HCl (30 to 60 mg), a peripheral vasodilator, may assist in the determination of the existence of a critical stenosis. The vasodilation results in decreased outflow resistance, which increases flow rates (Ascer & Veith, 1996).

A basic vascular setup is needed (see Chapter 8). Because the surgery is performed via two groin incisions, one or two Travers retractors for each groin are required. A long Kelly clamp or aortic DeBakey clamp makes an adequate device for tunneling the graft from one side to the other. An adequate inventory of vascular prosthetic grafts is needed. Six mm PTFE grafts, with or without external ring support, are most frequently used but some surgeons may select Dacron.

Be prepared for additional procedures that may be performed. The basic vascular setup should always include an endarterectomy spatula for performing an endarterectomy. Balloon angioplasty on the donor iliac artery may be indicated by the measurement of a critical stenosis (see Chapter 10 for details of supplies and technique).

RNFA CONSIDERATIONS

Knowledge of relevant anatomy
Use care in placing forceps and retractors so as not to cause trauma to axillary vein, subclavian vein, femoral vein, or femoral nerve
Avoid brachial plexus, located superior to axillary artery
"Follow" the vascular suture during anastomosis to prevent suture from catching on clamp, tangling, or knotting and to assist correct placement on suture line

Procedural Steps

The patient is positioned supine and lower abdomen, perineum and thighs prepped and draped. Ideally, two teams work simultaneously, one on each side.

1. Make vertical incisions over the common femoral arteries up to the inguinal ligaments.

STEP **1-1**

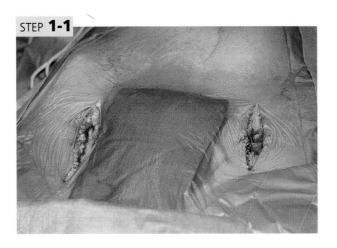

2. Divide the fascia, open the vessel sheath, and insert the Travers retractor as shown in right groin incision.

3. Identify the superficial femoral, common femoral, and deep femoral arteries. Place vessel loops around them as shown in left groin incision.

STEP **3-1**

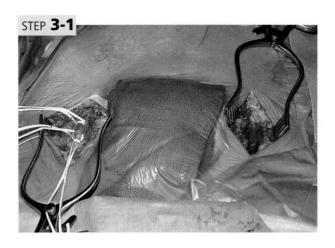

4. Encircle side branches with silk ligatures but do not divide them.

5. Create a suprapubic tunnel with finger or clamp to connect the two incisions. Tunnel the selected graft.

STEP **5-1**

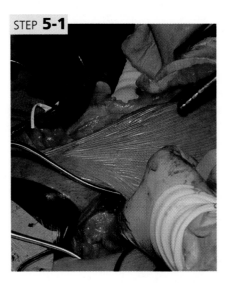

6. Heparinize the patient systemically. Clamp the three vessels on the *donor side* with vascular clamps (Calne & Pollard, 1992). (Veith & Ascer, 1996, prefer the reverse order, i.e., recipient first, to decrease needle hole leakage during normal pressures of donor side and decrease clamp time of donor leg).

7. Make an arteriotomy with a #11 blade on the common femoral; enlarge with an angled Potts scissors.

STEP **7-1**

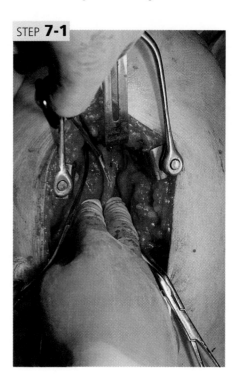

8. Angle cut the graft and make side-to-end anastomosis. Check the integrity of the suture line by releasing the clamps and allowing the graft to fill. Apply a Fogarty clamp to the free end of the graft.

STEP **8-1**

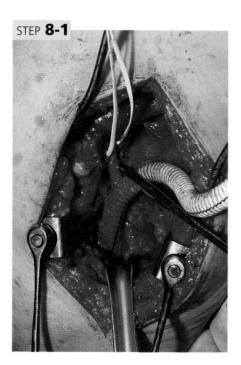

9. Select the anastomosis site on the second side; follow the above routine for the second anastomosis. Release the clamps to flush any air or debris from the graft just before the last stitch.

STEP **9-1**

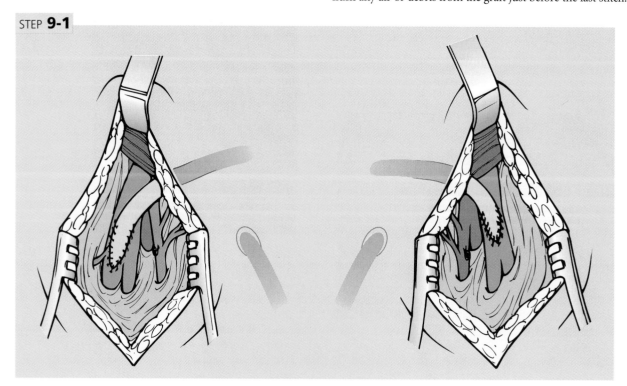

10. Ensure hemostasis, close routinely, and apply a dressing (Calne & Pollard, 1992).

Postoperative care and discharge planning

As with any vascular procedure, routine surveillance of neurovascular status is performed. It is rare that the donor side is placed at risk but the donor side and recipient side must be assessed for adequate perfusion. Any changes should be reported immediately to the surgical team. As cited previously (Chapter 10, Fundamentals of Vascular Surgery), meticulous wound care is needed to prevent infection since this is the most likely complication of the groin incision. Graft infection can cause anastomotic disruption and hemorrhage.

AXILLOFEMORAL GRAFTS

Description

A supraclavicular incision is made to access the axillary artery and a groin incision is made to access the femoral artery (these are on the same side of the body). A subcutaneous tunnel is made to connect the two sites. It may be necessary to make a third incision, inferior to the costal margin, to assist in graft placement. A synthetic graft (vein graft is rarely long enough) is tunneled and anastomosed at the axillary and femoral arteries. The procedure may be performed using local anesthesia but is often better tolerated under general anesthesia (Bergentz, 1989).

Indications and pathophysiology

The primary indication for axillofemoral bypass is severe ischemic disease of the lower extremity in a high risk patient. The occlusive disease is usually a chronic condition caused by atherosclerosis but may be acute in the case of iliac artery dissection or occlusion caused by cardiopulmonary bypass or intraaortic balloon pump insertion. Indications for axillofemoral bypass include the presence of an infected aortic graft, aortoenteric fistula, the need for revascularization of a threatened lower extremity, and aortoiliac occlusive disease in patients too ill to tolerate a major abdominal surgery (Brener, Brief, & Veith, 1994). Other reasons for avoiding the aorta for providing blood flow to the lower extremity include inoperable abdominal cancer, previous irradiation, and obesity. Patients with severe cardiac disease, pulmonary disease, or other systemic conditions that place them at high risk for abdominal surgery may be candidates for an extraanatomic procedure (Ascer & Veith, 1996). Axillofemoral bypass may also be performed in patients who need dialysis access when other sites have already been used and failed. The patient must have a patent femoral artery, either superficial or deep. Subclavian or axillary artery occlusion is a contraindication for surgery (Bergentz, 1989).

Preoperative planning

The blood pressure in both arms is measured to determine adequate flow. The subclavian and axillary arteries are auscultated to check for the presence of bruits. If the blood pressure is low or bruits are noted, an aortic arch arteriogram is performed to establish adequate patency of the intended inflow vessel (Bergentz, 1989). Adequate femoral artery patency is established through ultrasound or arteriogram. The results of the arteriogram are usually the basis for determining the placement of the distal anastomosis. If the profunda femoris (deep femoral artery) is stenotic, it will be included in the anastomosis in a patching technique (Ascer & Veith, 1996). Cardiac and pulmonary function are evaluated. Preoperative antibiotics are given (Calne & Pollard, 1992).

Equipment, instrumentation, medications, and solutions

As for most vascular surgeries, a radiopaque OR bed should be used. The appropriate supplies for angiography should be available (x-ray contrast, syringe, sterile cover for x-ray machine, lead protection for patient and staff as needed). A basic vascular instrument tray is needed, including four Travers self-retaining retractors for the axillary and femoral access sites. In addition, a vascular tunneler is needed to create a tunnel and carry the selected vascular graft. Vein graft is rarely long enough for this procedure and would add to the surgical time. Therefore, a synthetic graft, usually PTFE, with or without rings, is used. A sterile measuring device, such as a paper tape measure may be helpful in determining the correct graft length. If the procedure is performed under local anesthesia, the anesthetic of choice is provided.

Procedural Steps

The patient is positioned supine (on a radiopaque OR bed) with the arms abducted less than 90 degrees on arm rests. The patient's trunk is prepped from the neck to the knees and draped to exclude the groin area. Local anesthetic is injected around the incision sites as indicated.

1. Make a vertical incision over the femoral artery and a horizontal incision inferior to the middle third of the clavicle.

2. Incise the axillary artery sheath and mobilize the artery, dividing branches. Place vessel loops around the artery.

3. Expose the femoral artery, and place vessel loops around it.

4. Create a subcutaneous tunnel between the two incisions. It may be necessary to make a third incision below the costal margin to assist passage of the tunneler.

STEP **4-1**

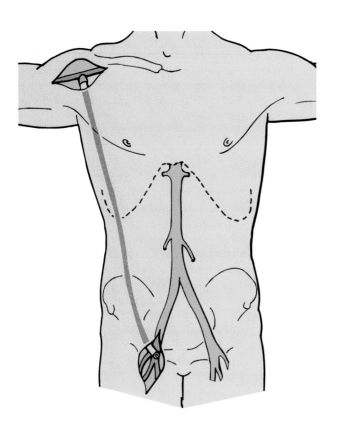

5. Heparinize the patient systemically. Place vascular clamps on the axillary artery, make an arteriotomy (#11 or #15 blade followed by enlargement with Potts scissors).

6. Anastomose the graft to the artery. Release the clamps and flush the graft. This tests the anastomosis site for leakage. Additional sutures are placed as needed.

STEP **6-1**

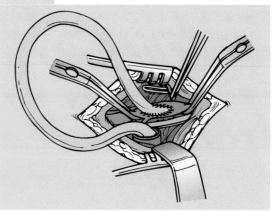

7. Place vascular clamps on the femoral artery. Make an arteriotomy and anastomose the distal end of the graft to the femoral artery.

8. Assess the anastomosis for hemostasis. Close the wounds and apply dressings.

COMPLICATIONS

Thrombosis of the graft as a result of technical error that causes graft kinking
Hemorrhage or infection
Late graft occlusion caused by constrictive clothing
Distal arterial occlusion caused by embolization of atherosclerotic material during manipulation of femoral artery (Calne & Pollard, 1992; Ascer & Veith, 1996).

POSTOPERATIVE

Care and Discharge Planning for Extraanatomic Bypass

POSTOPERATIVE CARE

Perform routine neurovascular assessment of arm and leg. (Axillary artery is prone to vasospasm.)

Assess incisions or dressings for bleeding or hematoma formation.

Monitor intake and output.

Activity as tolerated.

Advance diet as tolerated.

Observe for sudden loss of pulses or Doppler signal that may indicate graft occlusion, requiring immediate surgical intervention (wound exploration and possible thrombectomy).

Assess for pain; provide analgesics as needed.

DISCHARGE PLANNING AND PATIENT TEACHING

Provide written instructions to reinforce wound care, follow-up appointment, phone numbers for questions, and emergency care.

Instruct patient in routine wound care: Keep area clean and dry. Wash hands before touching dressing or area near incision. Do not use powders or lotions on incision.

The patient may shower after 24 hours, and should pat area dry gently with clean towel.

Instruct patient to report the onset of swelling, foul discharge, bleeding or drainage, fever, pain unrelieved by recommended analgesics, or any other change in the incision.

Instruct the patient to report any change in use, color, temperature, or sensation of toes, foot, or leg.

Instruct the patient to report any recurrence of preoperative symptoms.

When artificial graft material is used, prophylactic antibiotics are needed before any dental procedures or procedures requiring a "scope." Patient should notify dentists and other physicians of this need.

Instruct patients to avoid tight bras or belts that may contribute to graft obstruction.

Instruct the patient to avoid lying on operative side to prevent graft obstruction (Bergentz, 1989).

Instruct the patient to protect foot from trauma, and to avoid poor fitting shoes.

References

Ascer, E. & Veith, F. J. (1996). Extra-anatomic bypasses. In H. Haimovici (Ed.), *Vascular surgery: Principles and techniques* (4th ed., pp. 688-699). Cambridge, MA: Blackwell Science.

Bergentz, S. (1989). Axillofemoral bypass. In R. M. Greenhalgh (Ed.), *Vascular surgical techniques: An atlas* (2nd ed., pp. 173-179). Philadelphia: W. B. Saunders.

Brener, B. J., Brief, D. K., & Veith, F. J. (1994). Extraanatomic bypasses. In F. J. Veith, R. W. Hobson, R. A. Williams, & S. E. Wilson (Eds.), *Vascular surgery: Principles and practice* (2nd ed., pp. 485-499). New York: McGraw-Hill.

Brief, D. K., & Alpert, J. (1992). Crossover femorofemoral grafts. In L. M. Nyhus, & Baker, R. J. (Eds.) *Mastery of surgery* (2nd ed., pp. 1859-1864). Boston: Little, Brown.

Calne, R., & Pollard, S. G. (1992). Extra-anatomic bypass. In R. Calne, & S. G. Pollard (Eds.), *Slide atlas of operative surgery: Vascular surgery* (pp. 9.39-9.41). London: Gower.

Fiorani, P., et al (1989). Femorofemoral bypass. In R. M. Greenhalgh (Ed.), *Vascular surgical techniques: An atlas* (2nd ed., pp. 180-184). Philadelphia: W. B. Saunders.

18

Insertion of Vena Cava Filters

VENA CAVA FILTER INSERTION

Description

Vena cava filters are inserted percutaneously under fluoroscopic guidance using local or monitored anesthesia care. Some devices offer the option of jugular or femoral vein insertion and the insertion kit must be selected accordingly. The right femoral site is the most common (Nunnelee & Kurgan, 1993).

Pulmonary embolism (PE) has been reported to be responsible for approximately 50,000 to 200,000 deaths and 300,000 hospitalizations per year (Shortell, 1995; AJN, 1986; Greenfield & Proctor, 1996). PE is reported to be fatal within one hour for 11% of patients diagnosed with it (Greenfield & Proctor, 1996). The standard treatment to prevent PE is anticoagulation with heparin. Patients for whom heparin is contraindicated or ineffective may be candidates for insertion of a filter device. Vena cava interruption is a proven procedure for the prevention of pulmonary embolism.

The filter traps emboli that arise from the pelvis and lower extremities and thus prevents pulmonary emboli. Approximately 30,000 to 40,000 filters are inserted every year in the United States. Filters may be a cost-effective treatment compared with the costs and loss of life from PE and complications of long-term anticoagulation (Magnant, Walsh, Juravsky, & Cronenwett, 1992).

Attempts to interrupt the vena cava to prevent PE were reported as early as 1893. Later, suture plication and external clips were tried with varying success. These had the advantage of permitting limited blood flow through the vena cava (Becker, Philbrick, & Selby 1992). They had the major disadvantages of requiring a laparotomy and having a high rate of caval occlusion. One type of externally applied clip is the Adams-DeWeese vena cava clip. It is simply applied by spreading the plastic jaws, placing the clip around the vena cava, and tying the attached suture (Figure 18-1). Transvenous insertion of filtering devices such as the Mobin-Uddin umbrella and Hunter balloon led to many complications and their use was discontinued.

Several types of filters have been used successfully during the past 20 years. The Greenfield filter is the most successful and widely utilized device, and the associated mortality and morbidity rates have been extremely low (Person, 1989). The device has progressed from the earlier design that required an incision and venotomy to the percutaneous titanium and the current stainless steel vena cava filter (Figure 18-2). The filter maintains a patent vena cava but prevents PE by trapping the emboli at the apex of the device (Figure 18-3). The Greenfield vena cava filter (Medi-Tech, Watertown, Mass.) was introduced in 1973 for insertion transvenously by way of the jugular or femoral vein. Many other designs have entered the market. These include the Simon-Nitinol filter, the Gianturco-Roehm Bird's Nest filter (BNF), and Vena Tech filter (Figure 18-4). These three and the Greenfield, which is made in stainless steel, and titanium, are the five filters currently approved for insertion in the United States (Smith, 1994). The Gianturco-Roehm Bird's Nest filter (Cook, Bloomington, Ind.) was introduced in 1982 and modified in 1986 to prevent a problem with migration of the filter after placement. One advantage is the ability to insert this in larger vena cavae (up to 40 cm).

The Simon Nitinol filter (SNF) is made of a nickel titanium alloy that is flexible when cooled but converts to a rigid premolded shape when it is warmed to body temperature (Nitinol Medical Technologies, Woburn, Mass.). An IV set-up of refrigerated saline is infused into the carrier system during insertion. This allows the filter to remain in a small (9 Fr) delivery configuration. The cold saline is stopped when the filter has been correctly placed (Greenfield, 1992).

The Vena Tech device (L. G. Medical, Chasseneuil, France) is a 6-prong filter. It has had a number of problems with tilt, migration, and venous thromboembolism at the insertion site. The biggest concern with the Vena Tech is the unacceptable rate of caval occlusion (Shortell, 1995). These complications and the rate of recurrent PE are the basis for comparison for the devices.

Indications and pathophysiology

Patients at risk for PE usually have deep venous thrombosis. Acute venous thrombosis is caused by clot or thrombus in the deep venous system of the lower extremities. Patients present with a diagnosis of deep venous thrombosis (DVT), which may also be referred to as phlebitis, thrombophlebitis, or phlebo thrombosis. This merely indicates the existence of a clot, usually in the lower extremity. The patient may be asymptomatic or present with limb swelling, pain, and skin color change (Box 18-1). The danger lies in the potential for emboli migrating to the right ventricle and lodging in the lungs. PE can be fatal. Most of these originate in the lower extremities. The usual treatment is medical: heparin and bedrest. Thrombolytic agents (urokinase, streptokinase) have been used successfully.

Virchow, a pathologist, identified three conditions that cause vein clots. Dubbed Virchow's triangle, they are venous stasis, endothelial injury, and hypercoagulabililty. Endothelial injury may be due to direct trauma (catheter injury) or an existing or earlier venous thrombosis. Low-flow states may contribute to venous thrombosis. Surgical patients and patients on bedrest are prone to venous thrombosis (Verhaeghe & Verstraete, 1993).

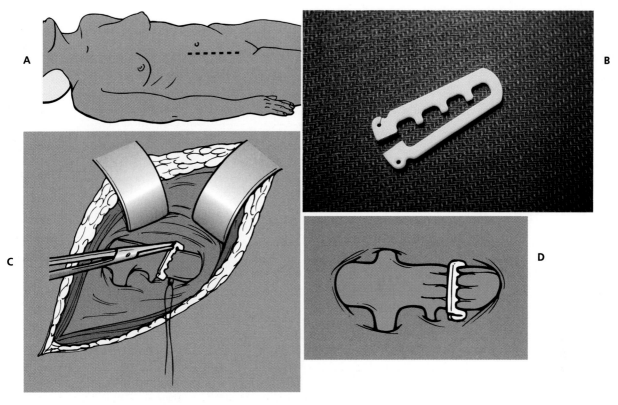

Fig. 18-1 Adams-DeWeese type externally applied, partial occluding vena cava clip. **A,** Patient position and incision. **B,** The vena cava clip. **C,** Application of the vena cava clip. **D,** Vena cava clip secured externally on vena cava with tie.

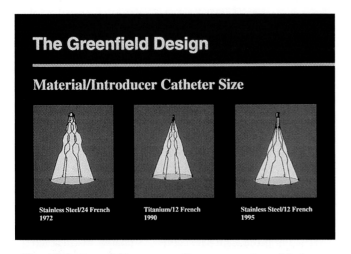

Fig. 18-2 Greenfield vena cava filter; progression of designs from 1972 to 1995. *(Courtesy Medi-Tech Division of Boston Scientific Corp., Watertown, MA.)*

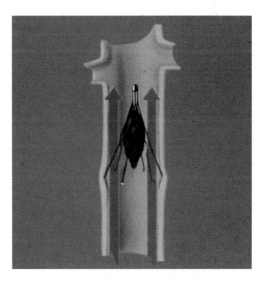

Fig. 18-3 Emboli trapped in filter in inferior vena cava. Arrows denote the continued flow of venous blood past the filter. *(Courtesy Medi-Tech Division of Boston Scientific Corp., Watertown, MA.)*

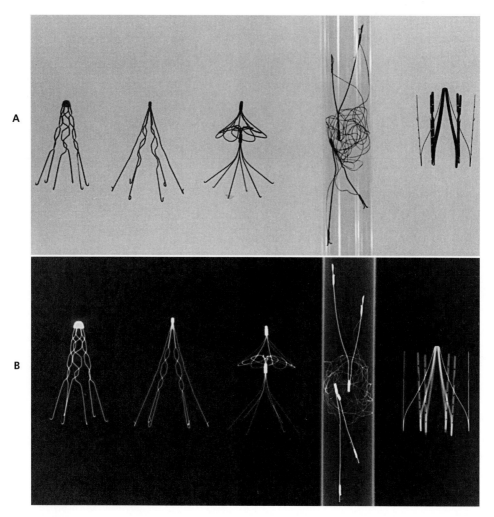

Fig. 18-4 Vena cava filters: *I,* Kimray-Greenfield; *II,* Titanium Greenfield; *III,* Simon-Nitinol; *IV,* Gianturco-Bird's Nest; *V,* Vena Tech. **A,** Actual filter. **B,** Radiographic images. *(From Ballinger, P. W. [1995]. Merrill's atlas of radiographic positions and radiologic procedures [8th ed.]. St. Louis: Mosby.)*

Box 18-1 Indications for Insertion of Vena Cava Filter

ABSOLUTE INDICATIONS
Pulmonary embolism with contraindication to anticoagulation
Pulmonary embolism on adequate dose of anticoagulation
Following pulmonary embolectomy

RELATIVE INDICATIONS
DVT with contraindication to anticoagulation
Patients who are noncompliant with anticoagulation therapy
Free-floating inferior vena cava clot
Patients at high risk of developing PE
Patients with severely compromised respiratory status who would not survive an episode of PE

The etiology of hypercoagulability is sometimes unknown but seen frequently in postoperative and cancer patients. Cancer patients, because of their hypercoagulable state, are at very high risk of DVT, perhaps as high as 40% (Cohen, Grella, & Citron, 1992). General surgical patients run a 20% to 30% chance of acute venous thrombosis, with orthopedic surgical patients and the elderly at even greater risk (Bright & Georgi, 1992). Other factors that contribute to thromboembolism and DVT because they may contribute to low-flow conditions include prolonged bedrest, any recent surgery, and impaired deep breathing (because of inadequate pain control). Smoking, vascular access devices, oral contraceptives, and some cancer therapies are risk factors for thromboembolism (Sticklin & Walkenstein, 1993). These factors may be responsible for endothelial injury.

PE are diagnosed by a variety of means and in many cases are not even suspected but subsequently diagnosed by autopsy. Patients may be diagnosed by a ventilation perfusion scan, pulmonary arteriography, or by clinical suspicion.

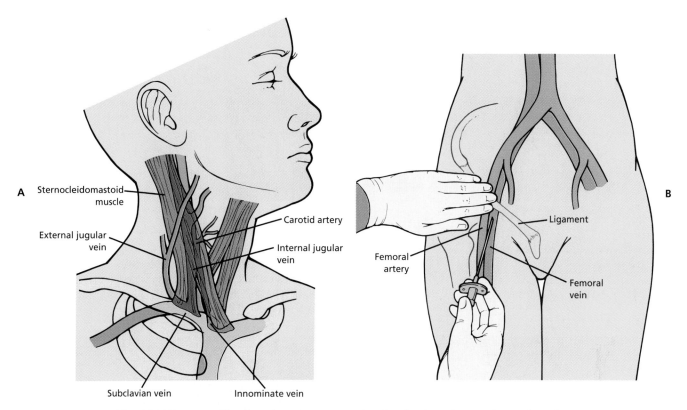

Fig. 18-5 Vena cava filter insertion. **A,** Anatomy of neck. Filter insertion may be via the right internal jugular vein or, **B,** the right femoral vein. *(From Meeker M. H., & Rothrock, J. C. [1995]. Alexander's care of the patient in surgery [10th ed.] St. Louis; Mosby.)*

Preoperative planning

Preoperative patient studies usually include a vena cavagram. This allows the surgical team to measure the diameter of the vena cava. Some filter devices are contraindicated for vena cavae that have a diameter of more than 28 mm because the device is too small to lodge in the vessel wall. In these instances, the filter could be placed in the iliac vein. Vena cavagrams reveal anatomic anomalies, show the level of the renal veins, and demonstrate patency of the IVC. Most filters are placed just below the renal vein and above the iliac vein bifurcation (Sticklin & Walkenstein, 1993). Ultrasonography also provides some anatomic information and shows the extent of the existing clot (Shortell, 1995). Thrombus at the femoral vein, iliac vein, or IVC may be a contraindication to femoral insertion (Sticklin & Walkenstein, 1993).

Equipment, instrumentation, medications, and solutions
Radiopaque OR bed
Lead aprons
Fluoroscopy unit
Sterile supplies
Drape towels (adhesive type avoids x-ray-visible metal towel clips)
Laparotomy sheet
Skin prep set

Gowns and gloves (optional)
Bowls and labels for solutions: local anesthetic, saline, heparinized saline, contrast
Local syringe and needle
10 cc or 20 cc syringe for flushing lumens with heparinized saline
20 or 30 cc syringe for contrast injection
Sponges
Filter and insertion kit of choice
Instrumentation
Usually none needed: Most filters have kits and are inserted percutaneously or via a 1 cm incision
Have instrumentation readily available for emergencies such as vessel perforation

Procedural Steps

The patient is placed in the supine position on a radiopaque OR bed to permit fluoroscopic visualization at the level of the renal veins. The head is turned to the left for jugular vein insertion or the groin is exposed for femoral vein insertion (Figure 18-5). The right femoral is preferred over the left because the anatomy of the left vein often makes threading the filter more difficult and may cause the sheath or delivery system to kink. Local anesthesia, heparinized saline to flush device lumens, and contrast medium should be available.

1. The right groin area is prepped and draped and infiltrated with local anesthesia.

2. An 18 gauge entry needle is used for right femoral venotomy.

STEP **2-1**

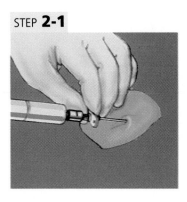

3. The guidewire is inserted and advanced to a level above the renal veins under fluoroscopic guidance.

STEP **3-1**

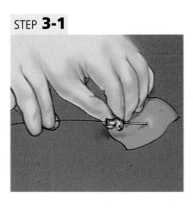

4. The sheathdilator is inserted over guidewire (flush all lumens with heparin solution before use).

STEP **4-1**

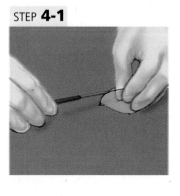

5. The sheath is removed and the introducer catheter is inserted and advanced to the implant site.

STEP **5-1**

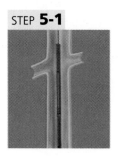

6. This catheter carries the preloaded radiopaque carrier capsule. The sheath is retracted, the filter discharged, and the sheath removed.

STEP **6-1**

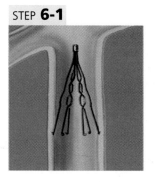

7. Pressure is applied to the puncture site for approximately 5 minutes or until hemostasis is achieved (Greenfield & Cho, 1990).

Complications

A number of complications occur with the insertion of the devices. Thrombosis of the vein used for insertion is "not uncommon" but usually not serious (Smith, 1994, p. 650). However, an extensive DVT may be serious. Technical errors may result in misplacement of a filter or failure of the device to attach properly to the vessel wall. This occurs less often as improvements are made in the delivery systems. A second filter may be introduced if necessary. Earlier designs resulted in occasional incorrect tilting that rendered the clot trapping function less effective (not a problem with the BNF). Vena caval occlusion may occur, causing lower extremity edema. Ideally, blood flow is maintained through the vena cava and when the underlying pathology is corrected, the trapped clot will be lysed. The anchoring mechanisms (tiny hooks) may rarely lead to caval perforation. Migration to the heart can cause arrhythmias, tamponade, or MI (Smith, 1994). Advances in radiologic techniques have improved the chances for successful retrieval but the risks must be carefully considered. The potential exists for an air embolism during insertion or the dislodgement of existing clot that could result in a massive, fatal pulmonary embolism. Perforation of the vena cava or adjacent structures is also uncommon but is a serious risk.

Documentation

Document medications used and amount of local anesthetic, sedation, and contrast injected. Complete the required implantation records according to FDA and institutional policy. Document that the device selection was confirmed by the surgeon. Provide the patient with the appropriate patient information card (if available) to be carried with them. Future health care providers may need to have the specific information provided on these cards. If a patient requires emergency care, some implants may not be compatible with the MRI scanner or may distort the resultant image (Nunnelee & Kurgan, 1993). However, the current Greenfield filter is known to give clear visualization on CT scan and be safe for use with MRI (Figure 18-6).

COMPLICATIONS

Hematoma at insertion site
Insertion site thrombosis
Total occlusion of vena cava
Placement failure leading to filter migration
Vessel perforation
PE caused by clot dislodgement
Air embolism
Infection at insertion site

RNFA CONSIDERATIONS

A primary role of the RNFA may be in the preoperative teaching. Review the purpose and provide diagrams of pertinent anatomy and of the type of device to be inserted.

Review the intraoperative experience including patient position, insertion site (jugular versus femoral vein), prepping, draping, injection of local anesthetic, use of fluoroscopy, injection of contrast and possible flushing from this, and immediate postoperative manual pressure on the entry site.

Intraoperatively: confer with the surgeon to prepare for correct entry site and select the appropriate device.

Assist in placing the patient on the radiopaque table for adequate fluoroscopy access.

Assist in prepping, draping, and infiltration of local anesthetic. Assist the surgeon in placement of entry needle, introducer sheath, guidewire, and carrier device as needed.

Inform the patient of the steps of the procedure as appropriate.

Apply 5 minutes of manual pressure to venipuncture site. Apply dressing.

Accompany patient from the OR (or radiology suite); reinforce postoperative teaching.

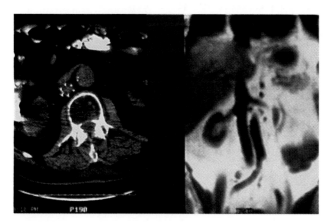

Fig. 18-6 Greenfield filter clearly visible on CT scan (left) and MRI image with no distortion (right). *(Courtesy Medi-Tech Division of Boston Scientific Corp., Watertown, MA.)*

POSTOPERATIVE

Care and Discharge Planning

POSTOPERATIVE CARE

A flat-plate abdominal film is usually taken immediately after insertion to confirm and document the filter location (Figure 18-7). This may be helpful for later comparisons and for determining if the filter has migrated.

Inspect and assess the insertion site for bleeding or hematoma formation.

Although the majority of patients have other reasons for remaining in the hospital, the insertion of a vena cava filter does not require hospitalization.

DISCHARGE PLANNING AND PATIENT TEACHING

Teach the signs and symptoms of local wound infection and hematoma formation.

Provide written instructions for wound care, follow-up appointments, and phone numbers for questions.

For a femoral vein insertion site; instruct the patient not to bend the leg for about 8 hours.

Instruct the patient to avoid strenuous activity or lifting more than 5 pounds.

Teach the patient that bruising of the insertion site is common (many patients are on or have been on anticoagulant therapy).

Teach a method to apply pressure if bleeding at insertion site occurs.

Instruct the patient to report signs of local infection or significant bleeding.

Teach the patient that lower extremity swelling may be a temporary side effect of the underlying DVT; relief may be obtained by elevating the effected leg and wearing elastic stockings.

Teach the purpose of and proper way to wear support stockings.

Instruct the patient to report sudden or severe leg swelling.

Patients may be on anticoagulant therapy concomitantly and must be instructed about bleeding precautions (see Chapter 4).

Reinforce the vena cava filter's purpose:

To trap clots before they reach the pulmonary circulation.

Filters do not cure the underlying cause of thromboembolism.

The filter remains in permanently (in rare instances it may migrate and need to be retrieved).

It will not set off a metal detector.

It is not rejected by the body.

No medications (antibiotics) are required by its presence.

Leg swelling is a result of the underlying venous thrombosis, not of the filter insertion, but the patient should report any sudden or severe swelling.

Some filter device manufacturers provide very good patient information booklets that answer the frequently asked questions for patients and family members.

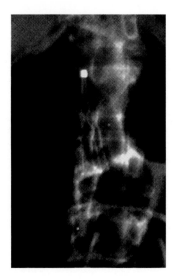

Fig. 18-7 X-ray confirming position of Greenfield vena cava filter. *(Courtesy Medi-Tech Division of Boston Scientific Corp., Watertown, MA.)*

References

Becker, D. M., Philbrick, J. T., & Selby, J. B. (1992). Inferior vena cava filters: Indications, safety, effectiveness. *Archives of Internal Medicine, 152*(10): 1985-1994.

Bright, L. D., & Georgi, S. (1992). Peripheral vascular disease: Is it venous or arterial? *American Journal of Nursing, 92*(9): 34-43.

Cohen, J. R., Grella, L., & Citron, M. (1992). Greenfield filter instead of heparin as primary treatment for deep venous thrombosis or pulmonary emboli in patients with cancer. *Cancer, 70*(7): 1993-1996.

Preventing thombosis/pulmonary embolism. *American Journal of Nursing* (6), 1986:648, 650.

Greenfield, L. J. (1992). Evolution of venous interruption for pulmonary thromboembolism. *Archives of Surgery, 127*(5): 622-626.

Greenfield, L. J., & Cho, K. J. (Ed.) (1990). *The Greenfield Vena Cava filter and 12 French introducer systems: Concept and technique.* Boston: Boston Scientific Corporation.

Greenfield, L. J., & Proctor, M. C. (1996). Venous interruption. In H. Haimovivi (Ed.), *Haimovici's vascular surgery: Principles and techniques* (4th ed., pp. 1210-1219). Cambridge: Blackwell Science.

Magnant, J. G., Walsh, D. B., Juravsky, L. I., & Cronenwett, J. L. (1992). Current use of inferior vena cava filters. *Journal of Vascular Surgery, 16*(5): 701-706.

Nunnelee, J. D., & Kurgan, A. (1993). Interruption of the inferior vena cava filter for venous thromboemboic disease. *Journal of Vascular Nursing, 11*(3): 80-82.

Persson, A. V. (1989). Acute deep venous thrombosis. In D. C. Brewster (Ed.), *Common problems in vascular surgery* (pp. 349-356). St. Louis: Mosby.

Reilly, K. M., & Salluzzo, R. (1990) Pulmonary embolism. *Resident & Staff Physician 36*(10): 43-48.

Shortell, C. K. (1995). Pulmonary embolism and vena caval interruption. In K. Ouriel (Ed.), *Lower extremity vascular disease* (pp. 409-415). Philadelphia: W. B. Saunders.

Smith, B. A. (1994). Vena caval filters. *Emergency Medicine Clinics of North America, 12*(3): 645-656.

Stocklin, L. A., & Walkenstein, M. (1993). Vena cava filters: A nursing perspective. *Oncology Nursing Forum, 20*(3): 507-513.

Understanding Your Greenfield Vena Cava Filter (patient teaching booklet). Medi-Tech Education Center, Watertown, MA.

Verhaeghe, R., & Verstraete, M. (1993). Hemostasis, thrombosis, and anti-thrombotic and thrombolytic therapy. In D. L. Clement, & J. T. Shepherd (Eds.), *Vascular diseases in the limbs: Mechanisms and principles of treatment* (pp. 133-152). St. Louis: Mosby.

19 Varicose Vein Surgery

VARICOSE VEIN SURGERY

Description

A patient with the diagnosis of varicose veins of one or both lower extremities presents for surgical removal by excision and ligation, which may or may not include stripping of the main trunk of the saphenous vein. The patient may be positioned either supine or prone, and in some degree of Trendelenburg. Multiple small incisions are made over the identified varicosities and the affected vein segments are removed. Stripping indicates removal of a long segment of vein by means of a special device.

Veins should have been marked, indelibly, with the patient standing to maximize visualization of the varicosities and ensure complete removal of the varicosities (Bergan, 1991; Johnson & Rutherford, 1995). A felt-tipped marker or a surgical skin marker may be used as long as the marks remain visible throughout the surgical procedure. Complete removal of varicosities is desirable from a cosmetic standpoint, for relief of symptoms, and to minimize recurrence (Hume, 1992). Recurrent varicosities may be due to an incomplete previous surgical procedure or inadequate sclerotherapy (Bergan, 1991).

Indications and pathophysiology

Varicose veins are usually found in the lower extremities. They appear as elongated, dilated, tortuous vessels readily visible and usually recognized by most patients. Patients complain of feelings of limb heaviness and fatigue, itching, and swelling. The discomfort is caused by increased venous volume and may result in neuralgia pain caused by pressure on accessory nerves (Bergan, 1993). Some patients describe burning, throbbing, and bursting sensations. These symptoms may occur even before any visible evidence of varicosities. Exercise, prolonged standing, and warm temperatures may exacerbate symptoms through nociceptor stimulation from venous distension, increased interstitial tissue pressure, or from the byproducts of exercise (Cockett & Thomas, 1965). Symptoms also have a hormonal association. Many occur for the first time during pregnancy; menses is also associated with increased varicose vein discomfort (Goldman, Weiss, & Bergan, 1994). In rare instances, patients will report bleeding from erosion of a superficial vein through the skin. Considered a benign process (Sumner, 1989), interestingly, there have been numerous deaths from spontaneous varicose vein hemorrhage (Morrow, et al, 1994). The majority of patients describe their symptoms as most evident at the end of the day with relief found by leg elevation (Johnson & Rutherford, 1995) or wearing support hose (Nordestgaard & Williams, 1994). Besides the discomfort, the unsightly appearance alone is enough to cause patients to seek treatment.

The pathophysiology of venous disease is the same whether discussing varicose veins or venous insufficiency (Bergan, 1993). There are four basic physical components of the venous system of the lower extremity:

- deep veins
- perforating or communicating veins
- superficial veins
- valves (Figure 19-1).

The components function together and a disturbance in one leads to dysfunction of the system. Competence of one-way valves serves to direct the blood from the superficial to the deep veins by way of the perforators (Goldman, Weiss, & Bergan, 1994). The valves of the venous system protect the veins below them. Valves are bombarded with increased pressure caused by standing, lifting, coughing, or straining (Nordestgaard & Williams, 1994). Since the main function of the venous system is to return blood to the heart, competent valves are essential (Bishara, et al, 1986).

Venous flow is primarily determined by three factors:

- an unobstructed pathway
- competent valves
- the calf muscle pump or "venous heart" (Jamieson, 1993).

It was a long-held belief that the deep and superficial veins of the leg filled alternately and the muscle contraction compressed deep veins that filled during relaxation through the perforators. Stegall (1966) studied the venous blood flow and determined the major contribution of the calf muscle pump. Pressure, flow velocity, and blood volume changes were measured in running adult subjects. He found that the abdominal contractions of runners served to impede venous return by the increased vena cava pressure. However, the leg muscles were able to overcome this and provide 30% of the energy needs for blood flow circulation demands of exercise. There is a consensus that pressure changes in the abdominal and thoracic cavities caused by breathing also contribute to the energy demanded during heavy exercise. At rest the heart provides 100% of the needed energy. The calf muscle is a much better blood pump than the muscle of the thigh. The power of the calf muscle pump is attributed to the fascial sheath that surrounds it, allowing the development of high compartment pressures during muscle contraction. The calf muscle contraction squeezes the venules and generates a pressure as high as 250 mmHg. Thigh pressures are lower. During relaxation, the pressure is slightly higher in the superficial veins and the flow is directed from muscles of distal veins to the deeper vessels (Nordestgaard & Williams, 1994). In the healthy leg 90% of venous blood is routed through the deep veins of the muscle pump (Goldman, Weiss, & Bergan, 1994) (Figure 19-2).

When valves become incompetent, they permit the reversal of blood flow from the deep to the superficial system. This reversal of flow is a major cause of pathology. Distal and proximal obstructions contribute to venous hypertension. The distal factors are incompetent perforating vein valves, arteriovenous anastomoses, and intraluminal blockage such as a thrombus. Proximal factors are intraabdominal pressure from straining or exercise, obesity, prolonged sitting, intraluminal blockages, and pelvic masses, e.g., pelvic tumors or the gravid uterus. Venous hypertension is the product of gravity and alteration in the functioning of the muscle pump (Bergan, 1993).

Varicose veins are described as primary or secondary. Primary varicose veins are more prevalent and are not associated with pathology of the deeper venous system, e.g., postthrombotic syndrome or a history of deep venous thrombosis (DVT). Secondary varicose veins are thought to be a result of insufficiency of the deep venous system. Differentiating between the two may not be possible by history and physical examination (Criado & Johnson, 1991). Villavicencio (1991) uses the terms *primary, essential,* and *familial* interchangeably. Secondary varicose veins are postphlebitic in nature. He also includes the congenital venous malformations of Klippel-Trenaunay syndrome. Klippel-Trenaunay syndrome is usually noted shortly after birth and involves abnormalities of the soft tissue, bones, cutaneous nevi, and varicose veins. The varicosities may not be evident until the child starts walking (Wilson & Browse, 1993). This is a rare entity but occasionally requires surgical intervention during childhood (Greenfield, 1994).

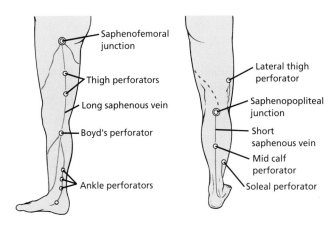

Fig. 19-1 Clinically important veins of the leg: medial view (*left*) and posterolateral view (*right*).

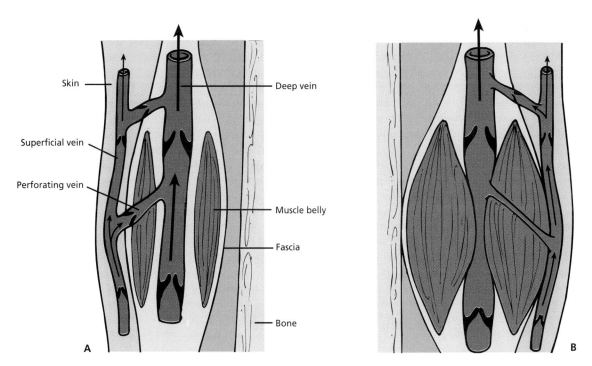

Fig. 19-2 Schematic diagram of calf muscle pump. **A,** Relaxed state. **B,** With muscle contraction the perforating veins are squeezed closed.

Among chronic diseases in the United States, varicose veins rank seventh in frequency (Villavicencio, 1991). The etiology has been difficult to pinpoint. Numerous theories abound but there is a consensus that alteration in the venous valves is the common denominator. Older theories ascribed the cause as the absence of valves in the veins. Normal iliac veins lack valves in 70% of the population, which may contribute to the occurrence of varicosities (Jamieson, 1991). Classic causes of varicose veins such as gender (female), obesity, pregnancy, occupations, diet, geographical location, age, race, and family history have been cited (Criado & Johnson, 1991; Greenfield, 1994). More recent evidence indicates the problem is multifactorial. Metabolic disturbances from the venous hypertension may lead to vein wall fibrosis. The fibrotic process leads to the collagen replacing muscle fibers, resulting in poor contraction, which causes stasis and incomplete valve closure (Jamieson, 1991). However, Callan (1993), in an extensive review of the literature, reports the following as risk factors: female gender, increased age, pregnancy, geographic location, and race (more prevalent in Caucasians). Obesity and family history are *not* risk factors. Conclusions are difficult to reach because of the varied criteria used to study the disease. However, it appears that lifestyle may play an important role. Criado and Johnson (1991) found that "chair sitting" with its resultant increase in ankle venous pressure may be worse than "ground sitting." This may imply that industrial versus nonindustrialized societies are at greater risk. Family history has not been substantiated in well-controlled studies but this impression has existed because patients with varicose veins are more likely to be asked about relatives with similar symptoms. Climate has been ruled out as a cause. Different populations, when moved to an industrial lifestyle, develop associated health problems. Affluence, diet, exercise, and environmental variables seem to be contributing factors (Geelhoed & Burkitt, 1991). The Framingham study points to the same risk factors for cardiac disease as are being implicated in venous disease. Associated with lower extremity venous varicosities are fiber-depleted diets, diverticular disease, DVT, and hemorrhoids. He suggests that it is an acquired disease and recommends weight and blood pressure control and dietary modifications to decrease refined sugar, saturated fats, salt, cholesterol, and alcohol. Geelhoed and Burkitt (1991) cite a study by Folse that verified the hypothesis that valves fail progressively downward on the lower extremities. This is induced by abdominal pressure.

Varicose veins in pregnancy. There is an increase in the incidence of varicose veins in pregnant women in industrialized countries. This is the only time that varicose veins may resolve without intervention (Villavicencio, 1991). Regression may take up to 3 months after delivery and surgery or sclerotherapy should be postponed until then. Valve incompetence in pregnant women is due to the increased blood volume and the obstruction of venous flow caused by the enlarged uterus. Estrogen relaxes smooth muscle cells of the vein, allowing increased distension and softens collagen fibers (Goldman, Weiss, & Bergan, 1994). Venous hypertension leads to edema.

Because the distension of the vessels is seen for 6 months after delivery, factors other than the size of the uterus are probably involved. Forty percent of pregnant women report symptoms of aching and throbbing of the legs (Skudder & Farrington, 1993). Varicosities of the saphenous, vulvar, and hemorrhoidal veins occur in 40% of pregnancies because of increased venous pressure in femoral and pelvic vessels from the gravid uterus (Dotz & Berman, 1991). In early pregnancy, increased levels of progesterone and estradiol cause the relaxation of smooth muscle tone, resulting in decreased venous tone. The gravid uterus obstructions usually occur in the third trimester (Jacobson & Haimov, 1991).

As varicose veins begin to appear, the first level of treatment is aimed at relieving symptoms by wearing lower leg graduated pressure stockings (Karp & Fahey, 1994). Patients complain of aching, heaviness, itching, swelling, and unsightly appearance. Bleeding is a rare reason for surgery (Criado & Johnson, 1991). Some patients describe the appearance of tender "knots" (Johnson & Rutherford, 1995). These symptoms are usually worse at the end of day and after prolonged periods of standing or sitting. Typically relief is obtained by leg elevation. (It is recommended that differentiation be made between primary and secondary varicose veins; secondary is often found in conjunction with stasis dermatitis and ulceration.) Diagnosis is usually made by inspection and the previously described patient complaints. Diagnosis is augmented with Doppler ultrasound and venous reflux plethysmography. Mild edema may be caused by the resultant venous hypertension of varicose veins, but cardiac or renal disease must be ruled out. "The usual distribution of varicose veins is below the knee in branches of the lesser saphenous vein" (Greenfield, 1994, p. 1004).

Preoperative planning

Preoperative tests are relatively benign for diagnosing and delineating varicose vein procedures. There are two widely used tests to locate any incompetent valves, the Trendelenburg test and the Perthes test (see Chapter 5).

Duplex ultrasonography is a noninvasive test that can determine whether the deep veins are patent or valves are competent (Karp & Fahey, 1994). This can be more useful than a simple Doppler examination but is more time consuming and costly and may not be helpful in the morbidly obese patient (Johnson & Rutherford, 1995). A variety of noninvasive tests or studies may be performed to quantify and locate the underlying pathology depending on the physician and available equipment. Doppler examination to locate incompetent valves and inspection are the required evaluations before surgical intervention (Bergan, 1991). Shah, et al (1986) studied the anatomy of the greater saphenous vein. They found there is a *single* trunk in the thigh in 65% of patients and in the calf in 45% of patients. The remainder had a double system by phlebography.

Their conclusion was that the anatomy of the saphenous system should be determined preoperatively by phlebography. The anatomy of double systems, cross connections, and perforator branches was considered to be helpful for surgical planning. Most surgeons do not advocate the use of phlebography routinely because of the expense, discomfort, and potential complications that an invasive study involves (Bergquist & Bergentz, 1990).

Ambulatory setting considerations. Patients who have lengthy or extensive varicose vein stripping and ligation procedures on their lower extremities or those who have medical conditions or an intraoperative complication that is best observed in an inpatient setting may not be candidates for discharge on the day of surgery. This is decided by the surgeon and anesthesiologist. However, many patients are ideal candidates for ambulatory settings.

The trend is to discharge patients on the day of surgery unless there is extensive surgery resulting in a large blood loss, prolonged recovery time, or if anticipated problems of home pain management are identified.

As more surgical procedures are performed on an outpatient basis, the opportunities for teaching may occur when the preoperative evaluation is performed. Patients usually need to be assessed for knowledge deficits regarding the basic anatomy, surgical goals, and postoperative planning. The majority of patients cannot differentiate between arterial and venous problems (Sumner, 1989). Patients benefit by having the opportunity to ask questions and express concerns. The nurse provides answers and emotional support and facilitates responses from other health team members as indicated. Written diagrams and instructions that the patient and family can keep as a reference are helpful.

Equipment, instrumentation, medications, and solutions

If the patient needs to be prone for access to posterior veins, the appropriate positioning devices should be immediately available. Some patients are positioned supine for part of the procedure and then turned to the prone position for completion. The nurse must plan for the provision of any additional prepping, draping, and other sterile items so there is no delay.

A minor basic instrument set is needed for the universal knife handles, towel clips, scissors, mosquito hemostats, and needle holders (see Box 8-8). Retractors such as deep Weitlaners for groin incisions, small Weitlaners for ankle incisions, skin hooks, and Senns should be available. Vein strippers with various tips may be disposable or nondisposable (see Figure 8-35). Some surgeons use specially designed crochet hooks or nerve hooks to lift the varicose vein for excision. Muller hooks, Graefe iridectomy forceps, and Oesch hooks are used for the minivenectomy techniques (Figures 19-3 through 19-6).

The surgeon may use a tourniquet on the prepped skin. It should be sterile and preferably disposable since the hook and latch (Velcro) fastener is difficult to clean (see Figure 8-36). Tourniquet boxes require either an air line or electric outlet for use. Additional supplies include sterile padding to protect the patient's skin from the tourniquet cuff (such as cotton webril), an appropriately sized sterile tourniquet cuff, and sterile extension tubing (optional) (Box 19-1).

Sutures are selected according to surgeon preference and may include nonabsorbable skin closing sutures or absorbable sutures for subcuticular closure. Small incisions and minivenectomy procedures may only require adhesive strip application. Elastic bandages or compression stockings are usually applied before the patient is taken out of Trendelenburg position to minimize venous congestion.

Local anesthetics with epinephrine may be requested for the hemostatic properties of the epinephrine. Furuya, Tada, and Sato (1992) described a procedure for reducing the incidence of bleeding complications from saphenous vein stripping. They filled a nasogastric tube with a dilute epinephrine solution, attached this to the stripper, and instilled the drug during the movement of the stripper (Figures 19-7 and 19-8). Compression was applied for 10 minutes. No adverse reactions were observed.

Box 19-1 **Research**

Corbett and Jayakumar (1989) reported a small, controlled, randomized study of excision and ligation of varicose veins with and without the use of a pneumatic tourniquet. They concluded there is no time savings or increase in the amount of veins collected, but they did save 100 cc of blood loss per leg when using the tourniquet. Thompson, et al (1990) studied 100 patients undergoing varicose vein excision with and without the use of a tourniquet and found a significantly better cosmetic result. They hypothesized that this may have been the result of better visibility of veins from operating in a bloodless field.

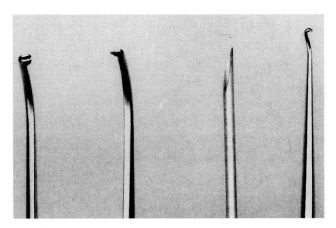

Fig. 19-3 Tips of a Graefe forceps on the left and a Muller hook (#1) on the right, with an 18 gauge needle (1.2 mm diameter) in the middle for comparison. *(From Ricci, S., Georgiev, M., & Goldman, M. P. [1995]. Ambulatory phlebectomy: A practical guide for treating varicose veins. St. Louis: Mosby.)*

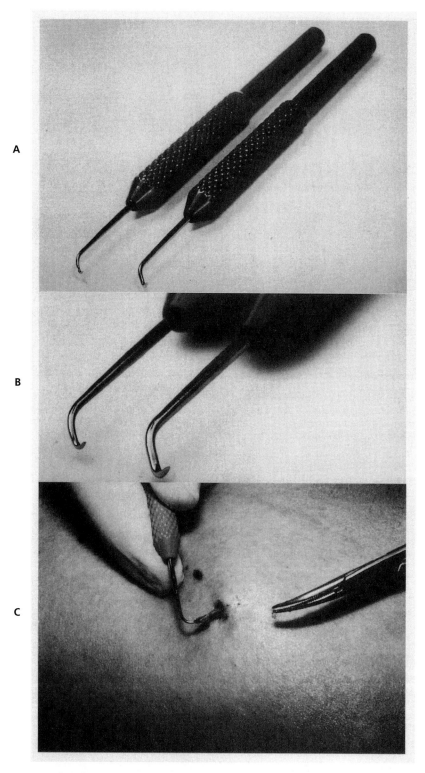

Fig. 19-4 A phlebectomy hook designed by Ramelet. **A,** Two different sized hooks. **B,** Magnification of the tips of the hooks. **C,** Appearance of the vein on the hook. *(From Ramelet, A. A. [1991]. Journal of Dermatologic Surgery and Oncology, 17:814-816.)*

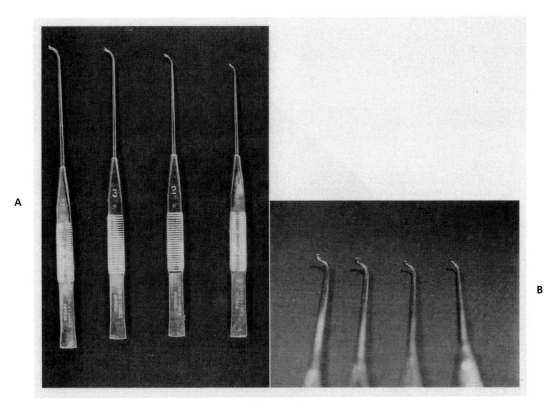

Fig. 19-5 Four sizes of Muller hooks. **A,** Overall appearance. **B,** Magnified view of specially designed curved end. *(From Bergan, J. J. [1992]. Surgical procedures for varicose veins: Axial striping and stab avulsion. In Bergan, J. J., & Kistner, R. L. [Eds.],* Atlas of venous surgery. *Philadelphia: W.B. Saunders.)*

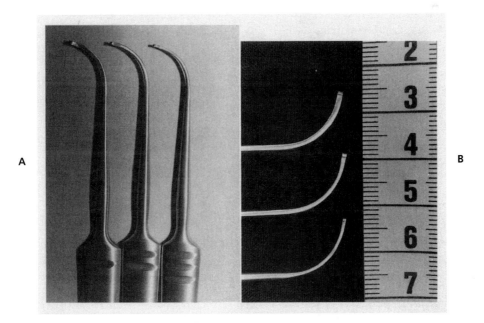

Fig. 19-6 Oesch hooks of various sizes. **A,** Overall appearance. **B,** Magnified view of specially designed "grasping" end. *(From Bergan, J. J. [1992]. Surgical procedures for varicose veins: Axial striping and stab avulsion. In Bergan, J. J., & Kistner, R. L. [Eds.],* Atlas of venous surgery. *Philadelphia: W.B. Saunders.)*

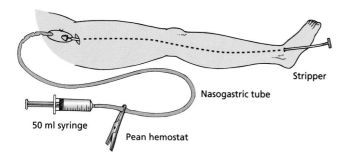

Fig. 19-7 A 14 Fr nasogastric tube and a 50 ml syringe filled with x 200,000 diluted epinephrine saline solution is connected to the head of the stripper.

RNFA CONSIDERATIONS

Mark the patient's veins with indelible marker on the day of surgery.
Assist with prepping and draping.
Assist in passing the stripper if stripping is performed.
    Apply manual pressure with a folded towel for 5 minutes over the area from which the vein was stripped. This provides homeostasis and minimizes the formation of a hematoma or bruising.
Excise varicose veins, making the smallest incisions possible.
Tie veins. Close wounds with suture or steri-strips.
Wash the leg before the application of dressings.
Apply dressings and elastic bandage in a figure-of-eight technique.
Reinforce postoperative and discharge instructions.
    Demonstrate the correct method of elastic bandage application.

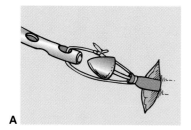
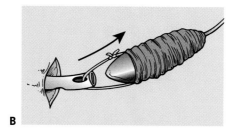
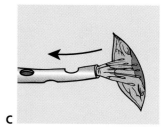

Fig. 19-8 A, Tube is tied to the stripper with 20 silk suture. **B,** Stripper is pulled out in the peripheral direction and connecting suture is cut outside the distal wound. **C,** Then the tube is drawn back, applying the solution into the subcutaneous route where the great saphenous vein was, followed by tight and wide compression for 10 minutes on the stripped area. *(From Furuya. T., Tada. Y., & Sato, O. [1992]. Letters to the editor.* Journal of Vascular Surgery, *16(3): 493-494.*

Procedural Steps

1. The skin is prepped with the appropriate antiseptic, usually from the foot to above the groin and the leg circumferentially. Sterile drapes are applied. The patient is usually placed in Trendelenburg to reduce bleeding.

2. One method of excision is to make **mini-venectomies.** One to two mm incisions are made over a varicosity, the vein is grasped with a small hook to remove clusters, and the veins ligated and excised. Great care must be taken excising veins of the lower saphenous system because of the close association of the sural nerve (Bergan, 1993).

Another technique for excision is called **stab wound avulsion.** The surgeon identifies the points of valve reflux with a Doppler to mark the incision sites. A tiny incision is made with a #11 blade point or an 18 gauge needle. Using blunt dissection technique and a crochet hook, small clamp, or specially designed instrument the vein is avulsed without ligation. Continual bleeding is an indication that the incompetent perforator has not been identified.

The perforator is identified by applying pressure to locate the bleeding stop point. "Vertical incisions give the best cosmetic results." (Johnson & Rutherford, 1995, p. 1827). This is debatable and many surgeons use horizontal incisions.

3. **Stripping of the long saphenous vein** is performed after high ligation. One incision is made just below and parallel to the inguinal crease and over the fossa ovalis.

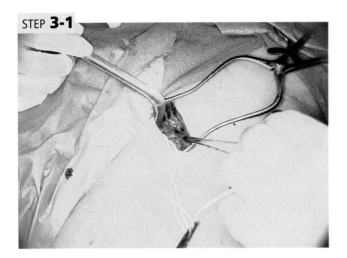

STEP **3-1**

4. A second incision is made at the ankle with a vertical incision just anterior to the medial malleolus. At the ankle the vein is divided and ligated.

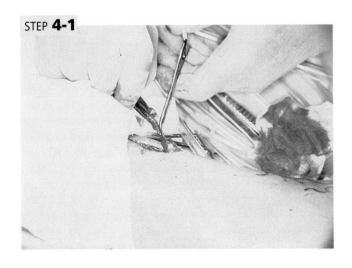

STEP **4-1**

5. A stripping device is inserted into the vein to be removed and advanced to the groin incision. Sometimes another skin incision is needed midway along the path of the stripper to allow free passage. The branches of the vessel are identified, ligated, and divided.

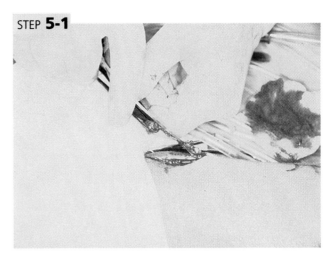

STEP **5-1**

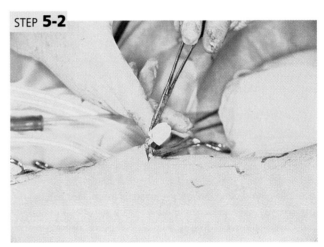

STEP **5-2**

6. The saphenofemoral junction is divided only after the stripper is verified as being in the saphenous vein to prevent inadvertent ligation of the superficial saphenous vein or femoral artery. A clamp is placed on the saphenous vein to protect the common femoral vein and the stripper is passed up from below. The vein is divided above.

7. The vein is secured to the stripper, a "head" is placed on the stripper, and the stripper is pulled from the groin to the ankle.

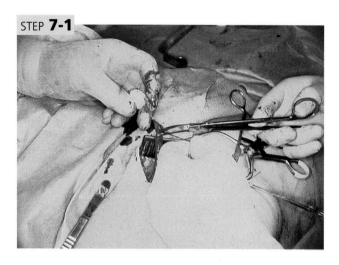

STEP **7-1**

8. Pressure is applied for 5 minutes and any residual clots are milked out. Incisions are closed with subcuticular suture and compression bandages are firmly applied (Johnson & Rutherford, 1995).

Sclerotherapy

Another approach to surgery is to combine it with adjuvant **sclerotherapy**. Greenfield (1994) believes the majority of patients can be treated conservatively. Treatment can be ablative surgery and injection sclerotherapy. Ablative surgery redirects the venous flow through veins with competent valves and improves leg appearance by removal of varicosities. Greenfield also cites the current trends to avoid stripping procedures to preserve normal segments of saphenous vein and avoidance of below-knee stripping to prevent sural nerve complications. Injection of a sclerosing agent destroys the vessel endothelium and promotes obliteration by the creation of scar tissue. Sclerotherapy can produce allergic reactions, DVT, and inflammatory responses. Skin sloughing can occur if the sclerosant leaks from a vein. Sclerotherapy is sometimes used postoperatively to remove persistent or recurrent small varicosities (and in cases that do not require surgery).

Controversy

Hume (1992) suggests that stripping is the "simplest part of what is otherwise a very tedious operation" (p. 949). The Physician's Current Procedural Terminology (CPT) codes for reimbursement suggest that procedures less radical than stripping are practically unmentioned although the trend indicates less radical procedures have good results and save the main trunk of the saphenous vein for arterial conduits. Treatment is more recently directed away from the older method of stripping the long saphenous vein. This saves any normal vein for future use in arterial bypass surgery and prevents complications associated with below knee stripping (Greenfield, 1994).

Bergan (conference, NYC, 1995) believes that vein sparing procedures are not necessarily in the patient's best interests. They should receive the operation *that they need at the time* rather than assuming that they will necessarily require cardiovascular surgery.

Complications

Complications are considered rare and include trauma to deep arteries or veins, DVT, and saphenous or sural nerve damage. Infection, bleeding, ecchymosis, and wound separation are possible in any procedure (Johnson & Rutherford, 1995). Patients with extensive bilateral varicose veins may have a significant blood loss intraoperatively, but rarely is transfusion necessary and postoperative bleeding is rare. Many patients choose surgical intervention primarily for the cosmetic result. Subcuticular closure or adhesive strip closure may improve the cosmetic result. Hematoma formation can occur but can be prevented by immediate compression bandages with a firm figure-of-eight wrap. Properly applied ace bandages are less likely to act as a tourniquet, but they do lose pressure in a matter of hours. Consequently, some surgeons order the application of compression stockings on the first postoperative day, with instructions that they be worn for several weeks. Compliance may be poor, especially during warm weather.

Because sensory nerves and veins occur in close proximity, nerves may be damaged during varicose vein surgery. Small nerves and empty veins may be confused and the nerve excised. This results in a loss of skin sensation. A traumatized nerve may have a transient anesthesia. Patients with a history of phlebitis or previous interventions are at greater risk for nerve trauma (Ricci, Georgiev, & Goldman, 1995). Nerve injuries can occur both with and without stripping. Major complications are rare and saphenous (sensory) nerve injury is usually only seen with stripping below the knee and can be minimized by using a small stripper head (Johnson & Rutherford, 1995). Saphenous nerve injury may be prevented by stripping caudally from the lower incision toward the upper (Criado & Johnson, 1991), although this is debatable. According to Ricci, Georgiev, and Goldman (1995), the distal segment of the long saphenous vein is best left intact because it is usually not diseased.

POSTOPERATIVE ▰▰▰▰▰▰

Care and Discharge Planning

There is usually no activity restriction other than the caution about driving or operating equipment until anesthetics or sedatives have been metabolized.

Discourage lengthy periods of sitting (Johnson & Rutherford, 1995).

Encourage early ambulation to assist in venous return.

Instruct the patient to avoid showering for the first day or until the surgeon allows this.

Many patients will have no visible sutures; those who have sutures that must be removed are instructed when to return to the physician's office.

Instruct the patient in routine wound care and signs and symptoms of infection.

Encourage the patient to elevate legs periodically to prevent pooling of blood and discomfort.

Reinforce the importance of keeping elastic compression stockings or ace bandage wraps on the legs to minimize discomfort, prevent hematoma formation, and maximize healing and cosmesis (Karp & Fahey, 1994). Criado and Johnson (1991) advocate the intraoperative application of figure-of-eight ace wrapping to prevent hematoma formation. This configuration has the advantage of providing good compression and stays in place longer. Most patients need to be taught the correct manner to apply an ace bandage.

THE PREGNANT PATIENT

The pregnant patient has special teaching needs despite the fact that surgery is either not needed or may be postponed. Surgery is advised for correction before subsequent pregnancies in patients whose varicose veins do not spontaneously resolve in the postpartum period. They need emotional support in dealing with this aggravating condition.

Elastic leotards may be helpful in relieving any vulvar varicosities in addition to leg varicosities.

Teaching patients to elevate legs and wear compressive stockings that fit properly may prevent thrombosis by collapsing the veins when stasis is most pronounced (Dotz & Berman, 1991).

One hour of bed rest every 4 hours is recommended for relief in severe cases.

It may be necessary to place the patient's bed on 8-inch blocks for leg elevation without hip flexion that could impede venous return (Cruikshank, 1994).

Advise pregnant patients to avoid standing motionless and to avoid crossing their legs.

References

Baker, R. J. (1992). Editorial comment (p1884). In L. M. Nyhus, & R. J. Baker (Eds.) *Mastery of surgery: Volume II* (2nd ed.). Boston: Little, Brown.

Bergen, J. J. (1993). New developments in the surgical treatment of venous disease. *Cardiovascular surgery, 1*(6): 624-630.

Bergen, J. J. (1991). Surgical procedures for varicose veins. In J. J. Bergan, & S. T. Yao (Eds.), *Venous disorders* (pp. 201-216). Philadelphia: W. B. Saunders.

Bergqvist, D., & Bergentz, S. (1990). Diagnosis of deep venous thrombosis. *World Journal of Surgery, 14*: 679-687.

Bishara, R. A., et al (1986). Deterioration of venous function in normal lower extremities during daily activity. *Journal of Vascular Surgery, 3*(5): 700-706.

Callam, M. J. (1994). Epidemiology of varicose veins. *British Journal of Surgery, 81*: 167-173.

Christopoulos, D., et al (1989). Pathogenesis of venous ulceration in relation to the calf muscle pump function. *Surgery, 106*(5): 829-835.

Cockett, F. B., & Thomas, M. L. (1965). The iliac compression syndrome. *British Journal of Surgery, 52*: 816-821.

Corbett, R., & Jayakumar, J. N. (1989). Clean up varicose vein surgery-use a tourniquet. *Annals of the Royal College of Surgeons, England, 71*(1): 57-58.

Criado, E., & Johnson, Jr., G. (1991). Venous disease. *Current Problems in Surgery, 28*(5): 335-400.

Cruikshank, D. P. (1994). Cardiovascular, pulmonary, renal, and hematological diseases in pregnancy. In J. R. Scott, P. J. DiSaia, C. B. Hammond, & W. N. Spellacy (Eds.), *Danforth's obstetrics and gynecology* (7th ed.). Philadelphia: J. B. Lippincott.

Docherty, J. G., Morrice, J. J., & Bell G. (1994). Saphenous neuritis following varicose vein surgery. *British Journal of Surgery, 81*(5): 698.

Dotz, W., & Berman, B. (1991). Dermatologic problems of pregnancy. In S. H. Cherry, & I. R. MerKatz (Eds.), *Complications of pregnancy: Medical, surgical, gynocological, psychosocial, and perinatal* (pp. 562-587). Baltimore: Williams & Wilkins.

Eldrup-Jorgensen, J. (1992). Local management of superficial varicosities and excision of lower extremity varicosities. In L. M. Nyhus, & R. J. Baker (Eds.), *Mastery of surgery: Volume II* (2nd ed., pp. 1877-1884). Boston: Little, Brown.

Furuya, T., Tada, Y., & Sato, O. (1992). Letters to the editor. *Journal of Vascular Surgery, 16*(3): 493-494.

Geelhoed, G. W., & Burkitt, D. P. (1991). Varicose veins: A reappraisal from a global perspective. *Southern Medical Journal, 84*(9): 1131-1134.

Greenfield, L. J. (1994). Venous and lymphatic disease. In S. I. Schwarz, G. T. Shires, & F. C. Spencer (Eds.), *Principles of surgery* (pp. 989-1014). New York: McGraw-Hill.

Goldman, M. P., Weiss, R. A., & Bergan, J. J. (1994). Diagnosis and treatment of varicose veins: A review. *Journal of the American Academy of Dermatology, 31*(3): 393-413.

Hobbs, J. T. (1991). Varicose veins. *British Journal of Medicine, 303*(6804): 707-710.

Hume, M. (1992). A venous renaissance? *Journal of Vascular Surgery, 15*(6): 947-951.

Jacobson, J. H. & Haimov, M. (1991). Treatment of venous disease in pregnancy. In S. H. Cherry, & I. R. MerKatz (Eds.), *Complications of pregnancy: Medical, surgical, gynocological, psychosocial, perinatal* (pp. 495-500). Baltimore: Williams & Wilkins.

Jamieson, W. G. (1993). State of the art of venous investigation and treatment. *Canandian Journal of Surgery, 36*(2): 119-128.

Johnson, Jr., G, & Rutherford, R. B. (1995). Varicose veins: Patient selection and treatment. In R. B. Rutherford (Ed.), *Vascular surgery* (4th ed., pp. 1825-1828). Philadelphia: W. B. Saunders.

Karp, D. L., & Fahey, V. A. (1994). Chronic venous disease (pp. 432-455). In V. A. Fahey (Ed.), *Vascular nursing* (2nd ed.). Philadelphia: W. B. Saunders.

Lofgren, E. P., & Lofgren, K. A. (1971). Recurrence of varicose veins after the stripping operation. *Archives of Surgery, 102*: 111-114.

Lotti, T., Fabbri, P., & Panconensi, E. (1987). The pathogenesis of venous ulcers. *Journal of the American Academy of Dermatology, 16*(4): 877-879.

Ludbrook, J. (1986). Primary great saphenous veins revisited. *World Journal of Surgery, 10*: 954-958.

Morrow, P. L., et al (1994). Fatal hemorrhage caused by varicose veins. *American Journal of Forensic Medicine and Pathology, 15*(2): 100-104.

Nordestgaard, A. G., & Williams, R. A. (1994). Varicose veins. In F. R. Veith, R. W. Hobson, R. A. Williams, & S. E. Wilson (Eds.), *Vascular surgery: Principles and practices* (2nd ed.) New York: McGraw-Hill.

Nyhus, L. M., & Baker, R. J. (Eds.) (1992). *Mastery of surgery: Volume II* (2nd ed.). Boston: Little, Brown.

Ricci, S., Georgiev, M., & Goldman, M. P. (1995). *Ambulatory phlebectomy: A practical guide for treating varicose veins.* St. Louis: Mosby.

Shah, D. M. et al (1986). The anatomy of the greater saphenous venous system. *Journal of Vascular Surgery, 3*(2): 273-281.

Shepherd, J. T. (1966). Role of the veins in the circulation. *Circulation, 33*: 484-491.

Skudder, P. A., & Farrington, D. T. (1993). Venous conditions associated with pregnancy. *Seminars in Dermatology, 12*(2): 72-77.

Stegall, H. F. (1966). Muscle pumping in the dependent leg. *Circulation Research, 19*: 180-190.

Sumner, D. J. (1995). Hemodynamics and pathophysiology of venous disease. In R. B. Rutherford (Ed.), *Vascular surgery* (4th ed., pp. 1673-1695). Philadelphia: W. B. Saunders.

Thompson, J. F., et al (1990). Varicose vein surgery using a pneumatic tourniquet: Reduced blood loss and improved cosmesis. *Annals of the Royal College of Surgeons of England, 72*(2): 119-122.

Van Rij, A. A, Solomon, C., & Christie, R. (1994). Anatomic and physiologic characteristics of venous ulceration. *Journal of Vascular Surgery, 20*(5): 759-764.

Villavincencio, J. L. (1991). Excision of varicose veins. In C. B. Ernst & J. C. Stanley (Eds.), *Current therapy in vascular surgery* (2nd ed.). St. Louis: Mosby.

Wilson, N. M., & Browse, N. L. (1993). Venous disease. In D. L. Clement, & J. T. Shepherd (Eds.), *Vascular diseases in the limbs: Mechanisms and principles of treatment* (pp. 199-220). St. Louis: Mosby.

20 Amputations

AMPUTATIONS

Description

Amputations involving the lower extremity are performed to eliminate ischemic, gangrenous, necrotic, or infected tissue, to relieve pain, and to promote maximum independence. *Primary* amputation is performed instead of revascularization. *Secondary* amputation is performed after revascularizatiion (Krajewski & Olin, 1996). Minor amputations include amputation of individual toes or midfoot, transmetatarsal. Major amputations of the lower extremity include the below-knee amputation (BKA), which is done at the midcalf level and above knee amputation (AKA) done at the distal thigh. The Syme amputation, through the ankle, is seldom performed because of improved prosthetics and rehabilitation that favor midcalf amputation (Krajewski & Olin, 1996). Upper extremity amputation is rare and will not be addressed.

Indications and pathophysiology

Urgent amputation may be indicated when extensive tissue necrosis precludes successful revascularization or infection with systemic sepsis is present. The notion that amputation is more cost effective than arterial reconstruction has been a long-standing assumption that has proved to be untrue. Perler (1995) reviewed the costs of amputation versus revascularization. Mortality rates were higher for amputation in the more debilitated population. Increased length of stay was influenced by complication rate and found to be greater in the amputation patients. Including rehabilitation and prosthetics in the cost of an amputation made the costs similar to revascularization. However, some patients do not successfully ambulate after amputation and therefore may need more costly long-term institutionalization, which significantly adds to the cost of amputation. Patients with diabetes, those of advanced age, those living alone, and those who have already had one limb amputated are less likely to have a successful course of rehabilitation and regain independence. Hospitalization after amputation is longer than after revascularization. These patients are also the most likely to need a contralateral amputation (Serletti & Ouriel, 1996). Vascular patients who have had one amputation have a 50% chance of contralateral amputation within 2 years, which further decreases their chances of maintaining independence (Bodily & Burgess, 1983).

Of the patients who undergo leg amputation, more than half are diabetics. They are prone to neurotrophic ulceration and neuropathies that cause bony malformations (Krajewski &

Olin, 1996). Diabetic patients may also be unaware of infection or injury until extensive changes have occurred. Diabetics benefit from support in maintaining good control of their diet and blood glucose. Nurses can assist by teaching and reinforcing proper foot care. Early referral to a vascular surgeon will ensure that these patients receive adequate evaluation and surgical interventions at a point where limb salvage is optimized (see Chapter 5 and Chapter 12)

Preoperative planning

Psychosocial aspects. At every stage of interaction with the patient having an amputation, emotional support is critical. Improved surgical interventions, anesthetic techniques, and rehabilitation have made revascularization a possibility for most patients, although there are some for whom this may not be a option and primary amputation is planned. Those patients who must have a secondary amputation have often undergone multiple surgical procedures to salvage the limb. It is sometimes difficult for patients and staff to accept that amputation does not mean failure (Helt, 1994). A goal of all members of the surgical team should be to provide support and assist in establishing realistic rehabilitation goals for the patient. A team approach that establishes a spirit of optimism and the expectation of successful rehabilitation is an important component to patient success (White, 1994). Patients are more accepting of amputation when they believe that it is not only inevitable but will provide positive outcomes, such as relief of pain, prevention of sepsis, discharge from the hospital, and optimal independence. Support groups and visits from patients who are close in age and activity level and who have successfully rehabilitated from amputation can provide invaluable hope for recovery. Both the volunteer support person and the new amputee can benefit from mutual support (Mikulaninec, 1992). Support group meetings can provide preoperative and postoperative information directly from people who have experienced the surgery. Patients can join together to share problem solving ideas, pool resources to advocate changes in the community (e.g., handicapped accessible buildings), inspire hope, and plan social activities. Information on the rehabilitation process and prosthetics can also assist the patient. Some patients have experienced chronic disability from ischemic ulcers that require daily wound care and other limitations that accompany severe lower extremity vascular disease. Patients have reported that the relief of pain and general feelings of well being were positive outcomes of amputation. Independence in performing activities of daily living was also reported to be more important than walking distance (Jones, Hall, & Schuld, 1993). The majority of vascular patients are candidates for a limb prosthesis even if it is for cosmetic effect alone. Mental status is more of a factor for successful rehabilitation than advanced age (Helt, 1994). Since the loss of a limb is a physical, symbolic, and functional loss, patients need assistance with the grieving process. Depression may need to be treated or it could interfere with the patient's ability to learn and maintain the motivation to adapt. The elderly have been found to experience a high incidence of depression after amputation (Rudolphi, 1992).

The patient's and family members' fears should be elicited and addressed. The team approach will assist the recovery. Patients may need repetition of surgical information and request second opinions. This should be respected. Reassure the patient that the surgery is short and will not require admission to the intensive care unit. Negative and hostile expressions from the patient and family may be a part of grieving and denial. Patients need to be certain that the amputation is necessary. A visit with a physical therapist and a tour of a physical therapy department will provide a positive focus for the patient. The therapist may assess functional status and mobility and teach transfer techniques and exercises for postoperative rehabilitation (Mikulaninec, 1992). The remaining limb needs to be protected with sheepskin and meticulous foot care practiced. When in bed and using an overhead trapeze, it is possible that the ipsilateral heel can be abraded by "digging in" to move.

A social worker can assist in obtaining community resources. Patients may need assistance in modifying their home or car to adjust to the amputation and arrangements may need to be made for a walker and wheelchair. The nurse can assist in coordinating the various referrals and visits from other health care team members and provide information in a manner that does not overwhelm the patient. Assessment of the patient's usual coping mechanisms and reinforcement of those practices that may be helpful can assist the patient throughout the adjustment. Spiritual practices should be included as appropriate. It may be necessary to contact a minister or chaplain if the patient expresses an interest and does not have an established affiliation with a religious organization.

Phantom limb pain. Patients may be fearful of disfigurement and pain. Phantom limb pain or phantom sensations should be addressed since now approximately 85% of amputees report experiencing this. For many years these sensations were regarded as a means of seeking attention and many patients did not discuss them because they thought they were imaginary. These sensations vary and patients describe them as itching, warmth, cold, aching, stabbing pain, and burning that can be constant or intermittent. These sensations may be associated with other activities or "triggers," such as elimination, orgasm, or touching a corresponding spot on the remaining limb. Phantom sensations may occur in the immediate postoperative period and usually decrease over a period of 2 years (Patterson, 1994). Some patients continue to experience the same pain they had preoperatively (Sullivan, 1994). The etiology is unknown but probably involves physiologic and psychologic aspects (Patterson, 1994).

Severe pain should be communicated to the surgeon and the wound examined for infection, hematoma, or ischemia. Contractures from lack of exercise may contribute to limb pain (White, 1994). Phantom pain may be minimized by preventing the nerve from becoming incorporated into the scar and by immediate postoperative prosthesis (Schwartz, 1994). Neuromas, regrowth of nerve fibers causing a nerve mass, are frequently diagnosed but are in fact rare (Sullivan, 1994).

The discomfort from phantom sensations usually does not require treatment but occasionally antidepressants or narcotics are helpful (White, 1994). Although analgesics are seldom effective for relief of phantom pain, nurses can assist the patient in managing these sensations in a variety of ways. Discussion and reassurance are important for rehabilitation. Massaging or tapping the stump, warm soaks, and exercise may help (Patterson, 1994). Ultrasound has been used successfully as well as transcutaneous electrical nerve stimulator (TENS) units. TENS units may be used safely for long periods and work by blocking the pain impulses (Patterson, 1994; Sullivan, 1994).

Preoperative preparation includes stabilizing the patient medically. Patients with ulcers or gangrenous lesions are given appropriate antibiotics. Abscesses are treated aggressively with early drainage and debridement. Smokers should stop smoking as early as possible before surgery and until healing is completed. Diabetics are controlled on a sliding scale insulin regimen as needed. Pain control in the early postoperative period is imperative not only for comfort but to allow adequate nutrition, which is essential to wound healing and mobility to prevent muscle atrophy or contractures, which could hamper rehabilitation (White, 1994).

Determination of the level of amputation. The amputation is performed at the most distal point possible to optimize wound healing and limb function. An angiogram is ordered when the possibility of limb salvage is still an option or to ascertain if there is adequate blood flow to support healing of the amputation site. It is not the sole factor in determining the level of amputation (White, 1994). A variety of tests, e.g., plethysmography, thermography, and ultrasound, may be used to predict successful healing. However, none of the studies are adequate for prediction of healing and most surgeons rely on physical examination and clinical judgment to select the level of amputation (McCollum, 1989).

Anesthetic considerations. Assessment of cardiac, respiratory, and renal status is required before surgery. An IV is needed and often in place for intravenous antibiotics. An arterial line is started at the discretion of the anesthesiologist. Spinal or epidural anesthesia may be preferred for leg amputations in those patients with respiratory and cardiac disease. General anesthesia is also an option and some patients prefer it for psychologic reasons. However, even those patients who prefer to be unaware of the operation and may be distressed by the sounds of a saw and potential motion of the limb can be adequately sedated in conjunction with regional anesthesia. A nerve block of the foot is possible for toe or partial foot amputations but may be ineffective and therefore contraindicated in the patient with extensive tissue inflammation or infection.

Equipment, instrumentation, medications, and solutions

Also refer to Chapter 8, Equipment, Supplies, and Instrumentation.

Equipment for positioning patient supine with adequate protection of contralateral limb.

Leg holder (see Figure 8-14) or soft support (blankets, pillows, or bunion block) for supporting leg for prep and/or surgery

A tourniquet is *not* used in amputations for vascular disease because this could compromise the arterial supply to the stump

Instrumentation

Soft tissue set or basic laparotomy set (see Box 8-7)

Bone instruments for large bones

Sterile supplies

Laparotomy drape or extremity drape

Stockinette (optional)

8 cloth towels

Gowns and gloves

Prep kit, gloves, sponges

Sponges

Blades: 1 each #10, #15, #20

2-0 silk ties

3-0 silk ties

3-0 silk pop-offs

Surgical clips: small and medium

Suction tubing

Suction tips

Electrocautery pencil

Marking pen and labels

Sharps container

Asepto

50 cc syringe

Suture (2-0 absorbable, skin closure-staples, or nonabsorbable suture)

Saline for irrigation

Closed wound drain (optional, debated)

Stump sock or ace wrap

Procedural Steps
Above-Knee Amputation

Patients are positioned supine with adequate padding of pressure areas for all of the described levels of amputation. A sheepskin bootie or other means of protection should be considered for the contralateral foot. The limb is supported to allow skin preparation (Figure 20-1).

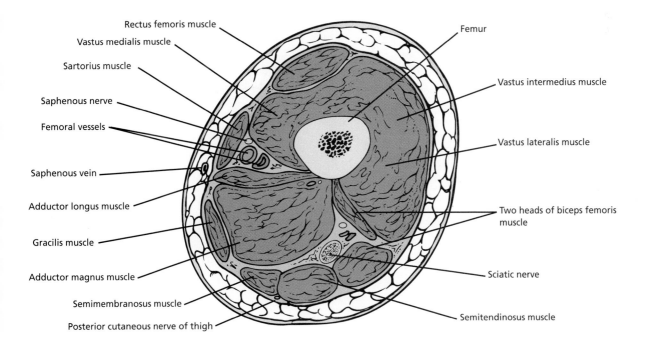

Fig. 20-1 Cross-section through the thigh for amputation. *(From Calne, R., & Pollard, S. G. [1992]. Operative surgery. London: Gower.)*

RNFA CONSIDERATIONS

Assist in the coordination of multiple team members that interact with the patient and family during the entire perioperative period.

Ensure timely communication for the intraoperative services of a prosthetist when needed.

Intraoperatively: ensure that the patient is spared from seeing the limb after amputation.

Ensure that the limb is handled appropriately and pertinent religious requirements are met, e.g., burial. Follow institutional policies for labeling and appropriate container or bag. The limb may go to pathology or ultimately to the morgue.

Because wound healing is so critical in these patients, meticulous surgical technique is demanded. Avoid undermining the skin when making a skin incision to prevent loss of blood supply. Prevent skin injury from electrocautery use. Provide hemostasis. Some surgeons do not allow forceps to be used on the skin edges.

Assess for adequate "cushioning" of the bone with muscle. Muscle and skin should be accurately apposed to promote healing. Avoid any suture tension on the skin. Assess skin perfusion before applying a dressing.

Insert a closed suction wound drain as needed, but adequate hemostasis to avoid a drain is preferred by some surgeons.

Apply dressings, either soft, bulky dressing with stockinette or roll bandage, bulky dressing with soft but tight "stump sock," or rigid plaster cast for immediate prosthesis.

1. The leg is supported by a limb holder (either mechanical or a person) and the skin is prepped circumferentially from the groin to the calf. The lower leg is draped to permit free motion. If the patient has dressings on the foot or lower leg, these are left intact to isolate and contain any drainage from the surgical area.

STEP **1-1**

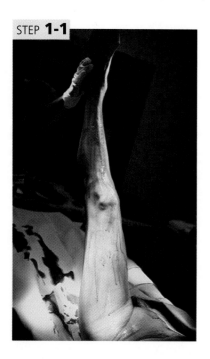

2. Mark the incisions with a skin mark to delineate the anterior and posterior flaps.

STEP **2-1**

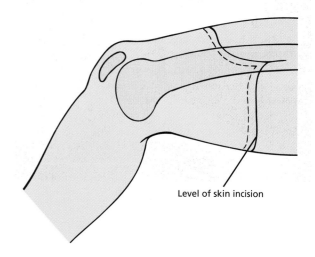

Level of skin incision

(The flaps may be equal or the dorsal flap may be shorter than the anterior flap.)

STEP **2-2**

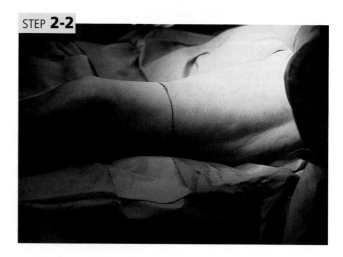

3. Incise to the deep fascia.

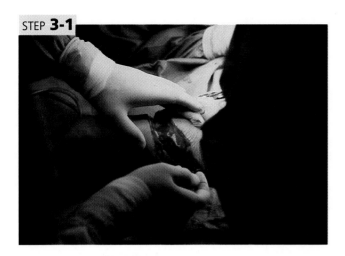

STEP **3-1**

4. Ligate and divide the long saphenous vein (if it is still intact).

5. Divide the sartorius muscle distally (muscle retracts more than skin and is therefore cut at the same level as the skin).

6. Ligate and divide the femoral artery and vein, avoiding the saphenous nerve. Incise the remaining muscles of the thigh. Identify the sciatic nerve and transect it above the level of the skin incision. Clamp vessels and continue the dissection to expose the femur.

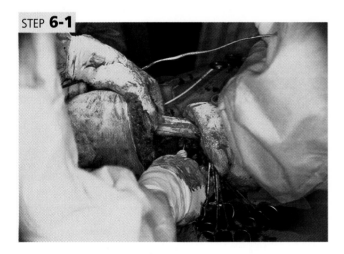

STEP **6-1**

7. Strip the periosteum of the femur proximally for 4 to 5 cm. Protecting the soft tissue, saw the femur with a Gigli saw.

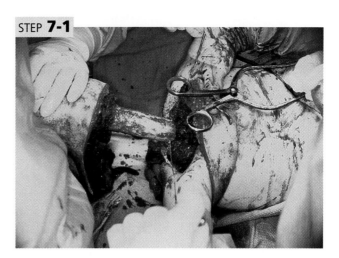

STEP **7-1**

STEP **7-2**

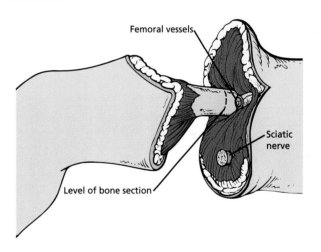

Femoral vessels

Sciatic nerve

Level of bone section

Smooth the bone edges with a rasp and irrigate with saline.

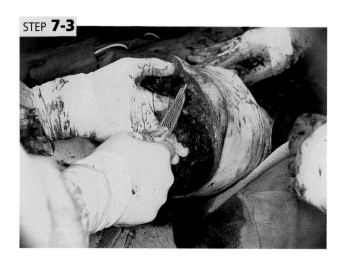

8. Pad the end of the femur well with muscle and close the wound with a 2-0 absorbable suture. (A drain may be inserted at this point but its use is debated.)

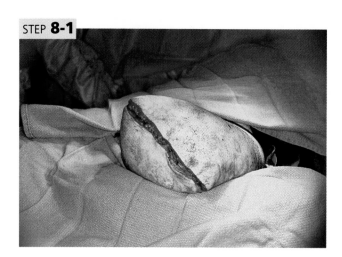

9. Close the skin with staples or a non-absorbable suture. Avoid forcep damage to skin edges.

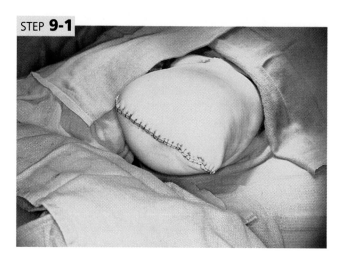

10. Assess the skin for adequate perfusion and tension. Apply a gauze dressing and elastic wrap or stump sock (Greatorex, 1992a; Van Urk, 1989).

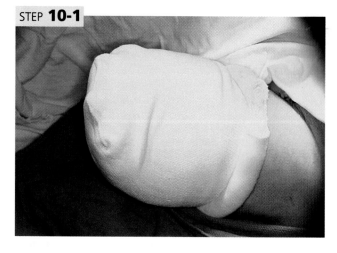

Procedural Steps
Below-Knee Amputation

The leg is supported by a mechanical limb holder or the foot supported by a soft support and the skin is prepped circumferentially from the groin to the ankle. The foot is draped in sterile towels to allow free movement of the leg (Figure 20-2).

1. Mark the incisions with a skin marker.

STEP **1-1**

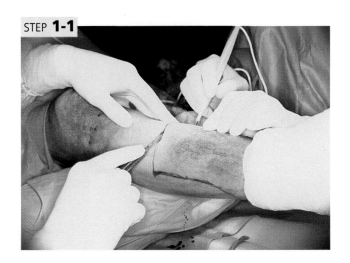

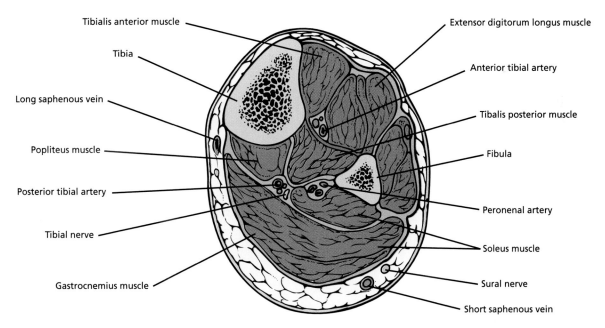

Fig. 20-2 Cross-section through calf for amputation. *(From Calne, R., & Pollard, S. G. [1992].* Operative surgery. *London: Gower.)*

CONSIDERATIONS Different methods of measuring for creation of the flap may be used: (A) The anterior incision is one half the calf circumference. The incision is continued distally at a length of 1 1/2 times the calf circumference. The posterior incision is the remaining half circumference. (B) Another method is depicted in the following figure. This uses measurements of one third and two thirds based on the circumference of the limb at the point of transection. (C) The surgeon may elect to make the transection incision and then create a long longitudinal incision distally. The flap is not transected distally until it has been brought up to cover the wound. It is tailored to fit and provide adequate padding of the bone.

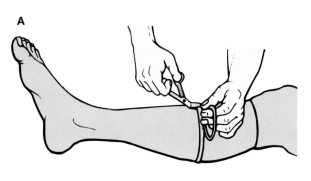

A

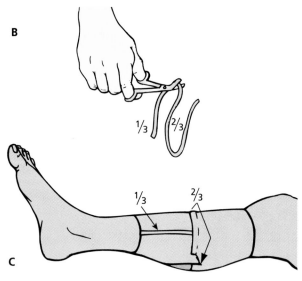

B

C

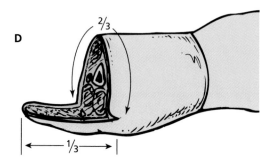

D

Skin flap measurement for below-knee amputation.

2. Assess the skin for adequate bleeding and modify the level if needed.

3. Ligate and divide the long saphenous vein, avoiding the saphenous nerve.

4. Incise the muscle to the tibia. Ligate and divide the tibial vessels.

5. Strip the periosteum proximally on the tibia to 2 cm above the planned amputation site.

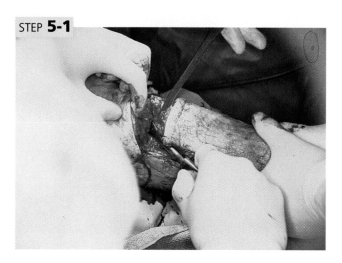

STEP **5-1**

6. Cut the tibia transversely with a Gigli saw. The first assistant stabilizes the limb to counteract the movement of the saw.

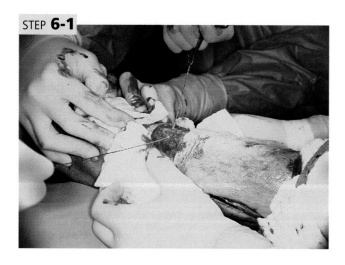

STEP **6-1**

7. Cut the fibula with a Gigli saw or bone cutter 2 cm above the cut end of the tibia.

STEP **7-1**

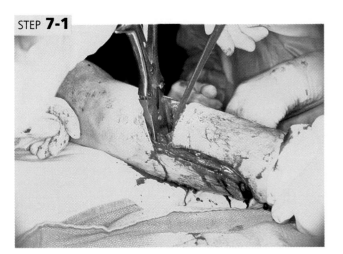

8. Continue the deep incision of muscle on the longitudinal markings through remaining muscle and tendons. Gently place the amputated limb on a table (out of sight of the patient) to be prepared for transport. Ensure hemostasis.

9. Identify and pull down on the sural nerve. Cut it with a knife so it retracts.

STEP **9-1**

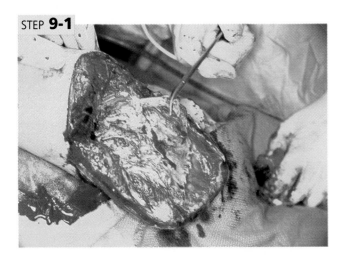

10. Smooth any rough bone edges with a rasp and irrigate with saline. Trim any excess muscle with an amputation knife.

STEP **10-1**

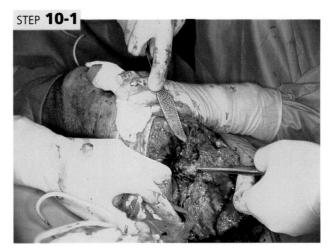

11. Irrigate the flap and assess for hemostasis and perfusion.

STEP **11-1**

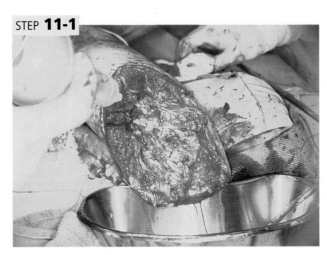

12. Bring the posterior flap over the bone, suture the muscle with 2-0 absorbable suture.

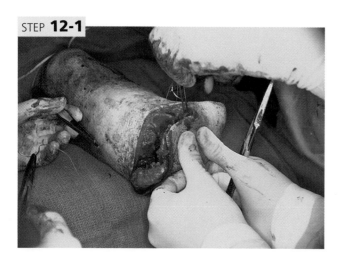

STEP **12-1**

13. Trim any excess skin to achieve good approximation of the tissues

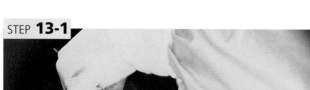
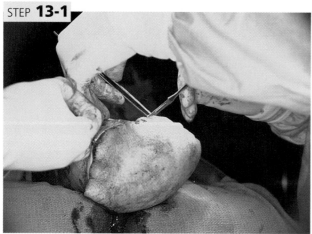

STEP **13-1**

14. Close the skin (staples or nonabsorbable suture).

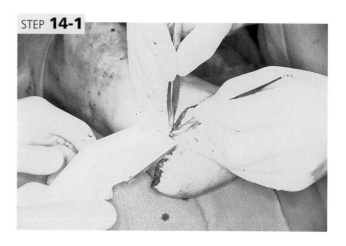

STEP **14-1**

15. Assess the perfusion to the skin edges.

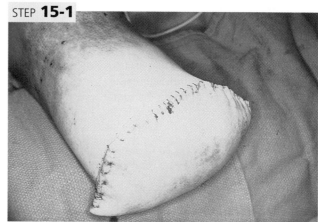

STEP **15-1**

16. Apply a gauze dressing and elastic wrap or stump sock (Greatorex, 1992b).

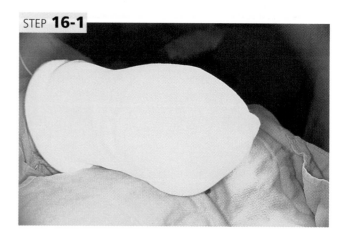

STEP **16-1**

Procedural Steps
Transmetatarsal Amputation

The upper leg and knee are supported on pillows to protect the knee from hyperextension and permit easy access to the entire foot. The skin is prepped to include the foot and above the ankle.

1. A skin incision is made on the dorsum of the foot as close to the toes as possible and perpendicular to the long axis of the metatarsals.

STEP **1-1**

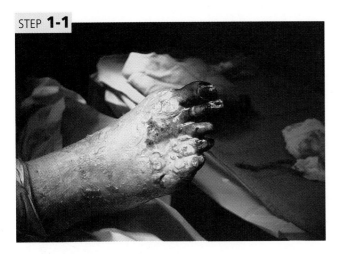

Gangrene of toes.

STEP **1-2**

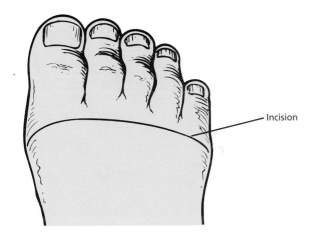

Incision for transmetatarsal amputation.

2. The metatarsals are cut individually with a bone cutter and smoothed with a rongeur or small rasp.

STEP **2-1**

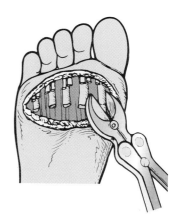

3. The tendons and other soft tissues are cut with a knife or scissors. The specimen is removed. The wound is rinsed with saline.

4. A flap is created from the plantar surface of the foot. The tissue under the metatarsals is left intact for padding.

5. The plantar flap is rotated into place and closed with interrupted 3-0 absorbable suture (fascia) and interrupted non-absorbable skin closure or steri-strips. A bulky gauze dressing is applied.

STEP **5-1**

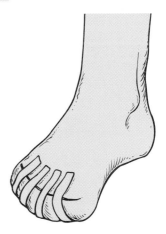

Weight bearing is avoided for 2 to 4 weeks. No prosthesis is needed and patients may wear a regular shoe filled with soft padding to fill the space (DeFrang, Taylor & Porter, 1991; McCollum, 1989; Green & Rob, 1985).

Procedural Steps
Toe Amputation

The upper leg and knee are supported on pillows to protect the knee from hyperextension and permit easy access to the entire foot. The skin is prepped to include the foot and above the ankle.

The uninvolved toes are retracted by placing gauze sponges around them and retracting outward.

1. A circular incision is made with a #15 blade.

STEP **1-1**

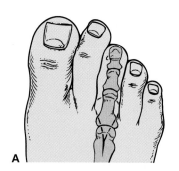

A

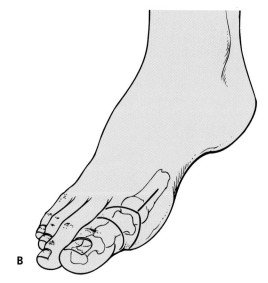

B

2. Divide the tendons. The distal metatarsalphalangeal head is removed with a rongeur and bone cutter. Soft tissue is divided with scissors and the wound irrigated.

STEP **2-1**

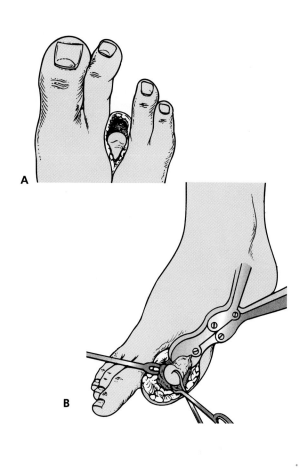

A

B

3. The wound is left open (not packed) or the skin closed loosely with interrupted nonabsorbable suture.

STEP **3-1**

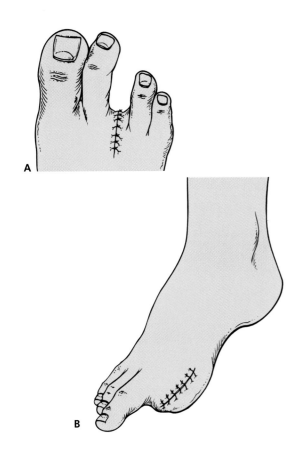

A

B

4. A loose gauze dressing is applied (Green & Rob, 1985).

COMPLICATIONS

Infection
Hematoma
Ischemia
Failure to heal stump wound
Contracture
Wound pain and phantom limb pain

POSTOPERATIVE

Care and Discharge Planning

POSTOPERATIVE CARE OF LIMB

Bleeding: Reinforce dressing, elevate on pillow for the first 24 hours.

Edema: Edema interferes with wound healing and should be prevented by elevation during the first 24 hours and with use of an ace wrap. Limb dangling is limited to minutes at a time.

Ischemia: Observe for signs of ischemia, e.g., poor capillary refill, pallor, cyanosis, or mottling. Increased pain may be an indication of ischemia. Keep the limb warm and protect it from trauma.

Infection: Observe for local signs of wound infection and fever.

PATIENT TEACHING

Reinforce that smoking should be stopped until healing is completed. Ideally, complete abstinence from smoking should be reinforced but this must be a realistic goal for the patient.

Discuss the possibility of phantom sensations.

Provide plan for rehabilitation.

Provide information on availability of social services for lifestyle modification (wheelchairs, ramps, car modifications).

Reinforce diabetic diet and foot care of contralateral limb as needed.

Describe postoperative care.

References

Bodily, K. C., & Burgess, E. M. (1983). Contralateral limb and patient survival after leg amputation. *American Journal of Surgery, 146*:280.

Greatorex, R. A. (1992a). Above knee amputation. In R. Calne, & S. G. Pollard (Eds.), *Slide atlas of operative surgery: Vascular surgery* (pp. 9.52-9.56). New York: Gower.

Greatorex, R. A. (1992b). Burgess-type below knee amputation. In R. Calne, & S. G. Pollard (Eds.), *Slide atlas of operative surgery: Vascular surgery* (pp. 9.57-9.60). New York: Gower.

Green, R. M., & Rob, C. G. (1985). Amputation. In J. A. DeWeese (Ed.), *Rob & Smith's operative surgery: Vascular surgery* (4th ed., pp. 398-414). Boston: Butterworth's.

Helt, J. (1994). Amputation in the vascular patient. In V. A. Fahey (Ed.), *Vascular nursing* (2nd ed., pp. 509-535). Philadelphia: W. B. Saunders.

Jones, L., Hall., & Schuld, W. (1993). Ability or disability? A study of the functional outcome of 65 consecutive lower limb amputees treated at the Royal South Syndey Hospital in 1988-1989. *Disability & Rehabilitation, 15*(4): 184-188.

Krajewski, L. P., & Olin, J. W. (1996). Atherosclerosis of the aorta and lower-extremity arteries. In J. R. Young, J. W. Olin, & J. R. Bartholomew (Eds.), *Peripheral vascular diseases* (2nd ed., pp. 208-233). St. Louis: Mosby.

McCollum, C. N. (1989). Posterior flap below-knee amputation. In R. M. Greenhalgh (Ed.), *Vascular surgical techniques: An atlas* (pp. 340-346). Philadelphia: W. B. Saunders.

Mikulaninec, C. E. (1992). An amputee critical path. *Journal of Vascular Nursing, 10*(2): 6-9.

Patterson, J. W. (1994). Banishing phantom limb pain. *Nursing 94, 24*(9): 64.

Perler, B. A. (1995). Cost-efficacy issues in the treatment of peripheral vascular disease: primary amputation or revascularization for limb-threatening ischemia. *Journal of Vascular and Interventional Radiology, 6*(6): 111S-115S.

Rudolphi, D. (1992). Limb loss in the elderly peripheral vascular patient. *Journal of Vascular Nursing, 10*(3): 8-13.

Schwartz, S. (1994). Amputations. In S. I. Schwarz, G. T., Shires, & F. C. Spencer (Eds.), *Principles of surgery* (pp. 1967-1884). New York: McGraw-Hill.

Serletti, J. M., & Ouriel, K. (1996). Free-tissue transfer in lower extremity ischemia. In K. Ouriel (Ed.), *Lower extremity vascular disease* (pp. 207-222). Philadelphia: W. B. Saunders.

Sullivan, R. A. (1994). Rehabilitation of the amputee. In F. J. Veith, R. W. Hobson, R. A. Williams, & S. E. Wilson (Eds.), *Vascular surgery: Principles and practice* (2nd ed., pp. 1109-1119). New York: McGraw-Hill.

Van Urk, H. (1989). Above-knee amputations. In R. M. Greenhalgh (Ed.), *Vascular surgical techniques: An atlas* (pp. 333-335). Philadelphia: W. B. Saunders.

White, G. H. (1994). Amputation in the dysvascular patient. In F. J. Veith, R. W. Hobson, R. A. Williams, & S. E. Wilson (Eds.), *Vascular surgery: Principles and practice* (2nd ed., pp. 1090-1107). New York: McGraw-Hill.

Index